The Pediatric Upper Limb

The Pediatric Upper Limb

Edited by

Steven ER Hovius MD PhD
Professor of Plastic and Reconstructive Surgery
University Hospital Rotterdam
Rotterdam, The Netherlands

in collaboration with
Guy Foucher
Piero L Raimondi

Published in association with the
Federation of European Societies
for Surgery of the Hand

CRC Press
Taylor & Francis Group
Boca Raton London New York

CRC Press is an imprint of the
Taylor & Francis Group, an **informa** business

First published in the United Kingdom in 2002 by
Martin Dunitz Ltd, The Livery House, 7--9 Pratt Street, London NW1 0AE

Tel.:   +44 (0) 20 74822202
Fax.:   +44 (0) 20 72670159
E-mail: info@dunitz.co.uk
Website: http:/+/www.dunitz.co.uk

Although every effort has been made to ensure that drug doses and other information are presented accurately in this publication, the ultimate responsibility rests with the prescribing physician. Neither the publishers nor the authors can be held responsible for errors or for any consequences arising from the use of information contained herein. For detailed prescribing information or instructions on the use of any product or procedure discussed herein, please consult the prescribing information or instructional material issued by the manufacturer.

A CIP record for this book is available from the British Library.

ISBN 1 84184 134 X

Distributed in the USA by
Fulfilment Center
Taylor & Francis
7625 Empire Drive
Florence, KY 41042, USA
Toll Free Tel.: +1 800 634 7064
E-mail: cserve@routledge_ny.com

Distributed in Canada by
Taylor & Francis
74 Rolark Drive
Scarborough, Ontario M1R 4G2, Canada
Toll Free Tel.: +1 877 226 2237
E-mail: tal_fran@istar.ca

Distributed in the rest of the world by
ITPS Limited
Cheriton House
North Way
Andover, Hampshire SP10 5BE, UK
Tel.:   +44 (0)1264 332424
E-mail: reception@itps.co.uk

Composition by Scribe Design, Gillingham, Kent, UK
Printed and bound in Spain by Grafos, S.A. Arte sobre papel

CONTENTS

LIST OF CONTRIBUTORS

Alexandros E Beris
Professor of Orthopaedics
Department of Orthopaedic Surgery
School of Medicine
University of Ioannina
15 C. Trikoupi str,
Ioannina 45332, Greece

Eileen Bradbury
Alexandra Hospital
Mill Lane
Cheadle
Cheshire SK8 2PX, UK

Maurizio Calcagni
Hand Surgery Unit
Multimedica Hospital, Milan, Italy

Roberto M Cavallazzi
Reparto di Chirurgia Plastica e della Mano
Ospedale di Legnano
20025 Legnano, Italy

Bruno C Coessens
Centre Hospitalier Universitaire Brugmann
Place a Van Gehuchten 4
1020 Bruxelles, Belgium

Jole Colombelli
Hand Surgery Unit
Multimedica Hospital, Milan, Italy

David M Evans
The Hand Clinic
Oakley Green
Windsor SL4 4LH, UK

Guy Foucher
Professor, Department of Orthopedics
Las Palmas University
Gran Canaria, Spain

Alain Gilbert
Institut de la Main
6, square Jouvenet
75016 Paris, France

Esther de Graaff
Department of Clinical Genetics
Erasmus University
PO Box 1738
3000 DR Rotterdam, The Netherlands

Rolf Habenicht
Abteilung Handchirurgie
Kinderkrankenhaus Wilhelmstift
Liliencronstrasse 130
22149 Hamburg, Germany

Raoul CM Hennekam
Pediatrics and Clinical Genetics
Academisch Medisch Centrum
Meibergdreef 9
1105 AZ Amsterdam, The Netherlands

Peter Heutink
Department of Clinical Genetics
Erasmus University
PO Box 1738
3000 DR Rotterdam, The Netherlands

Chantal MAM van der Horst
Department of Plastic Surgery
Academisch Medisch Centrum
Meibergdreef 9
1105 AZ Amsterdam, The Netherlands

Steven ER Hovius
Department of Plastic and Reconstructive
Surgery
University Hospital Rotterdam
Dr. Molewaterplein 40
3015 GD Rotterdam, The Netherlands

Susanne Kall
Klinik für Plastische Hand- und
Wiederhestellungschirurgie
Klinikum Oststadt
Podbielskistrasse 380
30659 Hannover, Germany

M Jeltje van Baren
Department of Clinical Genetics
Erasmus University
PO Box 1738
3000 DR Rotterdam, The Netherlands

Simon PJ Kay
Department of Plastic Surgery
St James's University Hospital
Leeds, UK

Ulrich Lanz
Klinik f(r Handchirurgie
Salzburger Leite 1
97616 Bad Neustadt, Germany

Caroline Leclercq
Institut de la Main
6, square Jouvenet
75016 Paris, France

Teun JM Luijsterburg
Research Institute Plastic and Reconstructive
Surgery
Erasmus University Rotterdam – HEE 1253
P.O. Box 1738
3000 DR Rotterdam, The Netherlands

Jose Medina
Hand Surgeon
Department of Orthopedics
Las Palmas
Gran Canaria, Spain

Ricardo Navarro
Professor of Orthopedics
Department of Orthopedics
Las Palmas University
Gran Canaria, Spain

Giorgio Pajardi
Head, Department of Hand Surgery
Milan University - Plastic Surgery Institut
Multimedica Hospital, Milan, Italy

Piero L Raimondi
Casa di Cura S Maria – Multimedica
Viale Piemonte, 70
21053 Castellanza, Italy

Margreet ter Schegget
European Federation of Hand Therapists
Zuideinde 6
9497 PS Donderen, The Netherlands

Hans-Martin Schmidt
Anatomisches Institut der Universität Bonn
Nussallee 10
53115 Bonn, Germany

Luc de Smet
Universitaire Ziekenhuizen Leuven
UZ Pellenberg
Weligerveld 1
3212 Lubbeck (Pellenberg), Belgium

Gillian D Smith
Clinical Hand Fellow
Department of Plastic and Reconstructive
Surgery
Great Ormond Street Hospital for Children
Great Ormond Street
London WC1 3JH, UK

Paul J Smith
Consultant Hand Surgeon
Department of Plastic and Reconstructive
Surgery
Great Ormond Street Hospital for Children
Great Ormond Street
London WC1 3JH, UK

Panayotis N Soucacos
Professor, Department of Orthopaedic Surgery
University of Ioannina
Ioannina 45110, Greece

Michael A Tonkin
Department of Hand Surgery and Peripheral
Nerve Surgery
Royal North Shore Medical Centre
St. Leonards, NSW 2065, Australia

Marios Vekris
Lecturer of Orthopaedics
Department of Orthopaedic Surgery
School of Medicine
University of Ioannina
Ioannina, Greece

Christl Vermeij-Keers
Research Institute Plastic and Reconstructive
Surgery
Erasmus University Rotterdam – HEE 1253
P.O. Box 1738
3000 DR Rotterdam, The Netherlands

Paolo Zerbinati
Hand Surgery Unit
Multimedica Hospital, Milan, Italy

INTRODUCTION

It has become a tradition to publish a book that includes papers of the presentations from the instructional courses of every meeting of the Federation of European Societies for Surgery of the Hand (FESSH). This series has already covered the subjects of wrist instability, stiff joints, finger bone and joint injuries, and brachial plexus injuries. The eighth FESSH meeting in 2002 in Amsterdam is devoted to the subject of the 'Pediatric Upper Limb'.

An intriguing part of any problem concerning the upper extremities encountered in childhood is the influence of growth and the great variety in congenital differences. Treatment is particularly challenging in the latter group and creativity is a necessity. It is also clear that a sound knowledge of pathoembryology, pathological anatomy, grip development and psychosocial behaviour is necessary in order to guide these children, with the help of their parents, through their developing years. The emphasis on early treatment in these children requires an insight into multifarious and complex problems, and one is constantly having to justify and re-evaluation one's desire to help and treat a patient—'primum nil nocere'— and in view of this, renowned experts were invited to participate in this book.

With respect to congenital differences, the topics of syndromology, clinical genetics, pathoembryology, grip development, psychological behaviour and the approach to the child at the first consultation, are touched on. Clearly it is impossible to cover all subjects. Therefore we have chosen to present the more common problems together with case presentations and discussions. In this way this instructional course book distinguishes itself from the classical textbook, in that it does not purport to be 'complete', although there are some insightful and in-depth presentations on technique.

The selected subjects are syndactyly, polydactyly, thumb hypoplasia, camptodactyly, symbrachydactyly and radial dysplasia. Diseases that are less common and quite difficult to treat, such as cerebral palsy, Volkmann's ischemic contracture and replantations and revascularizations in children are subjects that cannot be omitted when dealing with the paediatric upper extremity. Fractures in children and obstetrical brachial plexus injuries have been dealt with in earlier books in this series and are therefore not included here. A logical closing to the book, as stated earlier, covers the problems encountered with growth in the paediatric upper limb.

This book took a little more than a year to complete and to this end the editors wish to express their gratitude to the authors for their continued support, commitment and splendid contributions and without the help of the publishers—Martin Dunitz—particularly that of Robert Peden and Clive Lawson, the production of this book would never have been possible.

Steven ER Hovius

1

Syndromic hand anomalies

Raoul CM Hennekam

An isolated hand anomaly is a frequently occurring finding in daily practical care, and often forms a challenge for the clinician in reaching the right diagnosis, and inherent to this, the right prognosis, therapeutic regime and genetic counselling to both the patient and their relatives—a diagnostic process that often depends solely on localized symptoms and the expertise of the investigator.

However, a high percentage of patients with congenital hand anomalies also show symptoms elsewhere, mainly in the craniofacies, which can be extremely helpful in reaching the right diagnosis. As with the limbs, the craniofacies share a greater susceptibility to any kind of congenital anomaly, not only as malformations, but also disruptions, deformations and morphological variations (Gorlin et al 2001). This can be attributed in part to their developmental complexity, the extended period of morphogenesis, and the exposure of the craniofacies and limbs beyond the protection of the body wall (Stevenson and Meyer 1993). Nearly all human teratogens and chromosome anomalies affect both the limbs and the outer parts of the body and the same holds for single gene mutations—Winter and Baraitser's *London Dysmorphology Database* (1999) lists 1889 dysmorphologic entities that have at least one limb symptom.

A complete overview of all syndromic limb defects cannot be provided in a single chapter and this necessitates a choice in subjects. In the past such a review would have been based on an anatomical classification such as that of Temtamy and McKusick (1978), the International Clearinghouse for Birth Defects Monitoring Systems (Rosano et al 2000), or the EUROCAT registration (Stoll et al 1998). However, the recent advances in molecular biology, not only in limb development but also within the field of syndromology, and the application of knowledge from cell biology and developmental biology in the field should allow a classification of syndromic hand anomalies that is based on the pathogenesis. Such a classification has already been used for isolated cases of syndactylism and polydactylism by Winter and Tickle (1993), but can now be considerably expanded (Table 1). However, such a classification should be considered provisional due to the rapid further expansion of our knowledge on the subject.

Table 1 Provisional classification of syndromic hand anomalies by pathogenetic background

Pathogenic factor	Example
Vascular disturbance	Hypoglossia–hypodactyly
Apoptosis	Bartsocas–Papas syndrome
Signalling gene	Smith–Lemli–Opitz syndrome
Ligand	Spondylocostal dysostosis
Trans-membrane receptor	Gorlin syndrome
Tyrosine kinase	Apert syndrome
G protein	Allbright syndrome
Transcription factor	Greig syndrome
Structural gene	Marfan syndrome

Basic principles

Orthopaedic, plastic, and reconstructive surgeons are not always familiar with the terminology used in molecular and developmental biology, so a few basic principles are summarised for clarity. Furthermore, our increased understanding of the pathogenesis in congenital anomalies has revealed several unexpected relationships; these are also discussed.

Human genome

The entire human genome contains approximately three billion nucleotides (DNA base pairs) that together encode for 35 000–45 000 different genes. These genes are packed together in 23 pairs of chromosomes, in such a way that every human somatic cell nucleus contains the entire human genome. Every individual gene can produce one or more transcription products, namely, proteins that exhibit structural, regulatory or enzymatic activity. The original idea of a single gene producing a single protein with a single function, and thus any mutation of a single gene causing a specific single disorder has now been completely abandoned. We now know that a single gene may cause different disorders, that a single disorder may be caused by mutations in different genes, and that a single gene may have different functions with time, for instance acting prenatally as a developmental gene and postnatally as a tumour suppressor gene.

Gastrulation

During the embryonic development of most animals a complex and coordinated series of cellular movements occur at the end of cleavage. During gastrulation the three embryonic axes (dorso-ventral, cranio-caudal and medio-caudal) are established (or become apparent if they have been established before depending on the species). The details of these movements, called gastrulation, vary from species to species, but usually result in the formation of the three primary germ layers—the ectoderm, mesoderm, and the endoderm. The ectoderm gives rise to the surface epithelia and the nervous system, and the endoderm to the gut and related organs. The mesoderm is immediately patterned in an axial chord, the notochord, which leads to the formation of the neural tube (neurulation). On both sides of the notochord, the paraxial mesoderm segments in a cranio-caudal direction to form somites—epithelial spheres that later differentiate from the ventral sclerotome to form the axial skeleton, and from the dorsal dermo-myotome to form skeletal muscle and the dermis. Lateral to the somites, the intermediate mesoderm forms the urogenital system, and the lateral mesoderm gives rise to the blood, vasculature and heart.

Neurulation

Neurulation is the next stage in embryonic development following gastrulation and corresponds to the formation of the neural tube by closure of the neural plate, directed by the underlying notochord. The neural plate is a region of early embryonic ectodermal cells, known as the neuroectoderm that lies directly above the notochord. During neurulation, these neuroectodermal cells change shape, fold in on themselves (the neural fold) and fuse to form the neural tube. The neural tube gives rise to the brain, spinal chord, and the ganglia.

Limb bud

The limbs of vertebrates start as outgrowths of mesenchymal cells surrounded by a simple epithelium. The tip of the limb is thicker and is called the apical ectodermal ridge (AER). The distal region is referred to as the progress zone; it depends upon the AER and contains cells in active proliferation. There has been extensive study of positional information within the limb bud that has determined, for example, the proximal-distal pattern of bone development and the anterior-posterior specification of digits.

Organogenesis

Organogenesis is the formation of the organs as they appear in the adult. Initially one or more groups of cells occupy or migrate into a territory that will later form that specific organ (anlagen). These cells proliferate, undergo morphogenetic changes (morphogenesis) and then differentiate into the specialized cells that form the various tissues (histogenesis) of the organ.

Morphogenesis

Morphogenesis is the process of shape formation—a process that is responsible for producing the complex shapes of adults from a simple ball of cells that was derived from division of the fertilized egg.

Embryonic induction

Embryonic induction is the process by which differentiation in one tissue is influenced by its proximity to another tissue, arising for example during gastrulation. One of the best-known examples is the induction of the neural tube in the ectoderm by the underlying chordo-mesoderm. In order to respond to inducing signals (secreted or membrane-bound signalling molecules) responding cells must be competent, that is, they must express receptors and post-receptor intracellular signalling molecules that allow translation of the inducing signals to the nucleus.

Determination

Once a cell has committed to a particular path of differentiation, even though there may be no morphological features that reveal this move, determination is said to have occurred. Generally there is a first phase where, in response to inducing signals, responding cells activate the transcription of determination genes. If the induction signals are withdrawn, these genes may be deactivated; this phase of determination is thus reversible, but after a certain period (usually a few hours) determination genes act on other genes (and frequently on their own promoter) and determination becomes irreversible from the original inducing signals.

Differentiation

Differentiation is a process in the development of a multi-cellular organism in which cells become specialized for particular functions. Differentiation requires selective expression of portions of the genome and the fully differentiated state may be preceded by a stage in which the cell is already programmed for differentiation but is not yet expressing the characteristic phenotype (determination).

Trans-differentiation

Trans-differentiation is the change of a cell or tissue from one differentiated state to another. It is a rare event that can be more easily observed in cultured cells. In newts for example, the pigmented cells of the iris trans-differentiate to form lens cells if the existing lens is removed. In vertebrates, smooth cells of the oesophagus trans-differentiate to form skeletal muscle.

Signalling cells

Developmental processes are regulated by a network of signal transduction pathways that relay and integrate information from outside the cell through a receptor in the cell membrane to the nucleus to regulate the expression of target genes. These extracellular signals are usually 'ligands', such as diffusible growth factors or extracellular proteins, which bind to membrane receptors (Fig. 1). There is also a propagation of information from the nucleus outwards to alter structures in the cytoplasm, to modify the cell's responsiveness to signals from the outside and to affect the activities of neighbouring or distant cells.

Many receptors in cell membranes exhibit enzymatic kinase activity, which catalyzes the transfer of a phosphate group from adenosine triphosphate to the side chains of substrate amino acids. Such phosphorylation causes subtle changes in the conformation of the substrates altering their enzymatic activity or regulatory properties. With changes in such protein activity, signals are propagated into circuits or networks. The function of proteins can also be altered by conformational changes. Some proteins act as transcription factors, which increase or decrease transcription of specific genes within chromosomal DNA. This leads to qualitative and quantitative changes in protein synthesis. The overall effect of these signalling pathways and their regulation of gene expression is to control cell proliferation, migration, differentiation and programmed cell death (apoptosis). The coordinated control of groups of cells is fundamental in the formation of complex structures.

Cascades

In embryology genes seldom, if ever, function alone. Usually embryogenesis is regulated by

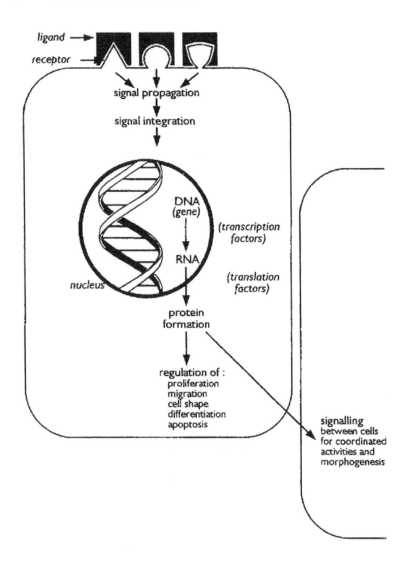

Figure 1

Developmental processes are regulated by networks of signal transduction pathways that relay and integrate information from outside the cell through a membrane receptor to the nucleus, thus regulating the expression of target genes (Breugem et al 2001).

complex signalling cascades, in which the function of one gene product (protein) is dependent on the function of another. It becomes increasingly clear that differences in phenotypic expression of mutated genes are at least in part determined by the functioning of the other genes involved in the cascade. Indeed in several disorders mutations have now been found in two or more different groups within the same cascade, which can explain the differences in clinical symptoms within families. Examples of such differences are mutations in genes *Sonic Hedgehog* (located on chromosome 7q36) and at the same time in *SIX3* (located on chromosome 2p21) and *ZIC2* (located on chromosome 13q32) in patients with holoprosencephaly (Muenke and Beachy 2001), and mutations in two different genes of the five genes (all located on different chromosomes) are known to cause Bardet-Biedl syndrome (Katsanis et al 2001). The occurrence of mutations in different genes on different chromosomes within the same patient was first regarded with disbelief, but now provides a new insight in the principle of monogenic entities; it may well be that monogenic entities are uncommon, and most entities are in fact polygenic.

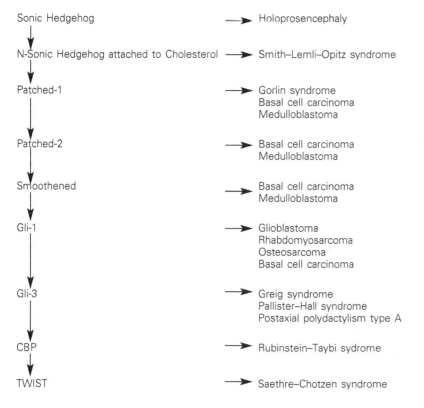

Figure 2

The human Sonic Hedgehog–Gli–CREB pathway and associated links to human disorders. The pathway has been simplified to those genes where human disorders are known. The regulatory mechanisms (such as the stimulation or suppression of genes) are not indicated. A more extensive review of the pathway can be found elsewhere (Villavicencio et al 2000).

A well-known example of a signalling cascade is the Sonic Hedgehog–Gli–CREB pathway (Fig. 2). Mutations in genes within this pathway often give rise to syndromes that are accompanied by limb defects. Indeed the phenotypes may resemble each other to a great extent, such as the hand and facial anomalies found in Greig syndrome, Rubinstein–Taybi syndrome, and Saethre– Chotzen syndrome (Fig. 3). The occurrence of these mutations in genes all acting within the same pathway may contribute to the apparent phenotypic resemblances.

Metabolic disorders and congenital anomalies

The prototypic symptoms of a metabolic disorder are a child who shows no symptoms at birth and who shows an increasing delay in development and/or physical problems in later life. It has become clear that many metabolic disorders can in fact cause congenital anomalies (Gorlin et al 2001). A major example is the Smith–Lemli–Opitz

syndrome, in which a disturbance of the cholesterol metabolism can give rise to different symptoms such as polydactylism, heart defects, absence of the callosal body, and sex reversal (Kelley and Hennekam 2000). A disturbance at another step of the same cholesterol metabolism can lead to a completely different clinical picture such as that found in desmosterolosis (Waterham et al 2001). The co-occurrence of congenital anomalies and a metabolic disorder has already been reported in other entities such as in Zellweger's syndrome (Goldfischer et al 1973), but at that time it was not realized that this was a general principle—that a congenital disorder can also be caused by a disturbance in human metabolism.

Cancer and congenital anomalies

In the past congenital anomalies and tumours were thought to belong to different groups and to be pathologically unrelated. In the last decade however, an increased incidence of specific

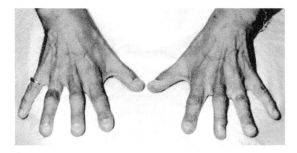

a

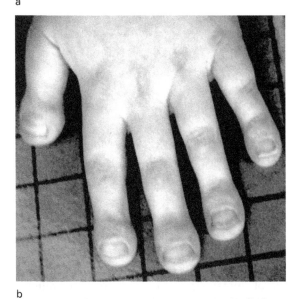

b

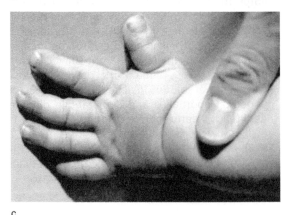

c

Figure 3

Three examples of syndromes resulting from a disturbance of different genes within the Sonic Hedgehog–Gli–CREB pathway. (a) Greig syndrome (mutation in Gli-3), (b) Rubinstein–Taybi syndrome (mutation in CBP), (c) Saethre–Chotzen syndrome (mutation in TWIST).

tumours in several syndromes has been reported, such as leukaemia in Noonan syndrome and CFC syndrome (Van de Berg and Hennekam 1999), medulloblastoma in Rubinstein–Taybi syndrome (Miller and Rubinstein 1995), and Wilms tumour in Beckwith–Wiedemann syndrome (Wiedemann 1997). Several entities that show both congenital anomalies and tumours were in fact already long known, such as Down syndrome (leukaemia), MEN2b syndrome (thyroid carcinoma), and Gorlin syndrome (basal cell carcinoma). In addition, in several pathways it has been found that mutations in one gene of the pathway can give rise to a tumour while mutations in another gene of that same pathway may cause a malformation syndrome. The Sonic Hedgehog–Gli–CREB pathway is a good example in this respect (Fig. 2).

This has all added proof to the general principle that a developmental gene has different functions at different moments in human life and thus mutations can cause different types of disorders depending on time. A mutated gene can cause a congenital anomaly if the function (or another related function) is disturbed in later life. This has had a great impact on the surveillance of children with congenital anomalies—the increased risk of developing cancer in several specific disorders has led to careful follow-up programmes and our growing awareness of such risks will undoubtedly have a knock-on effect when dealing with other disorders.

Conclusion

Modern molecular genetics and developmental biology have provided us with better tools to understand the symptoms displayed in children and adults with congenital anomalies. It has also provided us with unexpected insights into the pathogenesis of the disorders and revealed relationships that were considered unlikely to exist in the past.

We should not forget, however, that careful clinical observations are crucial. In patients with congenital hand anomalies this means that the surgeon will investigate the hands of the child or adult carefully and keep detailed systematic records. It also means that everyone with a congenital hand anomaly deserves a careful investigation of other parts of the body by someone (usually a pediatrician or clinical geneticist) who is aware of the symptoms that might be present. Without this the affected person will not obtain what we all pursue—optimal care.

References

Breugem C, Van der Horst CC, Hennekam RCM (2001) Towards the understanding of vascular malformations, *Plastic Reconstr Surg* **107**:1509–23.

Goldfischer S, Moore CL, Johnson AB et al (1973) Peroxisomal and mitochondrial defects in the cerebro-hepatorenal syndrome, *Science* **182**:62–64.

Gorlin RJ, Cohen MM Jr, Hennekam RCM (2001) *Syndromes of the Head and Neck*, 4th edn (Oxford University Press: New York).

Katsanis N, Ansley SJ, Badano JL et al (2001) Triallelic inheritance in Bardet–Biedl syndrome, a Mendelian recessive disorder, *Science* **293**:2256–59.

Kelley RI, Hennekam RCM (2000) The Smith–Lemli–Opitz syndrome, *J Med Genet* **37**:321–35.

Miller RW, Rubinstein JH (1995) Tumours in Rubinstein–Taybi syndrome, *Am J Med Genet* **56**:112–15.

Muenke M, Beachy PA (2001) Holoprosencephaly. In: Scriver CR, Beaudet AL, Sly WS, Valle D, Childs B, Kinzler KW, Vogelstein B, eds, *Metabolic and Molecular Bases of Inherited Disease* (McGraw-Hill Publishers: New York) 6203–30.

Rosano A, Botto LD, Olney RS et al (2000) Limb defects associated with major congenital anomalies: clinical and epidemiological study from the International Clearinghouse for Birth Defects Monitoring Systems, *Am J Med Genet* **93**:110–16.

Stevenson RE, Meyer LC (1993) The Limbs. In: Stevenson RE, Hall JG, Goodman RM, eds, *Human Malformations and Related Anomalies* (Oxford University Press: New York) 699–804.

Stoll C (1998) Classification of limb defects, *Am J Med Genet* **77**:439–41.

Temtamy SA, McKusick VA (1978) *The Genetics of Hand Anomalies* (Alan R Liss: New York).

Van den Berg H, Hennekam RCM (1999) Acute lymphoblastic leukaemia in a patient with cardiofacio-cutaneous syndrome, *J Med Genet* **36**:799–800.

Villavicencio EH, Walterhouse DO, Iannaccone PM (2000) The Sonic Hedgehog–Patched–Gli pathway in human development and disease, *Am J Hum Genet* **67**:1047–54.

Waterham HR, Koster J, Romeijn GJ et al (2001) Mutations in the 3beta-hydroxysterol delta24-reductase gene cause desmosterolosis, an autosomal recessive disorder of cholesterol biosynthesis, *Am J Hum Genet* **69**:685–94.

Wiedemann HR (1997) Frequency of Wiedemann–Beckwith syndrome in Germany; rate of hemihyperplasia and of tumours in affected children, *Eur J Pediatr* **156**:251.

Winter RM, Baraitser M (1999) *The London Dysmorphology Database* (Oxford University Press: Oxford).

Winter RM, Tickle C (1993) Syndactylies and polydactylies: embryological overview and suggested classification, *Eur J Hum Genet* **1**:96–104.

2
Clinical genetics of the upper limb

Esther de Graaff, M Jeltje van Baren and Peter Heutink

Introduction

In the past decade rapid advances have been made in the identification of human genes that play a role in upper limb malformations. It is only 10 years ago that the first gene associated with a human limb malformation was identified—in the Greig cephalopolysyndactyly syndrome, characterized by digital malformations and a peculiar skull shape; mutations were detected in the *GLI3* gene (Vortkamp et al 1991). Now, many more mutations responsible for upper limb malformations have been found in a large number of genes, elucidating the understanding of normal limb development.

In humans, malformations of the upper limb occur in approximately 1 in 626 new-borns (Flatt 1994). These malformations occur isolated, meaning that no other abnormalities are seen in the patient, or they are found in combination with other hand and/or foot malformations, or as part of a syndrome. In all cases, the cause of the malformation(s) may be genetic, environmental, or a combination of these factors. Although most inherited hand malformations are single gene disorders, patients from a single family often show a range of phenotypes indicating that other genes and/or the environment play a role in the phenotypic variability of the disorder.

Defects in limb formation are not always due to genetic causes. Restriction of blood flow to the developing limb, for instance, leads to limb reduction abnormalities such as truncation or oligodactyly. A well-known cause of limb truncations and other defects was the use of thalidomide, better known as Softenon, in the 1970s. Thalidomide is an inhibitor of angiogenesis (blood vessel formation) and this inhibition was probably the cause of the limb malformations.

Many of the genes involved in limb formation have been identified in the chicken and mouse. These organisms have been used extensively to study embryonic development and much insight has been gathered from manipulation of limb development. However, our insight in limb development is far from complete.

To identify new genes involved in limb formation, several approaches can be used, such as interaction studies with known proteins to identify their binding partners. One of the most powerful methods of finding genes involved in limb development is the identification of genes responsible for hereditary limb malformations.

The most frequently used strategy for the identification of disease-causing genes in humans is positional cloning. In this procedure, the chromosomal localization of the disease gene is determined first. Some diseases are associated with gene defects caused by chromosomal abnormalities, which can be detected with a microscope. Unfortunately, only a minority of cases shows these obvious abnormalities. Therefore, the genomic localization of the disease is more frequently done by linkage analysis. This method is based on the rationale that all affected family members must share a genomic region, which contains the mutated gene, whereas the unaffected individuals are less likely to share this region. The exact procedure of linkage analysis falls outside the scope of this chapter; excellent reviews can be found in most textbooks on human genetics (e.g. *Human Molecular Genetics* by Strachan and Read 1999). The disease region identified by linkage analysis often contains more than one gene. Mutation analysis of these genes in patients is performed to identify the mutation causing the limb malformation. Such a positional cloning project is a considerable task, which involves close cooperation of GPs, clinical geneticists and molecular biologists in order to find as many affected and unaffected family members as possible, obtain blood samples for DNA analysis and perform the study.

In order to understand how genetic alterations can lead to malformations of the upper limb, an overview will be given of the genetics of normal limb development.

Development of the limb

Development of the human upper limb initiates approximately 26–28 days after fertilization, when a thickening, the limb bud, becomes visible at the flank of the embryo (Fig. 1a). At around 52–54 days of gestation the upper arm and hand are almost fully patterned and developed, with full separation of the digits (Fig. 1d). Therefore, in a 25-day interval a large cascade of genetic and cellular interactions results in the patterning and development of the limb. Patterning is the term used to describe the emergence of spatial biological organization during development— 'telling' the cells to become a radius, phalanx, tendon, or muscle. It should be noted that the development of the lower limb resembles that of the upper limb, albeit with a two-day delay. The majority of factors involved in development of the upper and lower limbs are shared and it is therefore not surprising that malformations of the hand are frequently accompanied by similar malformations of the feet.

It is generally believed that the three-dimensional organization of the upper arm is determined by the skeletal pattern laid out early during limb development. The patterning of the muscles, blood vessels, and nerves occurs slightly later and follows the skeletal pattern (Chevallier et al 1977, Christ et al 1982).

The signals involved in the patterning are derived from three different signalling centres. The combination of these signals results in a three-dimensional coordinate system, telling each individual cell its positional information and what specific cell type to become. The growth of this three-dimensional structure is coordinated through three different axes, which will each be discussed later (D'Amato et al 1994).

The proximodistal axis

Human transversal limb malformations are most likely caused by defects in differentiation along the proximodistal axis. Cells at the tip of the limb bud form the apical ectodermal ridge (AER)—a thin, tightly packed band of epithelial cells which signals to the underlying mesoderm to promote outgrowth of the limb. The AER runs along the boundary between the dorsal and ventral side of the limb (Fig. 1a) and it specifies the proximodistal outgrowth. The AER keeps the underlying mesenchymal cells in an undifferentiated and highly proliferative state—the progress zone. As outgrowth continues, cells at the proximal side leave this zone and differentiate (Fig. 1b). By this time, their fate is specified: cells that leave the zone first, specialize and condense to form the primordia of the humerus. In contrast, cells that leave the zone later differentiate into the primordia of the radius and ulna, the wrist bones, and lastly the digits (Figs 1b and c) (Summerbell et al 1973).

The importance of the AER in the proximodistal development of the limb has been demonstrated in chick embryo experiments. Removal of the AER from chicken limb buds, and subsequent culturing of these embryos to allow further development, resulted in transverse limb malformations. Earlier removal of the AER results in the absence of most of the upper limb, whereas later removal only resulted in absent hands, with normal formation of the humerus and ulna/radius (Saunders 1948).

The most likely candidate molecules regulating limb bud outgrowth are members of the fibroblast growth factors (FGF) family. Several FGFs are expressed in the site important for proximodistal outgrowth—the AER. Fibroblast growth factor-8 and FGF-2 are expressed throughout the AER and FGF-4 is expressed in the posterior two-thirds of the ridge (for a review see Cohn and Tickle 1996). Fibroblast growth factor-8 is first expressed prior to the formation of the AER, in a broad strip of cells along the distal end of the limb and later becomes restricted to the ridge (Fig. 2a). Removal of FGF-8 in knockout mice results in the transverse limb malformation as was seen with removal of the AER. Most importantly, when removal of the AER is followed by application of any of these FGFs, outgrowth is restored. Thus, FGFs are both sufficient and essential for limb outgrowth (Moon and Capecchi 2000, Lewandoski et al 2000 and references therein).

The anteroposterior axis

The anteroposterior (A/P; thumb-little finger) axis in the developing limb is established by another signalling centre, the zone of polarizing activity (ZPA), located at the posterior side of the limb bud (Fig. 1a). When cells from this side of a chick limb were transplanted to the opposite side of another bud, an entire set of additional digits developed, in approximately a mirror image of the normal set (Saunders and Gasseling 1968). This outcome indicates that digit patterning involves a morphogen—a secreted molecule whose concentration varies along the AP-axis and cells exposed to a high concentration (i.e. near the site of expression) respond differently than cells exposed to a lower concentration (i.e. cells further away). This hypothesis was supported by the finding that when the ZPA was separated from the rest of the limb by an impenetrable barrier, preventing the diffusion of the morphogen, the anterior structures did not form. At first it was thought that this morphogen was retinoic acid, as application of retinoic acid could substitute for the ZPA, inducing mirror image duplications when applied to the anterior side of the limb bud. However, the ZPA does not contain retinoic acid in concentrations high enough to activate downstream patterning genes. The ZPA secrete Sonic hedgehog (*SHH*), and application of *SHH* protein to the anterior margin of the limb bud leads to polydactyly of the anterior digits. In addition, in mouse mutants with preaxial polydactyly, *SHH* is not only expressed by cells in the ZPA posteriorly, but also in the anterior site of the developing limb. This shows that *SHH* has polarizing activity and that it can take over the ZPA function. Notably, high concentrations of retinoic acid induce *SHH* expression, which explains the polarizing results of retinoic acid (reviewed in Johnson and Tabin 1997). Loss of *SHH* function mutations results in severe truncations of the limb in mice, further suggesting that *SHH* is crucial for limb outgrowth (Chiang et al 1996).

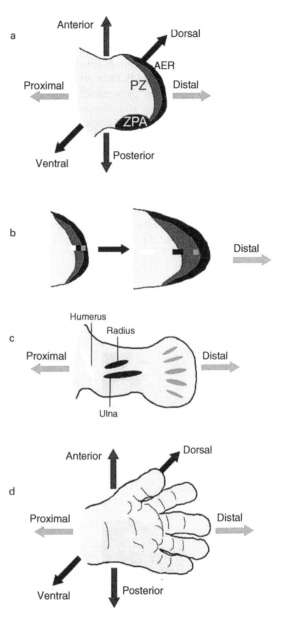

Figure 1

Schematic overview of upper arm development. (a) The progress zone (PZ) is specified at the distal end of the bud by the apical ectodermal ridge (AER). Anteroposterior information is acquired through the zone of polarizing activity (ZPA). Cartilaginous elements are laid out as the limb bud grows (b, c). The cartilage of the humerus is laid out first (white), followed by the radius and ulna (black), wrist elements and digits (grey). (d) Human hand, 56 days after fertilization. At this stage the digits are fully separated. In b and c: dark grey is precartilage, black is cartilage.

The dorsoventral axis

As described above, the AER forms at the border between the dorsal and ventral ectoderm. On the dorsal (back of the hand) side of this border, Radical fringe (*Rfng*) is expressed, whereas on the ventral (palm) side, the transcription factor Engrailed 1 (*En-1*) gene is detected (Fig. 2b). Engrailed 1 expression restricts *Rfng* expression, so that a sharp boundary is maintained in which the AER is formed. Engrailed 1 also restricts expression of *Wnt-7a*, another gene expressed in the dorsal ectoderm (Fig. 2b). Ectopic expression of *Wnt-7a* on the ventral side of the developing limb bud leads to dorsalization of the mesoderm, and absence of *Wnt-7a* in mice results in limb buds with a double ventral phenotype (Logan et al 1997 and references therein). In these mutants, the AER is formed in the proper place, indicating that *Wnt-7a* is not necessary for the formation of the AER.

Interestingly, the *Wnt-7a* mouse mutants also lack posterior digits, indicating a role for *Wnt-7a* in anteroposterior patterning. Indeed, there appears to be a mutual dependence between the three signalling axes: expression of *SHH* in the posterior margin induces and maintains expression of FGFs in the apical ridge and *Wnt-7a* expression in the dorsal mesenchyme together with these FGFs maintains *SHH* expression in the posterior mesenchyme. This feedback loop thus controls initial proliferation and differentiation of the limb (Tickle 1995).

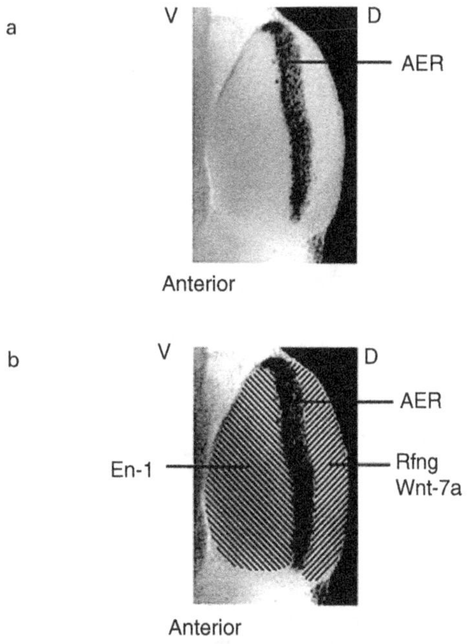

Figure 2

Formation of the AER. (a) In situ hybridization of FGF-8 on the upper limb of an E11.5 murine embryo. FGF-8 expression is restricted to the AER. (b) Schematic representation of the expression of *En-1* ventrally and *Rfng* and *Wnt7a* dorsally of the developing murine limb. Note the presence of the AER at the boundary.

HOX genes

How does a cell respond to the positional information? Candidates for recording these positional values are the *HOX* genes, which are expressed in overlapping patterns in many developing tissues. This gene family is named after the 'homeotic mutation', in which one body structure replaces another. A good example of this mutation is the *Drosophila* mutant *Antennapedia*, where legs sprout from a fly's head where antennae would normally be. The mechanical basis for this fly mutant is that the segment that normally harbours the antennae is now transformed in a segment that lies more posterior and normally produces a leg. This is important as it suggested the existence of control genes responsible for directing the development of large parts of the body (Lewis 1998).

HOX genes encode transcription factors, activating or repressing a large variety of downstream target genes. The structure of the genes differs considerably, but all *HOX* proteins contain a conserved motif, the homeodomain, which is a stretch of 60 amino acids that binds to specific DNA motifs in promoters of target genes.

In vertebrates, four *HOX* gene clusters are found, named *HOXA*, *HOXB*, *HOXC* and *HOXD*. The order of these genes in each genomic cluster corresponds to their timing and location of expression: a more 3' located gene like *HOXA1* is expressed earlier in development than the more 5' located gene *HOXA13*. There are 13 homology groups of *HOX* genes, but not every cluster contains a gene from every group. For example, *HOXA11* is homologous to *HOXC11* and *HOXD11*, but there is no *HOXB11*. In total, 39 *HOX* genes are known in mammals.

In the developing limb, *HOXA* and *HOXD* genes are expressed. The *HOXA* cluster is expressed in overlapping patterns that run from proximal to distal (Fig. 3). The transcript domain of a gene is contained within the domain of the gene located 3', in such a way that *HOXA9* is expressed almost throughout the limb bud while *HOXA13* is expressed only in the posterior part.

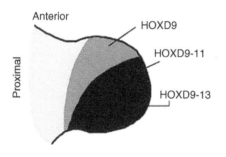

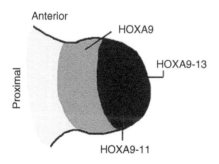

Figure 3

Pattern of *HOX* gene expression in the limb bud. Schematic representation of *HOXA* and *HOXD* expression in the limb bud. The *HOXD* genes are expressed in an anteroposterior pattern whereas the *HOXA* genes are expressed in a similar pattern along the proximodistal axis. *HOXA13* and *HOXD13* expression are more restricted than *HOXA9* and *HOXD9*, respectively.

The *HOXD* cluster is expressed in an anteroposterior way, with *HOXD9* expression throughout the limb and *HOXD13* in the distal part only (Fig. 3; for review see Krumlauf 1994).

Genetics of hand malformations

There is a wide variety of upper limb malformations and a number of classification systems for these phenotypes are available. Classification based on phenotype is the most common system, but this does not always reflect the molecular basis of the malformation: in families with the same mutation, the phenotype may differ considerably. However, a complete molecular classification system is not yet available, and we will discuss the genetics of hand malformations using the classification by Temtamy and McKusick (1978). This classification is generally used in clinical genetic studies, and therefore also in molecular biology.

The signalling effects of the AER and ZPA in the development of the limb have been known for several decades (Saunders 1948), but it is only in the past decade that the molecular basis of these signals became known. This information was mostly obtained by experimental work on mouse and chicken embryos. The explosive development in molecular understanding in these experimental systems has recently been followed by an increasing amount of studies on human limb malformations. As a result, several genes responsible for human hand malformations have been identified in the past few years (Table 1), some of which will be discussed below. For a detailed description of the different limb malformations we refer to the cases described further in this book.

Polydactyly

One of the most frequently observed hand malformations is polydactyly, with a prevalence of between 5 and 17 per 10,000 live births (de Walle et al 1992, EUROCAT 1991). Depending on the location of the extra digit, polydactyly is divided in preaxial, postaxial, and central polydactyly, although it is not clear whether central

Table 1 Selection of genes responsible for human congenital malformations that have been localized or identified.

Disorder/syndrome	Localization	Gene	(MIM entry)
Reduction anomalies-isolated			
Acheiropody	7q36	LMBR1	200500
Split hand split foot 1	7q21.2–21.3	?	183600
Split hand split foot 2	Xq26	?	313350
Split hand split foot 3	10q24	(Dactylin)	600095
Split hand split foot 4	3q27	Tumor protein63	605289
Reduction anomalies-associated			
Holt-Oram	12q24.1	TBX5	142900
Schinzel (Ulnar-Mammary)	12q24.1	TBX3	181450
EEC 1	7q11.2–q21.3	?	129900
EEC 3	3q27	Tumor protein63	604292
Hypoplasia of several segments			
Hunter-Thompson dysplasia	20q11.2	CDMP1	201250
Grebe's chondrodysplasia	20q11.2	CDMP1	200700
Brachydactylies-isolated			
Brachydactyly A1	2q35–36	IHH	112500
Brachydactyly B1	9q22	ROR2	113000
Brachydactyly C-Haws type	12q24	?	113100
Barchydactyly C-Robin type	20q11,2	CDMP1	113100
Brachydactylies-associated			
Hand-Foot-Genital	7p15–14.2	HOXA13	140000
Trichorhinophalangeal	8q24.12	TRPS	190350
Syndactylies-isolated			
Syndactyly I	2q34–36	?	185900
Syndactyly II (synpolydactyly)	2q31–32	HOXD13	186000
Syndactyly III	6q22–23	?	186100
Syndactylies-associated			
Apert	10q26	FGFR-2	101200
Pfeiffer	10q26	FGFR-2	101600
Pfeiffer	8p11	FGFR-1	101600
Oculodentodigital dysplasia	6q22–23	?	164200
Polydactylies-isolated			
Postaxial polydactyly A1	7p13	GLI3	174200
Postaxial polydactyly A2	13q21	?	602085
Postaxial polydactyly B	?	GLI3	?
Preaxial polydactyly type II	7q36	?	174500
Preaxial polydactyly type III	7q36	?	190605
Preaxial polydactyly type IV	7q36	?	190605
Preaxial polydactyly type IV	7p13	GLI3	174700
Polydactylies-associated			
Smith-Lemli-Opitz type I	11q12–13	DHCR7	270400
Smith-Lemli-Opitz type II	11q12–13	DHCR7	268670
Ellis-van Creveld syndrome	4p16	EVC	225500
Weyers acrofacial dysostosis	4p16	EVC	193530
Bardet-Biedl	16q21		209900
Simpson-Golabi-Behmel	Xq26	glypican-3	312870
OFD1	Xp22.3–22.2	CXORF5	311200
McKusick-Kaufman syndrome	20p12	MKKS	236700
Meckel type I	7q22–23	?	249000
Meckel type II	11q13	?	603194
Pallister-Hall syndrome	7p13	GLI3	146510
Greig cephalopolysyndactyly syndrome	7p13	GLI3	175700
Acropectoral syndrome	7q36	?	605967
Townes-Brocks syndrome	16q12.1	SALL1	107480

polydactyly represents a separate entity. In preax-ial polydactyly, or PPD, the extra digit is located on the thumb side of the hand, with extra thumbs and/or index fingers. Postaxial polydactyly (PAP) is a duplication of the little finger.

Temtamy and McKusick (1978) subdivided the postaxial polydactyly in two types. In postaxial polydactyly type A, the extra digit is well formed and articulates with the fifth or an extra metacarpal, whereas in type B a rudimentary extra fifth digit (pedunculated postminimus) is present that is usually represented by an extra skin tag without any bone. Using linkage analy-sis, the disease gene was localized to a locus on *7p13*, and later mutations were detected in the transcription factor *GLI3* (Radhakrishna et al 1997, 1999). Another family did not link to the *7p13* locus, but to chromosome *13q21-32*, and was on this genetic basis reclassified as type A2 (Akarsu et al 1996). No locus has been described for the type B PAP alone. Recently however, a family was described in which type A and B was found on different limbs of the same individual, which demonstrates that the same gene, *GLI3*, is responsible for both types A and B. So-called modifying genes most likely cause the different phenotype, with PAP B being a milder manifes-tation of the type A phenotype (Radhakrishna et al 1999). The finding of mutations in *GLI3* in PAP is not entirely surprising, as *GLI3* is one of the genes downstream of *SHH*, the molecule involved in determining the anteroposterior axis in the developing limb.

Following the classification of Temtamy and McKusick (1978) again, preaxial polydactyly is subdivided into four types: Type I/thumb polydactyly compromises various degrees of duplication of biphalangeal thumbs. This type of PPD is usually sporadic and often unilateral, and so far it is unclear whether the malformation is caused by a single gene with reduced penetra-tion, or by a combination of several genes (Orioli and Castilla 1999). Preaxial polydactyly type II (polydactyly of a triphalangeal thumb), type III (polydactyly of an index finger) and type IV (polysyndactyly, extra digits which are partially fused) are usually inherited as autosomal dominant traits (Temtamy and McKusick 1978). In 1994, two independent studies reported linkage of the PPD type II/III (both also called triphalangeal thumb) and type IV to chromosome *7q36* (Heutink et al 1994, Tsukurov et al 1994).

Interestingly, all PPD type II/III families mapped so far, are linked to this *7q36* locus, despite their large variability in phenotype (Hing et al 1995). Recently, two more limb disorders were mapped to this region: acheiropody and an acropectoral syndrome (Dundar et al 2001, Escamilla et al 2000). Acheiropody is characterized by bilateral congenital absence of the upper and lower extremities and aplasia of the hands and feet, with no other systemic manifestations; patients with the acropectoral syndrome have complex polysyndactyly, in combination with vertebral malformations. Linkage of all these separate phenotypes to the same locus suggested that they could be caused by different mutations in the same gene (allelic heterogeneity) or by mutations in different but closely linked genes (locus heterogeneity).

The critical region, shared by all affected individuals of the PPD type II/III family, was recently reduced to an interval of 450 kb (Heus et al 1999). Of all phenotypes linked to this locus, a mutation has only been detected in the family with acheiropody. A deletion of the fourth exon of the *LMBR1* gene was thought to result in the absence of this protein, of which the function is unknown (Ianakiev et al 2001). None of the genes identified in the critical 450 kb region seemed to harbour a mutation for any of the other limb malformations.

In the PPD and complex polysyndactyly pheno-types, human genetics is aided by mouse genet-ics. Preaxial polydactyly in a number of mouse mutants is caused by ectopic expression of *SHH* in the anterior (preaxial) side of the developing limb bud (as opposed to only in the posterior side). Interestingly, the *SHH* gene is located just outside the critical region containing the defects on *7q36*. One of the mouse mutants, *Hemimellic extra toe* (*Hx*) has also been mapped to the mouse chromosomal locus, harbouring approxi-mately the same genes as the human *7q36* locus. The limb deformity in this mouse mutant, PPD with tibial dysplasia, is very similar to the pheno-type described in one of the families. In addition, the disease gene for a second mouse mutant, *Hammertoe* (*Hm*), has been mapped very close to the *Hx* disease gene. The phenotype in *Hm* mice resembles the complex polysyndactyly phenotype mentioned earlier (Tsukurov et al 1994). In mice, *SHH* is also located in the vicin-ity of the murine locus of these *Hx* and *Hm* mutants as was found with the human disease gene and there appears to be a mutation in sequences upstream of *SHH* which causes its misexpression at the anterior side of the developing limb.

Syndactyly

According to Temtamy and McKusick (1978), the syndactyly phenotype has been divided into five different types of syndactyly, depending on the parts of digits not separated in the hand and/or feet. All forms are inherited as an autosomal dominant trait and usually there is uniformity of the type of syndactyly within a given pedigree. Both syndactyly type IV (complete syndactyly of all fingers but no bone fusion and associated with polydactyly) and type V (fusion of the metacarpals and metatarsals) are relatively rare, and no linkage to any chromosomal locus has been found.

The features of syndactyly type III are mainly complete and bilateral soft-tissue syndactyly of the fourth and fifth finger, with occasional fusion of the distal phalanges. This phenotype is also part of the craniofacial disorder oculodentodigital dysplasia, which is characterized by facial, dental, and digital anomalies. Interestingly, both disorders have been mapped to the same locus, on *6q22–23*, suggesting that syndactyly type III and oculodentodigital dysplasia may be caused by different mutations in the same gene (Boyadjiev et al 1999, Gladwin et al 1997).

Syndactyly type I is characterized by non-separation involving digits three and four (complete or partial) and may include fusion of the distal phalanges of the third and fourth digit and/or second and third toes. Linkage analysis in a large German family mapped the disease gene to *2q34–36* (Bosse et al 2000). Syndactyly type II or synpolydactyly (SPD), was mapped to the neighbouring locus *2q31–32*. Syndactyly type II or synpolydactyly is defined as syndactyly of the third and fourth fingers as well as syndactyly of toes four and five, associated with polydactyly of the same fingers and/or toes. Syndactyly type II or synpolydactyly was the first isolated congenital hand malformation in which a mutation was detected (Muragaki et al 1996).

Syndactyly type II or synpolydactyly is caused by mutations in the homeobox gene *HOXD13*, (Akarsu et al 1996, Muragaki et al 1996). The mutation in *HOXD13* does not cause the absence of the protein, but most likely results in a protein with an altered function. As mentioned before, *HOXD13* is the last *HOXD* gene activated in the developing limb and is mainly expressed in the most posterior distal part of the developing limb, where also *HOXD9–12* are expressed (see Fig. 3). This corresponds with the finding of poly- and syndactyly in the posterior part of the limb. Recently a similar mutation was found in a mouse mutant, which resulted in the same phenotype (Johnson et al 1998).

The similarity in both mutation and phenotype between human and mouse aided in the identification of mutations in the hand-feet-genital (HFG) syndrome. The hand-feet-genital (HFG) syndrome is characterized by short thumbs, small feet with short big toes and defects of the Mullerian duct or its derivatives. The limb malformations resembled the phenotype found in a mouse mutant in which a mutation was found in the *HOXA13* gene (Mortlock et al 1996) and this triggered the search for mutations in the human *HOXA13* gene. In HFG patients a mutation was detected at a crucial position for DNA binding, most likely producing a nonfunctional protein that cannot bind DNA (Mortlock and Innis 1997).

So far, mutations have only been found in three human *HOX* genes. Beside the *HOXA13* and *HOXD13* mutations described above, mutations have been found in the *HOXA11* gene. And whereas the previous two mutations affect digits and hands only, the mutations in *HOXA11* were found in patients with radio-ulnar synostosis associated with a blood platelet disorder (Thompson and Nguyen 2000). The involvement of radius and ulna as opposed to only digits is in agreement with the wider and earlier expression of *HOXA11* as compared to both *HOXA13* and *HOXD13*, of which the expression is restricted to the more distal part of the developing limb.

Brachydactyly

Brachydactyly (BD) denotes a group of malformations in which the common feature is shortening of the digits. All five types are highly variable both between and within families. Type A is characterized by shortening or absence of the middle phalanges. When accompanied by rudimentary or absent terminal phalanges the BD is called type B. Brachydactyly type C is noted for its widely variable clinical phenotype both within and between families, featuring shortness of the second and fifth middle phalanges and the first metacarpal. Type D is characterized by short and broad terminal phalanges of the thumbs and big toes. In type E, shortening of the fingers is mainly in the metacarpals and metatarsals.

Three different genes have been identified so far for three different types of BD (see Table 1). Interestingly, but not surprisingly, all three genes are involved in a later stage of limb development, namely the proliferation and differentiation of chondrocytes into bone. Mutation in *IHH* leads to a reduced proliferation of chondrocytes and this explains the shortening or absence of the middle phalanges in BD type A (Gao et al 2001). A receptor tyrosine kinase, *ROR2*, is mutated in the more severe type B. This gene is involved in both the initial growth and patterning, as well as the proliferating chondrocytes, which would explain the more severe phenotype (Oldridge et al 2000). Finally, in BD type C, mutations have been found in the *CDMP1* gene (cartilage-derived morphogenetic protein-1), which encodes a BMP-like protein (Polinkovsky et al 1997). These mutations were found to lead to the production of a protein that inhibits chondrogenesis. The *CDMP1* protein can initiate and promote chondrogenesis.

The different phenotypes seen in the three BDs can be explained by differences in spatial and temporal expression of the three genes. Since all three genes identified so far in BD are involved in chondrogenesis, the genes in the other loci for BD are likely to play a role in bone formation.

Conclusions

Despite the rapid advances made in human genetics of the upper limb, relatively few specific human mutations that cause limb abnormalities have been identified. Hand surgeons should be aware of the basic molecular pathways control-ling limb development because they are in a unique position to be able to identify affected patients and their families, which could be suitable for linkage analysis. In turn, detailed clinical descriptions of congenital anomalies affecting the upper extremities will advance the understanding of the cellular events controlled by the molecular pathways of limb development and may help in identifying new genes. With the identification of new genes we will increase our insight into the molecular basis of congenital upper arm anomalies, and functional analysis of these gene families and their pathways will reveal their role in patterning and (normal) embryogenesis. In the future, the current morphological classifications of congenital limb malformations may be supplemented with genetic ones, possibly providing explanations for the great clinical variability and overlapping phenotypes.

References

Akarsu AN, Stoilov I, Yilmaz E, et al (1996) Genomic structure of HOXD13 gene: a nine polyalanine duplication causes synpolydactyly in two unrelated families, *Hum Mol Genet* **5**:945–52.

Bosse K, Betz RC, Lee YA, et al (2000) Localization of a gene for syndactyly type 1 to chromosome 2q34–q36, *Am J Hum Genet* **67**:492–7.

Boyadjiev SA, Jabs EW, LaBuda M, et al (1999) Linkage analysis narrows the critical region for oculodentodigital dysplasia to chromosome 6q22–q23, *Genomics* **58**:34–40.

Chevallier A, Kieny M, Mauger A (1977) Limb-somite relationship: origin of the limb musculature, *J Embryol Exp Morphol* **41**:245–58.

Chiang C, Litingtung Y, Lee E, et al (1996) Cyclopia and defective axial patterning in mice lacking Sonic hedgehog gene function, *Nature* **383**:407–13.

Christ B, Jacob HJ, Jacob M, et al (1982) On the origin, distribution and determination of avian limb mesenchymal cells, *Prog Clin Biol Res* **110**:281–91.

Cohn MJ, Tickle C (1996) Limbs: a model for pattern formation within the vertebrate body plan, *Trends Genet* **12**:253–7.

D'Amato RJ, Loughnan MS, Flynn E, et al (1994) Thalidomide is an inhibitor of angiogenesis, *Proc Natl Acad Sci U S A* **91**:4082–5.

de Walle HEK, Cornel MC, Haverman TM, et al (1992) EUROCAT, registration of congenital anomalies North Netherlands, tables 1981–1990, Rijksuniversiteit, Department of Medical Genetics, Medical Faculty, Groningen.

Dundar M, Gordon TM, Ozyazgan I, et al (2001) A novel acropectoral syndrome maps to chromosome 7q36, *J Med Genet* **38**:304–9.

Escamilla, MA, DeMille, MC, Benavides E, et al (2000) A minimalist approach to gene mapping: locating the gene for acheiropodia, by homozygosity analysis, *Am J Hum Genet* **66,** 1995–2000.

EUROCAT (1991), Surveillance of congenital anomalies, 1980–1988 EUROCAT central registry, Brussels.

Flatt, AE(1994) The Care of Congenital Hand Anomalies, Quality Medical Publishing, St Louis.

Gao B, Guo J, She C et al (2001) Mutations in IHH, encoding Indian hedgehog, cause brachydactyly type A-1, *Nat Genet* **28**:386–8.

Gladwin A, Donnai D, Metcalfe K, et al (1997) Localization of a gene for oculodentodigital syndrome to human chromosome 6q22–q24, *Hum Mol Genet* **6**: 123–7.

Heus HC, Hing A, van Baren MJ, et al (1999) A physical and transcriptional map of the preaxial polydactyly locus on chromosome 7q36, *Genomics* **57**:342–51.

Heutink P, Zguricas J, van Oosterhout L, et al (1994) The gene for triphalangeal thumb maps to the subtelomeric region of chromosome 7q, *Nat Genet* **6**:287–92.

Hing AV, Helms C, Slaugh R, et al (1995) Linkage of preaxial polydactyly type 2 to 7q36, *Am J Med Genet* **58**:128–35.

Ianakiev P, van Baren MJ, Daly MJ, et al (2001) Acheiropodia Is Caused by a Genomic Deletion in C7orf2, the Human Orthologue of the Lmbr1 Gene, *Am J Hum Genet* **68**:38–45.

Johnson KR, Sweet HO, Donahue LR, et al (1998) A new spontaneous mouse mutation of Hoxd13 with a polyalanine expansion and phenotype similar to human synpolydactyly, *Hum Mol Genet* **7**:1033–8.

Johnson RL, Tabin CJ (1997) Molecular models for vertebrate limb development, *Cell* **90**:979–90.

Krumlauf R (1994) Hox genes in vertebrate development, *Cell* **78**:191–201.

Lewandoski M, Sun X, Martin GR (2000) Fgf8 signalling from the AER is essential for normal limb development, *Nat Genet* **26**:460–3.

Lewis EB (1998) The bithorax complex: the first fifty years, *Int J Dev Biol* **42**:403–15.

Logan C, Hornbruch A, Campbell I, et al (1997) The role of Engrailed in establishing the dorsoventral axis of the chick limb, *Development* **124**:2317–24.

Moon AM, Capecchi MR (2000) Fgf8 is required for outgrowth and patterning of the limbs, *Nat Genet* **26**:455–9.

Mortlock DP, Innis JW (1997) Mutation of HOXA13 in hand-foot-genital syndrome, *Nat Genet* **15**:179–80.

Mortlock DP, Post LC, Innis JW (1996) The molecular basis of hypodactyly (Hd): a deletion in Hoxa 13 leads to arrest of digital arch formation, *Nat Genet* **13**:284–9.

Muragaki Y, Mundlos S, Upton J, et al (1996) Altered growth and branching patterns in synpolydactyly caused by mutations in HOXD13, *Science* **272**:548–51.

Oldridge M, Fortuna AM, Maringa M, et al (2000) Dominant mutations in ROR2, encoding an orphan receptor tyrosine kinase, cause brachydactyly type B, *Nat Genet* **24**:275–8.

Orioli IM, Castilla EE (1999) Thumb/hallux duplication and preaxial polydactyly type I, *Am J Med Genet* **82**:219–24.

Polinkovsky A, Robin NH, Thomas JT, et al (1997) Mutations in CDMP1 cause autosomal dominant brachydactyly type C, *Nat Genet* **17**:18–9.

Radhakrishna U, Blouin JL, Mehenni H, et al (1997) Mapping one form of autosomal dominant postaxial polydactyly type A to chromosome 7p15–q11.23 by linkage analysis, *Am J Hum Genet* **60**:597–604.

Radhakrishna U, Bornholdt D, Scott HS, et al (1999) The phenotypic spectrum of GLI3 morphopathies includes autosomal dominant preaxial polydactyly type-IV and postaxial polydactyly type-A/B; No phenotype prediction from the position of GLI3 mutations, *Am J Hum Genet* **65**:645–55.

Saunders JWJ (1948) The proximo-distal sequence of origin of the parts of the chick wing and the role of the ectoderm, *J Exp Zool* **108**:363–403.

Saunders JWJ, Gasseling MT (1968) Ectodermal-mesodermal interactions in the origin of limb symmetry, In: Fleischmajer RE,, Billingham R, eds, *Epithlelial-Mesenchymal Interactions* (Williams and Wilkins: Baltimore) 78–97.

Strachan T, Read AP (1999) *Human Molecular Genetics* (BIOS Scientific Publishers, Oxford).

Summerbell D, Lewis JH, Wolpert L (1973) Positional information in chick limb morphogenesis, *Nature* **244**:492–6.

Temtamy SA, McKusick VA (1978) The genetics of hand malformations, *Birth Defects Orig Artic Ser* **14**, **i-xviii:**1–619.

Thompson AA, Nguyen LT (2000) Amegakaryocytic thrombocytopenia and radio-ulnar synostosis are associated with HOXA11 mutation, *Nature Genet* **26**:397–8.

Tickle C (1995) Vertebrate limb development, *Curr Opin Genet Dev* **5**:478–84.

Tsukurov O, Boehmer A, Flynn J (1994) A complex bilateral polysyndactyly disease locus maps to chromosome 7q36, *Nat Genet* **6**:282–6.

Vortkamp A, Gessler M, Grzeschik KH (1991) GLI3 zinc-finger gene interrupted by translocations in Greig syndrome families *Nature* **352**:539–40.

3

Classification and related pathoembryology of congenital upper limb differences

Teun JM Luijsterburg, Christl Vermeij-Keers and Steven ER Hovius

When a child is born with a congenital difference of the upper limb, the parents are concerned about the aetiology, treatment, and future prospects of their child. Frequently, aberrations of other body systems are involved, such as the heart, the craniofacial region, and the lower limbs. Explanation of the aetiology, including potential risks for offspring, may partially calm the parent's concerns. Unfortunately, the under-lying cause, i.e. a genetic defect and/or a terato-gen, is often not known. The condition of their child can often be clarified using knowledge about the mechanisms that may precede the difference, i.e. the pathogenesis.

To understand the pathogenesis, a thorough knowledge of normal embryonic and fetal devel-opment is required. Morphological changes during normal development are tightly orches-trated in time and space, and are influenced by genetic and environmental factors. If those changes do not appear at the right time and/or at the right place, or if they do not appear at all, aberrations will develop. Interpretation of these aberrations in general and those of the upper limbs in particular is rather confusing.

In order to assist with the interpretation of the observed differences, several classification systems regarding upper limb differences have been developed (Frantz and O'Rahilly 1961, Swanson et al 1983, Temtamy and McKusick 1978). The most frequently used classification, the classification of Swanson et al (1983), is based on clinical diagnosis and failure during embryogenesis. After establishment and classifi-cation of the clinical diagnosis, the underlying mechanism should be revealed. Therefore,

consistency of the classification is of paramount importance. The consistency of Swanson's classi-fication has been discussed by several authors (Cheng et al 1987, De Smet et al 1997, Flatt 1994, Luijsterburg et al 2000, Ogino et al 1986). For example, clinical relationships have been demon-strated between polydactyly, syndactyly and typical cleft hand (Ogino 1990), and between brachysyndactyly, symbrachydactyly, and trans-verse deficiency (Miura et al 1994). However, these overlapping diagnoses are currently placed into different categories using Swanson's classi-fication, and prevent consistent interpretation. For groups of hand differences, several clinical (sub) classifications have been developed in order to aid the physician in the choice of treat-ment strategy (Bayne and Klug 1987, Blauth 1967, Blauth and Olason 1988, Temtamy and McKusick 1978). Nevertheless, problems arise if more differences are present in one limb, such as radial polydactyly and syndactyly. To overcome these difficulties, a descriptive method has been devel-oped at the Department of Plastic and Reconstructive Surgery of the University Hospital Rotterdam in The Netherlands. Recording only individual aberrations along with knowledge of normal and abnormal embryogenesis, expressed in terms of morphology and topography, will enable consistent interpretation of the differ-ences.

After introducing the recording form, four cases (syndactyly, polydactyly, symbrachydactyly, and thumb hypoplasia and radial club) will be presented using this descriptive method. Normal embryogenesis will be briefly outlined, and serves as background to explain the cases on the

Hospital Institute of Plastic Surgery **Please fill in white boxes**

1. GENERAL

Date of this registration	
Patient identification number	
Date of birth	
Gender	Male Female Unknown
Name of physician	
Clinical genetics consulted	Yes No Unknown
If affirmative, please specify location	
Adoption or foster child	Yes No Unknown

Caucasian father	Yes No Unknown
Caucasian mother	Yes No Unknown
Consanguinity	Yes No Unknown
If affirmative, please specify	
Occurrence among relatives	Yes No Unknown
If affirmative, please specify	
Birth weight (grams)	
Gestational age (weeks)	
Remarks about pregnancy	Yes No Unknown
If affirmative, please specify	

2. ABERRATIONS OF THE UPPER LIMB

L = left
R = right

Columns: H* R* U* C* | Ray I (MC* P1 P2 P3 N*) | Ray II (MC* P1 P2 P3 N*) | Ray III (MC* P1 P2 P3 N*) | Ray IV (MC* P1 P2 P3 N*) | Ray V (MC* P1 P2 P3 N*)

Rows (each cell has L/R boxes):
- Absence
- Malformed [1]
- Hypoplasia [2]
- Hyperplasia [3]
- Synostosis
- Syndactyly / fusion
- Duplication / polydactyly
- Clinodactyly
- Camptodactyly
- Ring constriction sec
- Tumor
- Trigger (L / R)
- Flexion impairment sec
- Extension impairment sec

Abnormal shoulder   Left   Yes   No   Unknown   Right   Yes   No   Unknown

Other aberrations of the upper limb, not appropriate above   Left   Yes   No   Unknown   Right   Yes   No   Unknown

■ (Preliminary) diagnosis of the left arm   Yes   No   Unknown _____

■ (Preliminary) diagnosis of the right arm   Yes   No   Unknown _____

3. OTHER ABERRATIONS

Circulatory system	Yes No Unknown
Respiratory system	Yes No Unknown
Digestive system	Yes No Unknown
Urogenital system	Yes No Unknown
Central nervous system	Yes No Unknown
Vertebral column	Yes No Unknown
Body wall	Yes No Unknown
Head and neck area	Yes No Unknown
Skin	Yes No Unknown
Lower limbs	Yes No Unknown
(Preliminary) common diagnosis	Yes No Unknown

1 = present, wrong shape; appropriate configuration, undersized = 2, oversized = 3
* H = humerus; R = radius; U = ulna; C = carpal bones; MC = metacarpal; N = nail

Please send form to Mw Dr Chr. Vermeij-Keers; Institute of Plastic Surgery, EE 1251A;
Erasmus Universiteit Rotterdam; Postbus 1738; 3000 DR Rotterdam; The Netherlands

ISBN 90-76580-07-3

Figure 1

Recording form.

- One recording form for each un-operated patient.

- Please only use ball point to mark the white boxes and to write text.

- The bold terms in this manual concern terms in the recording form.

Ad **2. ABERRATIONS OF THE UPPER LIMB**

- Recording is based on a morphological description of the congenital differences. Roughly, these can be divided into bony and soft tissue defects.

- More than one aberration can be marked. If aberrations can not be recorded, please check the box **other aberrations of the upper limb, not appropriate above**, and specify the aberrations.

- Bony defects
  - ➢ The concerning bones are **absent** or present (normal, **malformed, hypoplastic** or **hyperplastic**). Furthermore, please note any nail aberrations. The terms **malformed, hypoplasia,** and **hyperplasia** are explained in the footnotes of the recording form, as well as the abbreviations.
  - ➢ Fusion of bones can exist in transverse and longitudinal direction. Both cases are described as **synostosis**, and the concerning bones are marked.
  - ➢ Triphalangeal thumbs are noted as **polydactyly** of **P2 of ray I**.

- Soft tissue defects
  - ➢ In soft tissue **syndactyly** the height is indicated by recording concerning bones, for example a complete syndactyly of ray 3 and 4 is marked as **syndactyly** of **P1, P2** and **P3 of ray III and IV**.
  - ➢ In clino- and camptodactyly the corresponding bones are noted. If for example a clinodactyly of the proximal interphalangeal joint of ray 5 exists because of a Δ P1, please mark **malformed P1 of ray V** and **clinodactyly of P1 and P2 of ray V**.
  - ➢ If constriction bands are present, **ring constriction sec** is *also* noted at the level of the corresponding bones. For example, a constriction band is present at the level of right fourth P2, and P3 and the nail are absent, **ring constriction sec of P2 of ray IV** and **absence of P3 and N of ray IV** are marked.
  - ➢ **Tumors** also include lymphatic and/or vascular tumors, and are marked at the level of the corresponding bones.
  - ➢ Trigger fingers and thumbs are only indicated by the involved ray.
  - ➢ **Flexion- and/or extension impairment sec** concerns flexion and/or extension impairments without primary bone defects. Flexion impairment resulting from for example synostotic phalanges are *not* marked under this heading.

- If a diagnosis of the aberrations of the *upper limb* has been established, specify it in the box **(preliminary) diagnosis of the left and/or right arm**, after checking the **Yes** box.
  Example: i) Poland's syndrome with a hypoplastic hand: please fill in hypoplastic hand (**not** Poland, see also *Ad 3*), ii) **absence** of **P1** and **P3** of **ray I**, please fill in absent thumb.

Ad **3. OTHER ABERRATIONS**

- **Body wall** concerns the thoracic and abdominal wall.

- Pelvic aberrations are marked in the box **lower limbs**.

- If for example the aberrations are part of Poland's syndrome, please check the box **(preliminary) common diagnosis, Yes**, and fill in Poland. If the aberrations are not part of any syndrome, association, sequention, please mark this box **No**.

Remarks about the recording form and this manual may be adressed to: Mrs Dr Vermeij-Keers, Institute of Plastic Surgery, Room EE-1251A, Erasmus University Rotterdam, P.O. Box 1738, 3000 DR Rotterdam, the Netherlands. Phone: +31-10-4087242, Fax: +31-10-4089410, Email: Vermeij@plch.fgg.eur.nl
ISBN: 90-76580-07-3

Figure 2

Manual for the recording form.

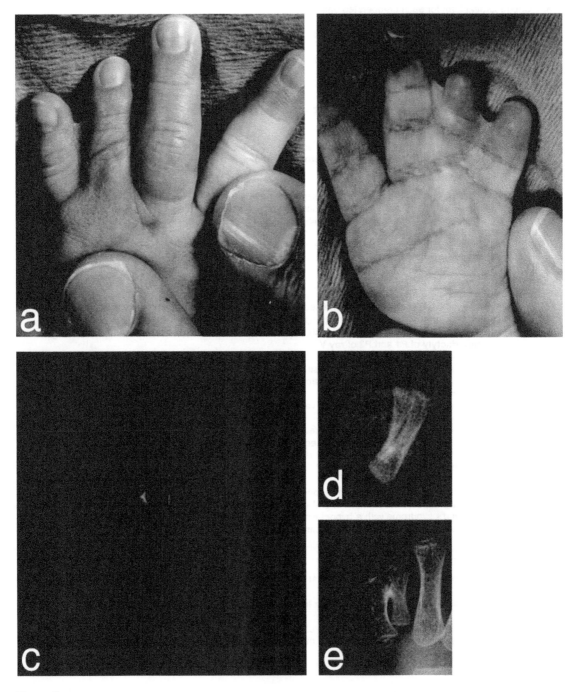

Figure 3

Case 1 Syndactyly. Dorsal (a) and palmar (b) view of the right hand, which displays an incomplete syndactyly between digits 1, 2 and 3, as well as an absent fifth ray. (c) Radiograph of the right hand showing absence of the fifth ray, and hypoplasia of P2 and P3 of ray 2. Detailed x-ray of the first and second metacarpals at the age of two months (d), and three years (e), which displays synostosis of the distal part of the first and second metacarpals. (f) Part 2 of the record displays all aberrations.

L = left / R = right	H*	R*	U*	C*	Ray I (MC* P1 P2 P3 N*)	Ray II (MC* P1 P2 P3 N*)	Ray III (MC* P1 P2 P3 N*)	Ray IV (MC* P1 P2 P3 N*)	Ray V (MC* P1 P2 P3 N*)	
Absence	L X	L X	X X	X X	L R, L R, L R, L R, L R	L R, L R, L R, L R, L R	L R, L R, L R, L R, L R	L R, L R, L R, L R, L R	L R, L R, L R, L R, L R	Absence
Malformed [1]	L R	L R	X R	L X	X R, L R, L R, L R, L R	L R, L R, L R, L R, L R	L R, L R, L R, L R, L R	L R, L R, L R, L R, L R	L R, L R, L R, L R, L R	Malformed [1]
Hypoplasia [2]	L R	L R	L R	L R	R X, L R, X X, L R, L R	L R, L R, L R, L R, L R	L R, L R, L R, L R, L R	L R, L R, L R, L R, L R	L R, L R, L R, L R, L R	Hypoplasia [2]
Hyperplasia [3]	L R	L R	L R	L R	L R, L R, L R, L R, L R	L R, L R, L R, L R, L R	L R, L R, L R, L R, L R	L R, L R, L R, L R, L R	L R, L R, L R, L R, L R	Hyperplasia [3]
Synostosis	L R	L R	L R	L R	L R, L R, L R, L R	L R, L R, L R, L R	L R, L R, L R, L R	L R, L R, L R, L R	L R, L R, L R, L R	Synostosis
Syndactyly / fusion					L R, L R, L R, L R	L R, L R, L R, L R	L R, L R, L R, L R	L R, L R, L R, L R	L R, L R, L R, L R	Syndactyly / fusion
Duplication / polydactyly	L R	L R	L R	L R	L R, L R, L R, L R, L R	L R, L R, L R, L R, L R	L R, L R, L R, L R, L R	L R, L R, L R, L R, L R	L R, L R, L R, L R, L R	Duplication / polydactyly
Clinodactyly					L R, L R, L R, L R	L R, L R, L R, L R	L R, L R, L R, L R	L R, L R, L R, L R	L R, L R, L R, L R	Clinodactyly
Camptodactyly					L R, L R, L R, L R	L R, L R, L R, L R	L R, L R, L R, L R	L R, L R, L R, L R	L R, L R, L R, L R	Camptodactyly
Ring constriction sec	L R	L R	L R	L R	L R, L R, L R	L R, L R, L R	L R, L R, L R	L R, L R, L R	L R, L R, L R	Ring constriction sec
Tumor	L R	L R	L R	L R	L R, L R, L R	L R, L R, L R	L R, L R, L R	L R, L R, L R	L R, L R, L R	Tumor
Trigger					L R	L R	L R	L R	L R	Trigger
Flexion impairment sec	L R	L R	L R	L R	L R	L R	L R	L R	L R	Flexion impairment sec
Extension impairment sec	L R	L R	L R	L R	L R	L R	L R	L R	L R	Extension impairment sec

1 = present, wrong shape; appropriate configuration, undersized = 2, oversized = 3
* H = humerus; R = radius; U = ulna; C = carpal bones; MC = metacarpal; N = nail

basis of imbalanced cell biological mechanisms, i.e. the pathoembryology.

The recording form

Morphological aberrations of each bone of both arms are described on the Y-axis of the recording form (Fig. 1). Bones can be absent or malformed, i.e. having the wrong shape. Furthermore, bones may exhibit an undersized (hypoplastic) or oversized (hyperplastic) configuration. Longitudinal or transverse fusion of bones is indicated as synostosis. Non-separation of digits without bone involvement is called syndactyly. Synostosis and syndactyly are indicated between the bones concerned (Fig. 2). Bones may be duplicated (polydactyly/duplication). The deviation of fingers in the radioulnar and dorsoventral plane is designated as clinodactyly and camptodactyly, respectively. Annular ring constrictions, as present in the congenital ring constriction syndrome, can be noted as well as tumours. Flexion and extension may be limited, without bony aetiology. Trigger fingers and thumbs are described as a separate category. Also, nails are described by their absence, wrong shape, undersized or oversized shape, their fusion, and their duplication. Topography is indicated on the X-axis and concerns all bony structures in a proximodistal way, from humerus to distal phalanges, and in a radioulnar way, from the thumb to the little finger.

Combining morphology and topography a two-dimensional table emerges, and it should be possible to describe every combination of aberrations of the upper limb. If an aberration will not fit in this table, a description can be given in the box 'other aberrations of the upper limb, not appropriate above'.

In order to provide information about the history of the patient and his or her family, a 'general' section and a section concerning 'other aberrations' are included. In addition, a manual is provided (Fig. 2).

Case 1 Syndactyly

At the age of two months, a male infant was referred to our outpatient clinic. He was born after 39 weeks of gestation and had a birth weight of 2750 grams. Physical examination revealed an incomplete (soft tissue) syndactyly between digits 1, 2, and 3 of the right hand, and an absent little finger (Figs 3a and b). The syndactylies reached up to the distal interphalangeal joints. The x-ray showed an absent fifth ray, and hypoplastic P2 and P3 of the index finger (Fig. 3c). Furthermore, the distal parts of metacarpals 1 and 2 were fused (Figs 3d and e). The record of this patient is shown in Figure 3f.

Case 2 Polydactyly

A three-month-old female patient was referred with a congenital difference of the right upper limb. She had a hyperplastic first metacarpal, and a polydactyly of P1 and P3 of digit I (type IV; Blauth and Olason 1988), including a duplication of its nail (Figs 4a-c). The distal phalanx is recorded as P3 in order to allow P1, P2, and P3 in a triphalangeal thumb to be registered. No other aberrations were present. Congenital differences of the upper limbs did not occur among her relatives.

Case 3 Symbrachydactyly

A one-year-old female patient was referred with aberrations of upper and lower limbs, craniofacial and renal differences. Occurrence among relatives was not known. She was born after 32 weeks of gestation and her birth weight was 2650 grams. Her shoulders, upper arms, and forearms were normal, but her hands were extremely malformed (Figs 5a and c). The left hand displayed a hyperplastic first metacarpal, a phalanx duplication of ray 1, and a camptodactyly of the first metacarpophalangeal and interphalangeal joints (Figs 5a and b). On the recording form (Fig. 5e) the duplication was designated as P1, as no nail was observed. The digits 2 and 3 were absent, including their nails. Furthermore, a so-called transverse bone was present, which was fused with P1 of ray 4. On the form this bone was designated as the P1 of the third digit, because of the presence of a growth plate at the proximal side of this phalanx. Lastly, a clinodactyly of the fourth metacarpophalangeal joint was observed.

The right hand displayed a duplication of the first metacarpal (Figs 5c and d). The first interphalangeal joint showed a camptodactyly. The second and third digits were absent, as were their nails. The metacarpals of rays 2 and 3 were hypoplastic. A clinodactyly was present on the metacarpophalangeal joints of rays 4 and 5.

Her feet also showed symbrachydactyly. Moreover, she had a bilateral cleft lip and palate, and renal cysts. Since the combination of the complex hand differences, symbrachydactyly of both feet, cleft and renal aberrations may originate from a genetic disorder, this patient was referred to the clinical genetics department for assessment.

Case 4 Thumb hypoplasia and radial club

A young female was first referred to our outpatient clinic at the age of 12. Physical examination and x-rays showed differences of both upper limbs. Both limbs had no aberrations of the shoulder and upper arm. The left limb showed an absent radius (type IV; Bayne and Klug 1987) and a malformed ulna (Fig. 6c), thereby causing a severe radial deviation (Fig. 6a), and an absent thumb (Type V; Blauth 1967) (Figs 6a and c). Also, radial carpals were absent. The right limb displayed malformed radial carpals. The first ray exhibited a malformed metacarpal, and hypoplasia of P1, P3, and the

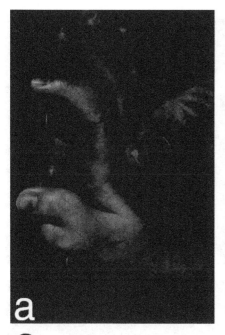

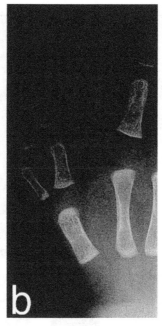

Figure 4

Case 2 Polydactyly. (a) Dorsal view of the right hand, which shows a duplicated thumb. Its nail was also duplicated (not visible). (b) The x-ray shows a hyperplastic first metacarpal, and a duplicated P1 and P3. (c) Part 2 of the record of this patient.

c

L = left / R = right	H*	R*	U*	C*	Ray I MC*	P1	P2	P3	N*	Ray II MC*	P1	P2	P3	N*	Ray III MC*	P1	P2	P3	N*	Ray IV MC*	P1	P2	P3	N*	Ray V MC*	P1	P2	P3	N*	
Absence	L/R	L/R	L/R	L/R	L/R	L/R		L/R	L/R	L/R	L/R	L/R	L/R	L/R	L/R	L/R	L/R	L/R	L/R	L/R	L/R	L/R	L/R	L/R	L/R	L/R	L/R	L/R	L/R	Absence
Malformed[1]	L/R	L/R	L/R	L/R	L/R	L/R		L/R	L/R	L/R	L/R	L/R	L/R	L/R	L/R	L/R	L/R	L/R	L/R	L/R	L/R	L/R	L/R	L/R	L/R	L/R	L/R	L/R	L/R	Malformed[1]
Hypoplasia[2]	L/R	L/R	L/R	L/R	L/R	L/R		L/R	L/R	L/R	L/R	L/R	L/R	L/R	L/R	L/R	L/R	L/R	L/R	L/R	L/R	L/R	L/R	L/R	L/R	L/R	L/R	L/R	L/R	Hypoplasia[2]
Hyperplasia[3]	L/R	L/R	L/R	L/R	L/X	L/R		L/R	L/R	L/R	L/R	L/R	L/R	L/R	L/R	L/R	L/R	L/R	L/R	L/R	L/R	L/R	L/R	L/R	L/R	L/R	L/R	L/R	L/R	Hyperplasia[3]
Synostosis	L/R	L/R	L/R	L/R	L/R	L/R	L/R	L/R		L/R	L/R	L/R	L/R		L/R	L/R	L/R	L/R		L/R	L/R	L/R	L/R		L/R	L/R	L/R	L/R		Synostosis
Syndactyly / fusion					L/R	L/R	L/R	L/R		L/R	L/R	L/R	L/R		L/R	L/R	L/R	L/R	L/R	L/R	L/R	L/R	L/R		L/R	L/R	L/R	L/R		Syndactyly / fusion
Duplication / polydactyly	L/R	L/R	L/R	L/R	L/R	L/X	L/R	L/X	L/X	L/R	L/R	L/R	L/R	L/R	L/R	L/R	L/R	L/R	L/R	L/R	L/R	L/R	L/R	L/R	L/R	L/R	L/R	L/R	L/R	Duplication / polydactyly
Clinodactyly					L/R	L/R		L/R		L/R	L/R	L/R	L/R		L/R	L/R	L/R	L/R		L/R	L/R	L/R	L/R		L/R	L/R	L/R	L/R		Clinodactyly
Camptodactyly					L/R	L/R		L/R		L/R	L/R	L/R	L/R		L/R	L/R	L/R	L/R		L/R	L/R	L/R	L/R		L/R	L/R	L/R	L/R		Camptodactyly
Ring constriction sec	L/R	L/R	L/R	L/R	L/R	L/R		L/R		L/R	L/R	L/R	L/R		L/R	L/R	L/R	L/R		L/R	L/R	L/R	L/R		L/R	L/R	L/R	L/R		Ring constriction sec
Tumor	L/R	L/R	L/R	L/R	L/R	L/R		L/R		L/R	L/R	L/R	L/R		L/R	L/R	L/R	L/R		L/R	L/R	L/R	L/R		L/R	L/R	L/R	L/R		Tumor
Trigger						L/R					L/R					L/R					L/R					L/R				Trigger
Flexion impairment sec	L/R	L/R	L/R	L/R		L/R					L/R					L/R					L/R					L/R				Flexion impairment sec
Extension impairment sec	L/R	L/R	L/R	L/R		L/R					L/R					L/R					L/R					L/R				Extension impairment sec

1 = present, wrong shape; appropriate configuration, undersized = 2, oversized = 3
* H = humerus; R = radius; U = ulna; C = carpal bones; MC = metacarpal; N = nail

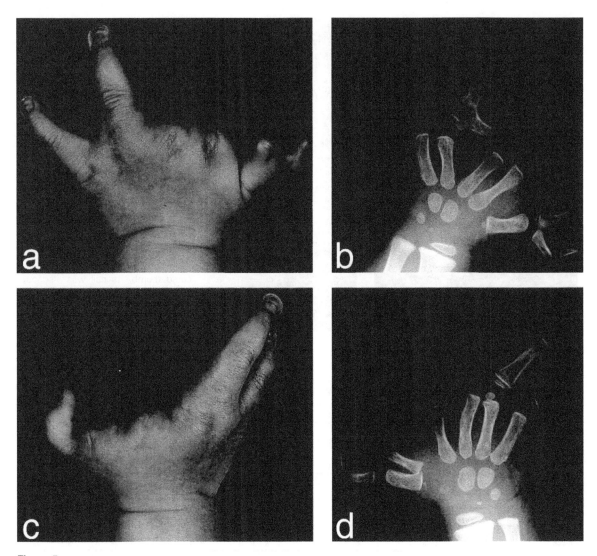

Figure 5

Case 3 Symbrachydactyly. Dorsal view of the left (a) and right (c) hand displaying absent rays and nails, camptodactyly, and clinodactyly. Radiographs of the left (b) and right (d) showing duplications, absent digits, camptodactylies, and clinodactylies. Note the proximal growth plate of the third P1. (e) The record demonstrates that these more complex differences can be described in part 2.

nail (type IIIB; Blauth 1967, Manske and McCarroll 1992) (Figs 6d and e). The function of the thumb was limited to translation at the carpometacarpal level. In addition, the thumb was unstable at the metacarpophalangeal joint. The record is shown in Figure 6f.

Previously, surgery was performed due to a tetralogy of Fallot and oesophageal atresia. These congenital differences can be diagnosed the VACTERL association (vertebral defects, anal atresia, cardiovascular defects, tracheo-oesophageal fistula, renal and limb defects).

L = left / R = right	H*	R*	U*	C*	Ray I					Ray II					Ray III					Ray IV					Ray V					
					MC*	P1	P2	P3	N*	MC*	P1	P2	P3	N*	MC*	P1	P2	P3	N*	MC*	P1	P2	P3	N*	MC*	P1	P2	P3	N*	
Absence	L/R	L/R	L/R	L/R	L/R	L/R		L/R	L/R	L/R	X	X	X	X	L/R	L	X	X	X	L/R	L/R	L/R	L/R	L/R	L/R	L/R	L/R	L/R	L/R	Absence
Malformed [1]	L/R	L/R	L/R	L/R	L/R	L/R		L/R	L/R	L/R	L/R	L/R	L/R	L/R	L/R	L/R	L/R	L/R	L/R	L/R	L/R	L/R	L/R	L/R	L/R	L/R	L/R	L/R	L/R	Malformed [1]
Hypoplasia [2]	L/R	L/R	L/R	L/R	L/R	L/R		L/R	L/R	L/X	L/R	L/R	L/R	L/R	L/X	L/R	L/R	L/R	L/R	L/R	L/R	L/R	L/R	L/R	L/R	L/R	L/R	L/R	L/R	Hypoplasia [2]
Hyperplasia [3]	L/R	L/R	L/R	L/R	X/R	L/R		L/R	L/R	L/R	L/R	L/R	L/R	L/R	L/R	L/R	L/R	L/R	L/R	L/R	L/R	L/R	L/R	L/R	L/R	L/R	L/R	L/R	L/R	Hyperplasia [3]
Synostosis	L/R	L/R	L/R	L/R	L/R	L/R	L/R	L		L/R	L/R	L/R	L		L/R	X	L	L		L/R	X	L	L		L/R	L/R	L/R	L		Synostosis
Syndactyly / fusion					L/R	L/R	L/R	L/R		L/R	L/R	L/R	L/R		L/R	L/R	L/R	L/R		L/R	L/R	L/R	L/R		L/R	L/R	L/R	L/R		Syndactyly / fusion
Duplication / polydactyly	L/R	L/R	L/R	L/R	L/X	X/R	L/R	L/R	L/R	L/R	L/R	L/R	L/R	L/R	L/R	L/R	L/R	L/R	L/R	L/R	L/R	L/R	L/R	L/R	L/R	L/R	L/R	L/R	L/R	Duplication / polydactyly
Clinodactyly					L/R	L/R		L/R		L/R	L/R	L/R	L/R		L/R	L/R	L/R	L/R		X/X	X/X	L/R	L/R		X/X	X/X	L/R	L/R		Clinodactyly
Camptodactyly					X/R	X/X		X/X		L/R	L/R	L/R	L/R		L/R	L/R	L/R	L/R		L/R	L/R	L/R	L/R		L/R	L/R	L/R	L/R		Camptodactyly
Ring constriction sec	L/R	L/R	L/R	L/R	L/R	L/R		L/R		L/R	L/R	L/R	L/R		L/R	L/R	L/R	L/R		L/R	L/R	L/R	L/R		L/R	L/R	L/R	L/R		Ring constriction sec
Tumor	L/R	L/R	L/R	L/R	L/R	L/R		L/R		L/R	L/R	L/R	L/R		L/R	L/R	L/R	L/R		L/R	L/R	L/R	L/R		L/R	L/R	L/R	L/R		Tumor
Trigger					L/R					L/R					L/R					L/R					L/R					Trigger
Flexion impairment sec	L/R	L/R	L/R	L/R	L/R					L/R					L/R					L/R					L/R					Flexion impairment sec
Extension impairment sec	L/R	L/R	L/R	L/R	L/R					L/R					L/R					L/R					L/R					Extension impairment sec

1 = present, wrong shape; appropriate configuration, undersized = 2, oversized = 3
* H = humerus; R = radius; U = ulna; C = carpal bones; MC = metacarpal; N = nail

Normal limb development

General principles

As genetic aspects of limb development are discussed elsewhere in this book, some basic processes during limb formation will be described here. Important cell biological processes for development of any tissue are cell proliferation, cell differentiation, and cell death. Forming a tissue or an organ requires cell proliferation, i.e. obtaining volume via mitosis. To provide a tissue with its future shape and function, cells differentiate and cells die as well. Differentiation means that a cell gets a more specialized function. For example, an undifferentiated mesodermal cell, i.e., this cell has the potential to become many cell types, loses some

potential, and is bound to differentiate into a chondroblast and eventually via an osteoblast into an osteocyte. Specific genes are switched on and off, thereby determining cell fate. Which genes are activated or repressed largely depends on their environment.

Besides mitosis, abundant cells die (apoptosis) to enable shaping of tissue. Apoptosis can be morphologically distinguished from necrosis (Kerr et al 1972, Wyllie et al 1980). A necrotic cell loses its plasma membrane integrity, thereby draining its contents into the extracellular space and provoking an inflammatory response. During this response the debris is removed by macrophages. In contrast, an apoptotic cell maintains its plasma membrane integrity, the cytoplasm shrinks, and the nucleus condensates and becomes pyknotic. Cells are removed by

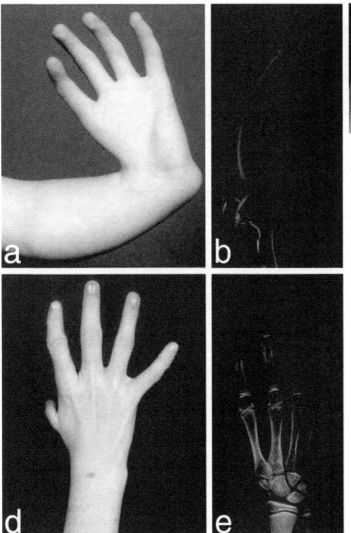

Figure 6

Case 4 Thumb hypoplasia and radial club. (a) Palmar view of the left forearm and hand showing severe radial deviation and an absent thumb. Radiographs of the left forearm (b) and hand (c) displaying absence of the radius and thumb. Dorsal view (d) and x-ray (e) of the right hand. The thumb is severely hypoplastic. (f) The patient's record (part 2).

phagocytosis of neighbouring cells or specialized phagocytes (Wood et al 2000). When a cell gets the signal to become apoptotic, it actively initiates an energy consuming 'death' cascade. Several cascades exist in each cell, and the choice of the cascade appears to be dependent on the trigger of death and/or of the cell type (Fesus 1993). Furthermore, an apoptotic cell has to signal to its environment that it is set to die in order to be recognized and removed by phagocytes (Savill et al 1993). One of these

signals is exposure of the phospholipid, phosphatidylserine (PS) at the outer leaflet of the plasma membrane and is a trigger for phagocytosis in vivo (Hamon et al 2000, Luciani and Chimini 1996, van den Eijnde et al 1997). Normally PS resides at the inner leaflet of the plasma membrane.

Obviously, the cell biological processes are tightly regulated in time and space and orchestrate the enormous morphological changes in a developing limb. The positional information of a

f

L = left / R = right	H*	R*	U*	C*	Ray I MC*	P1	P2	P3	N*	Ray II MC*	P1	P2	P3	N*	Ray III MC*	P1	P2	P3	N*	Ray IV MC*	P1	P2	P3	N*	Ray V MC*	P1	P2	P3	N*	
Absence	L/R	L/R	L/R	L/R	L/R	L/R		L/R	L/R	L/R	L/R	L/R	L/R	L/R	L/R	L/R	L/R	L/R	L/R	L/R	L/R	L/R	L/R	L/R	X	X	X	X	X	Absence
Malformed 1	L/R	L/R	L/R	L/R	L/R	L/R		L/R	L/R	L/R	L/R	L/R	L/R	L/R	L/R	L/R	L/R	L/R	L/R	L/R	L/R	L/R	L/R	L/R	L/R	L/R	L/R	L/R	L/R	Malformed 1
Hypoplasia 2	L/R	L/R	L/R	L/R	L/R	L/R		L/R	L/R	L/R	L/R	X	X	L/R	L/R	L/R	L/R	L/R	L/R	L/R	L/R	L/R	L/R	L/R	L/R	L/R	L/R	L/R	L/R	Hypoplasia 2
Hyperplasia 3	L/R	L/R	L/R	L/R	L/R	L/R		L/R	L/R	L/R	L/R	L/R	L/R	L/R	L/R	L/R	L/R	L/R	L/R	L/R	L/R	L/R	L/R	L/R	L/R	L/R	L/R	L/R	L/R	Hyperplasia 3
Synostosis	L/R	L/R	L/R	L/R	L/X	L/R	L/R	L/R		L/X	L/R	L/R			L/R	L/R	L/R	L/R		L/R	L/R	L/R	L/R		L/R	L/R	L/R	L/R		Synostosis
Syndactyly / fusion						L/X	L/R	L/X	L/R		L/X	L/X	L/R	L/R		L/X	L/X	L/R	L/R		L/R	L/R	L/R	L/R		L/R	L/R	L/R	L/R	Syndactyly / fusion
Duplication / polydactyly	L/R	L/R	L/R	L/R	L/R	L/R	L/R	L/R	L/R	L/R	L/R	L/R	L/R	L/R	L/R	L/R	L/R	L/R	L/R	L/R	L/R	L/R	L/R	L/R	L/R	L/R	L/R	L/R	L/R	Duplication / polydactyly
Clinodactyly					L/R	L/R		L/R		L/R	L/R	L/R	L/R		L/R	L/R	L/R	L/R		L/R	L/R	L/R	L/R		L/R	L/R	L/R	L/R		Clinodactyly
Camptodactyly					L/R	L/R		L/R		L/R	L/R	L/R	L/R		L/R	L/R	L/R	L/R		L/R	L/R	L/R	L/R		L/R	L/R	L/R	L/R		Camptodactyly
Ring constriction sec	L/R	L/R	L/R	L/R	L/R	L/R		L/R		L/R	L/R	L/R	L/R		L/R	L/R	L/R	L/R		L/R	L/R	L/R	L/R		L/R	L/R	L/R	L/R		Ring constriction sec
Tumor	L/R	L/R	L/R	L/R	L/R	L/R		L/R		L/R	L/R	L/R	L/R		L/R	L/R	L/R	L/R		L/R	L/R	L/R	L/R		L/R	L/R	L/R	L/R		Tumor
Trigger					L/R					L/R					L/R					L/R					L/R					Trigger
Flexion impairment sec	L/R	L/R	L/R	L/R	L/R					L/R					L/R					L/R					L/R					Flexion impairment sec
Extension impairment sec	L/R	L/R	L/R	L/R	L/R					L/R					L/R					L/R					L/R					Extension impairment sec

1 = present, wrong shape; appropriate configuration, undersized = 2, oversized = 3
* H = humerus; R = radius; U = ulna; C = carpal bones; MC = metacarpal; N = nail

cell at a certain time during development is considered to be the most important factor for proliferation, differentiation, and apoptosis. Here, morphological changes are related to the timing in mouse embryos. An overview of these changes in human embryos is shown in Table 1 (O'Rahilly et al 1959, O'Rahilly and Gardner 1972 and 1975, Vermeij-Keers C, personal communication).

Outgrowth and apoptosis

Forelimbs emerge from the lateral body wall in mouse embryos at nine days post coitum (dpc). The lower limbs develop slightly later than the upper limbs, and most factors controlling their morphogenesis are identical. This accounts for the often striking resemblance in phenotypes of the affected upper and lower limbs, of which the lower limbs often exhibit a more severe phenotype. Each limb bud consists of an undifferentiated proliferating core of mesodermal cells, covered by a single layer of ectoderm. At 10 dpc apoptotic cells are scattered across the mesenchyme and ectoderm of the limbs. On the border between the dorsal and palmar surfaces of the limb, a ridge of specialized ectoderm is formed, i.e. the apical ectodermal ridge (AER). This ridge consists of pseudostratified epithelium, which means that the nuclei are arranged in different layers, but each cell contacts the basal membrane. The AER is induced by factors

Table 1 Timing of morphological changes in the developing human upper limbs during embryogenesis (corresponding 12 weeks of development).

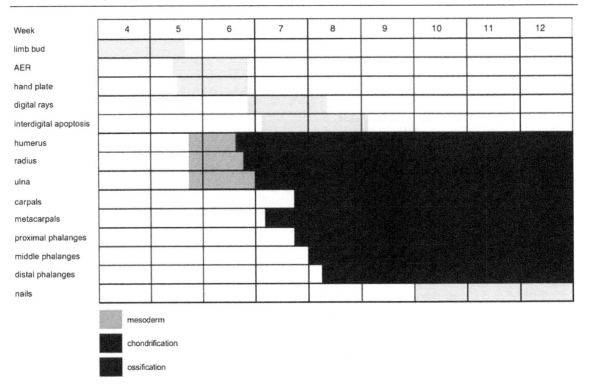

secreted by the underlying mesoderm, which is called the progress zone. This zone is bordered by the marginal sinus, which is part of the blood supply of the limb. The AER is considered to be essential for outgrowth in the proximodistal axis.

Two theories exist regarding this outgrowth. One theory is based on AER signals to the underlying mesoderm (Crackower et al 1998, Tabin 1995, Tickle 1996a and 1996b). The signals maintain the cells in the progress zone in an undifferentiated and highly proliferative state. In addition many cells die, thereby leading to indirect differential growth. The second theory postulates that the AER is directly involved in outgrowth. Apoptosis in the AER causes loss of cell contacts and disruption of the basal membrane. Subsequently, ectodermal cells are transferred to the progress zone and transform into mesodermal cells, i.e. epitheliomesodermal transformation. The apoptotic cells in the progress zone are thought to give passage to the transferred ectodermal cells (Boshart et al 2000, Hartwig et al 1990). This process is called appositional growth. As the outgrowth continues, cells that are located proximally leave the progress zone. Before they leave positional information is acquired. So cells in the future upper arm get their positional information earlier than cells in the forearm, and subsequently differentiation of proximal structures precedes distal structures (Summerbell et al 1973).

At 11 dpc the whole limb is present, i.e. the upper arm, the forearm, and hand plate are recognizable. Apoptosis is present in the AER, and in the lateral borders of the developing limb, i.e. preaxial (thumb side) and postaxial (little finger side) (Figs 7a-c). Pre- and postaxial apoptosis participates in the shaping of the forearm and hand plate. These patterns remain visible until 14 dpc (Hurle et al 1996, Kimura and Shiota 1996, Milaire and Rooze 1983).

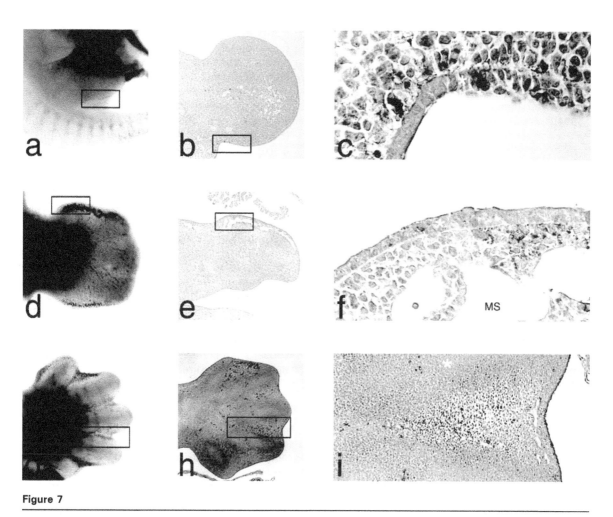

Figure 7

Limbs of 11 dpc mouse embryos. (a) Whole mount staining with the cell death marker Nile Blue sulphate. The postaxial side of the limb is the boxed area. (b and c) Frontal microscopic sections stained with the cell death marker, Annexin V biotin. Figure (c) is a magnification of the boxed area in Figure (b). Note that postaxially cells are dying both in the AER (*) and in the underlying mesoderm (#).

Limbs of 12 dpc mouse embryos. (d) Whole mount staining with Nile Blue sulphate. Note the preaxial and postaxial cell death regions. The marginal sinus is represented by the red staining. (e and f) Sagittal sections through the boxed area in Figure (d). Note the overwhelming cell death in the progress zone (#), and in the AER (*), visualized with Annexin V biotin. MS: marginal sinus.

Limbs of 13 dpc mouse embryos. (g and h) Massive interdigital cell death: Nile Blue sulphate (g), and Annexin V biotin (h). The boxed area in Figure (h) is magnified in Figure (i). (i) Interdigital cell death visualized with Annexin V biotin. *: digit; #: interdigital mesoderm.

Digital rays become visible at 12 dpc. Apoptosis is present in a triangular region between the upper arm and forearm, thereby forming the future elbow joint. In the mesodermal anlage of the forearm apoptosis is observed. This region, the opaque patch, divides the anlage into the presumptive radius and ulna (Milaire and Rooze 1983; Kimura and Shiota 1996). In the AER and progress zone, many apoptotic cells are observed and are related to the outgrowth (Figs 7d-f). At the end of the twelfth day, cells die in the proximal and distal interdigital regions.

Those apoptosis areas expand and reach each other, thereby causing the ectoderm and mesoderm of the whole V-shaped interdigital region to be abundant with apoptotic cells at 13 dpc (Figs 7g-i) (Mori et al 1995, Salas-Vidal et al 2001, van den Eijnde et al 1997, Zakeri et al 1994).

Differentiation and apoptosis

From 13 to 14 dpc, apoptosis is observed in specific regions of the 'solid' mesodermal condensations of the wrist and digits. The apoptotic cells are removed by phagocytosis, and the cavities created form the presumptive joints in the wrist region and the presumptive phalangeal joints (van den Eijnde et al 1997). This process is called luminization. The same process establishes separation of the digits.

Formation of the skeletal elements involves three differentiation steps, and is associated with apoptosis. Mesoderm differentiates into pre-cartilaginous condensed mesoderm, which turns into cartilage, and finally into bone. Pre-cartilaginous mesoderm formation starts on 11 dpc, and chondrification on 12 dpc in a proximodistal direction with a gradient from the preaxial to the postaxial side. Chondrification is completed at 14–15 dpc. Ossification starts on 14 dpc and finishes postnatally. The direction of the definitive differentiation in mouse bone centres is as follows: humerus, radius, ulna, scapula, metacarpals, distal phalanges, proximal phalanges, and middle phalanges. Finally the smaller carpals start to ossify (Kaufman 1992). Nails are formed during the first stages of the ossification of the distal phalanges (regarding human embryos, see Table 1).

Besides the above-mentioned cell death patterns, individual cells also die and are removed, especially during remodelling of muscles and nerves. Differentiation of the muscles starts with the formation of the cartilage and ossification.

Abnormal limb development

Regardless whether the differences originate from genetic and/or environmental factors, key roles appear to be present for the timing and the amount of cell proliferation, cell differentiation, and cell death.

If experimentally the AER is removed, no further outgrowth is possible, but more proximal structures are still capable of differentiation (Saunders 1948). The earlier the AER is disrupted, the more proximal structures fail to develop. If in the AER too much apoptosis is present, or if the onset of apoptosis is too early, a decrease in AER activity may follow, thereby impairing outgrowth. In humans, transverse reduction defects are believed to be the result of disruption of the AER. For example a transverse reduction defect at the level of the wrist is considered to originate later than a reduction at the level of the humerus. Note that the term reduction is not correct, since it implies that distal structures were formed and disappear later on. In contrast, increase in AER activity because of a delay and/or decrease in apoptosis may cause an increase in skeletal elements in the proximodistal direction (triphalangeal thumb). However, triphalangeal thumbs can also be the result of diminished apoptosis at preaxial sites. Diminished apoptosis at preaxial and postaxial sites may lead to polydactyly. Case 2 is an example of a 'straightforward' preaxial polydactyly, that could be the result of this mechanism, irrespective of its unknown inducer.

Separation of the precartilaginous mesodermal condensations can be disturbed by a decrease in apoptosis. This would give rise to transverse synostosis (Hoeven et al 1994). Increased cell death may result in (partial) loss of the mesodermal models and thereby give rise to absent or malformed bones. Abnormal chondrification and/or ossification will also lead to absent or malformed bone(s). Case 3 may serve as an example in which an increase of apoptosis in the central distal part of the hand plate results in the observed phenotype. The polydactyly of both first rays may originate from changed positional information, which tells the cells to differentiate into bone instead of telling them to die. An explanation for case 4, the patient with absence of the left radius and thumb and a hypoplastic right radius and thumb, is that a combination of too much apoptosis and subsequent diminished differentiation has led to the phenotype. Note, that in this patient the whole radial side is underdeveloped, and aberrant or absent nerves, muscles, and blood vessels are also observed.

If cell death is diminished in interdigital regions, (soft tissue) syndactyly results. Total absence of interdigital apoptosis leads to complete syndactyly (Knudsen and Kochhar 1981, Zakeri et al 1994). Incomplete syndactyly located distally, proximally or in the middle, can be explained by focal lack of cell death (case 1). Decreased cell death during joint formation may result in longitudinal synostosis of the phalanges of the same finger (symphalangism).

Considering the formation of the skeletal elements, derailments in all differentiation steps can occur. No ossification of the phalanges may result in finger buds. If for example the chondroblasts fail to differentiate into osteoblasts at 10 weeks of development in humans, the distal phalanx may be ossified and the middle and proximal phalanges of the same ray may be missing (see Table 1). Hypoplastic middle phalanges and normal proximal and distal phalanges (brachydactyly; Temtamy and McKusick 1978) may be explained by defective ossification of the middle phalanges, whereas the other phalanges have already ossified. As ossification of the distal phalanx is accompanied by nail formation, the presence of nails indicates that the distal phalanx has been formed.

It should be noted that the above-mentioned cases are relatively clear examples about the consequences of derailments in cell proliferation, cell differentiation, and cell death. However, in more complex differences of the upper limb these relationships cannot be readily reproduced.

Conclusions

Physicians, involved in treating patients with congenital differences of the upper limb, have also an important task to inform the patient and the parents about the difference. Only the results of developmental derailments can be observed in a child, and not the derailments themselves, because the morphological changes occurred during embryogenesis and fetal development. Therefore, the physician should be able to render the observed aberrations into the preceding mechanisms.

Support for this interpretation is provided by

several classification systems. However, these systems do not always allow a consistent interpretation. In the ideal situation, a classification should be straightforward and must give a full description of the differences, including more complex differences. These conditions are conflicting, and concessions have to be made. Consequently, every system has its limitations. Our new recording system allows consistent description of the aberrations, but very specific details cannot be noted (for example type III and IV radial polydactyly; Blauth and Olason 1988). No division is made based on diagnosis, because establishing diagnoses interprets the observed aberrations and causes loss of information about the aberrations (see for example the symbrachydactyly case). Our recording system combined with knowledge of normal and abnormal basic processes during embryogenesis, should allow an explanation in most cases of how the difference may have emerged. In the future, additional information will obviously be provided by the rapidly expanding knowledge regarding the genetic aspects of limb development.

Besides informing the patient and the parents about the difference, consistent classification is also very important to allow the pathogenesis to be studied. Furthermore, intra-centre and national and international inter-centre studies concerning frequency, treatment, and surveillance of the differences require consistent description of the differences. After recording, each difference can be categorized according to any classification. Finally, when diagnoses are modified because of new data about the pathogenesis, the same records can be used to implement these modifications without losing details about simple and complex differences.

References

Bayne LG, Klug MS (1987) Long-term review of the surgical treatment of radial deficiencies, *J Hand Surg [Am]* 12:169–79.

Blauth W (1967) The hypoplastic thumb, *Arch Orthop Unfallchir* **62**:225–46.

Blauth W, Olason AT (1988) Classification of polydactyly of the hands and feet, *Arch Orthop Trauma Surg* **107**:334–44.

Boshart L, Vlot AE, Vermeij-Keers C (2000) Epithelio-mesenchymal transformation in the embryonic face: implications for craniofacial malformations, *Eur J Plast Surg* **23**:217–23.

Cheng JC, Chow SK, Leung PC (1987) Classification of 578 cases of congenital upper limb anomalies with the IFSSH system—a 10 year experience, *J Hand Surg [Am]* **12**:1055–60.

Crackower MA, Motoyama J, Tsui LC (1998) Defect in the maintenance of the apical ectodermal ridge in the Dactylaplasia mouse, *Dev Biol* **201**:78–89.

De Smet L, Matton G, Monstrey S, et al (1997) Application of the IFSSH(3)-classification for congenital anomalies of the hand: results and problems, *Acta Orthop Belg* **63**:182–8.

Fesus L (1993) Biochemical events in naturally occurring forms of cell death, *FEBS Lett* **328**:1–5.

Flatt AE (1994) Classification and incidence. In: Flatt AE, ed, *The care of congenital hand anomalies*, 2nd edn (Quality Medical Publishing Inc: St Louis) 47–63.

Frantz CH, O'Rahilly R (1961) Congenital skeletal limb deficiencies, *J Bone Joint Surg* **43A**:1202–24.

Hamon Y, Broccardo C, Chambenoit O, et al (2000) ABC1 promotes engulfment of apoptotic cells and transbilayer redistribution of phosphatidylserine, *Nat Cell Biol* **2**:399–406.

Hartwig NG, Vermeij-Keers C, Smits-van Prooije AE (1990) Limb-bud placodes: sources of cells for developing limbs, *J Anat* **173**:229–30.

Hoeven FVD, Schimmang T, Volkmann A, et al (1994) Programmed cell death is affected in the novel mouse mutant fused toes (Ft), **120**:2601–7.

Hurle JM, Ros MA, Climent V, et al (1996) Morphology and significance of programmed cell death in the developing limb bud of the vertebrate embryo, *Microsc Res Tech* **34**:236–46.

Kaufman MH (1992) *The atlas of mouse development*, (Academic Press Limited: London).

Kerr JFR, Wyllie AH, Currie AR (1972) Apoptosis: a basic biological phenomenon with wide-ranging implications in tissue kinetics, *Br J Cancer* **26**:239–257.

Kimura S, Shiota K (1996) Sequential changes of programmed cell death in developing fetal mouse limbs and its possible roles in limb morphogenesis, *J Morphol* **229**:337–46.

Knudsen TB, Kochhar DM (1981) The role of morphogenetic cell death during abnormal limb-bud outgrowth in mice heterozygous for the dominant mutation Hemimelia-extra toe (Hmx), *J Embryol Exp Morphol* 65 Suppl:289–307.

Luciani MF, Chimini G (1996) The ATP binding cassette transporter ABC1, is required for the engulfment of corpses generated by apoptotic cell death, *EMBO J* **15**:226–35.

Luijsterburg AJ, van Huizum MA, Impelmans BE, et al (2000) Classification of congenital anomalies of the upper limb, *J Hand Surg [Br]* **25**:3–7.

Manske PR, McCarroll HR (1992) Reconstruction of the congenitally deficient thumb, *Hand Clin* **8**:177–96.

Milaire J, Rooze M (1983) Hereditary and induced modifications of the normal necrotic patterns in the developing limb buds of the rat and mouse: facts and hypotheses, **94**:459–90.

Miura T, Nakamura R, Horii E (1994) The position of symbrachydactyly in the classification of congenital hand anomalies, *J Hand Surg* **19B**:350–54.

Mori C, Nakamura N, Kimura S, et al (1995) Programmed cell death in the interdigital tissue of the fetal mouse limb is apoptosis with DNA fragmentation, *Anat Rec* **242**:103–10.

Ogino T (1990) Teratogenic relationship between polydactyly, syndactyly and cleft hand, *J Hand Surg [Br]* **15**:201–9.

Ogino T, Minami A, Fukuda K, et al (1986) Congenital anomalies of the upper limb among the Japanese in Sapporo, *J Hand Surg* **11B**:364–71.

O'Rahilly R, Gardner E (1972) The initial appearance of ossification in staged human embryos, *Am J Anat* **134**:291–301.

O'Rahilly R, Gardner E (1975) The timing and sequence of events in the development of the limbs in the human embryo, *Anat Embryol (Berl)* **148**:1–23.

O'Rahilly R, Gardner E, Gray DJ (1959) The skeletal development of the hand, *Clin Orthop* **13**:42–51.

Salas-Vidal E, Valencia C, Covarrubias L (2001) Differential tissue growth and patterns of cell death in mouse limb autopod morphogenesis, *Dev Dyn* **220**:295–306.

Saunders JWJ (1948) The proximodistal sequence of origin of the parts of the chick wing and the role of the ectoderm, *Exp J Zool* **108**:363–403.

Savill J, Fadok V, Henson P, et al (1993) Phagocyte recognition of cells undergoing apoptosis, *Immunol Today* **14**:131–36.

Summerbell D, Lewis JH, Wolpert L (1973) Positional information in chick limb morphogenesis, *Nature* **244**:492–96.

Swanson AB, DeGroot Swanson G, Tada K (1983) A classification for congenital limb malformation, *J Hand Surg [Am]* **8**:693–702.

Tabin C (1995) The initiation of the limb bud: growth factors, Hox genes, and retinoids, *Cell* **80**:671–74.

Temtamy SA, McKusick VA (1978) The genetics of hand malformations, *Birth Defects Orig Artic Ser* **14:i–xviii**, 1–619.

Tickle C (1996a) Genetics and limb development, *Dev Genet* **19**:1–8.

Tickle C (1996b) Vertebrate limb development, *Sem Cell Dev* **7**:137–143.

van den Eijnde S, Luijsterburg A, Boshart L, et al (1997) In situ detection of apoptosis during embryogenesis with annexin V: from whole mount to ultrastructure, *Cytometry* **29**:313–20.

Wood W, Turmaine M, Weber R, et al (2000) Mesenchymal cells engulf and clear apoptotic footplate cells in macrophageless PU.1 null mouse embryos, *Development* **127**:5245–52.

Wyllie AH, Kerr JFR, Currie AR (1980) Cell death: the significance of apoptosis, *Int Rev Cytol* **68**:251–306.

Zakeri Z, Quaglino D, Ahuja HS (1994) Apoptotic cell death in the mouse limb and its suppression in the hammertoe mutant, *Dev Biol* **165**:294–97.

4

Grip development in the growing child

Margreet ter Schegget

Many of our daily life activities can be performed without the use of our legs and feet, but only a few can be performed without the use of our arms and hands. From the very beginning of life, the infant's hands are intricately involved in every aspect of total development: motor, social, language, and cognitive (Erhardt 1994a). Gesell studied changes in function during development and he found these changes to depend primarily on neuromotor readiness. He considered the development of hand function like the development of other motor behaviour as an expansion of the total reflex system. At first it is dependent on postural positions, next it becomes more versatile and independent and at last it will be smoothly synergized (Gesell and Armatruda 1969). Gesell attributed variances among children to the differences in the mechanisms of self-regulation: the children change at a different rate but in the same sequence. He thought environmental factors not to be of essential importance. Bower (1979) concludes very much the same. He states that maturational processes use input from the environment but do not really need it. He also believes that maturing patterns depend primarily on intrinsic growth factors and neuromotor readiness rather than on environmental influences. Researchers like, for example, Ayres (1973, 1974) and Gilfoyle et al (1981) conclude that the environment itself demands interpretation of stimuli and adaptive responses and is therefore important for developmental growth. Erhardt (1994b) points to the fact that babies exhibit an indomitable urge to repeat emerging skills. This indicates that a fundamental need for repetition at an opportune time is essential for integration and perfection of new skills. If neuromotor readiness is present and if opportunities for practice are provided, critical new learning can take place.

For most activities it is necessary to be able to reach, to grasp, to hold, to carry and to release. For adequate use of these prehensile functions the hand must be placed in the correct position so the range of movement at the shoulder and elbow is important; the use of only the wrist and the hand is of limited functional value. For eye–hand coordination a stable cervical spine is important so the eyes can monitor the activities of the hand, as well as a stable shoulder girdle for guiding the arm and hand to its task and holding it there during manipulation. Equally important for functional prehension are both sensory qualities like touch, proprioception and vision, as well as sensorimotor qualities like praxis (the planning of an activity so that it can be smoothly performed).

The ontogenetic development of reaching and prehension is based on the integration of motor, sensory, and visual mechanisms and it includes the entire development from postural dependent to postural independent movements. Characteristic for this developmental process is that it proceeds from proximal to distal; from flexion to extension; from the ulnar side of the hand to the radial side of the hand; from pronation to supination, and from the unilateral side of the body to the contralateral side of the body. This last phenomenon is also known as crossing the body's midline. It marks the beginning of lateralization or dominance that is the conscious choice between the left and the right side of the body.

The sequence of grip development

The newborn

The newborn infant is not able to reach or grasp voluntarily. It shows gross, total motor patterns. The prevailing uterine physiological flexing posture that develops during the last 10 weeks in utero, influences all movements. The humerus and scapula function as one unit, so at rest the arms are usually flexed, adducted and internally rotated. There is no differentiation between the head and the shoulder girdle. The shoulders are elevated so it looks as if the baby has no neck. The hands are mostly held in a fist with the thumb in the palm.

Movements of the hand are mostly reflexive, triggered by a variety of stimuli. These reflexes originate from the lower part of the brain (brain stem and spinal cord), and the motor cortex is not yet involved. The tactile grasping reflex is dominant. Touching the palmar ulnar side of the hand combined with some traction causes it to close in a strong fist with synergistic flexion of the entire extremity. Since this is a tonic reflex, the response will be present as long as the stimulus is provided. This means that a newborn cannot release voluntarily.

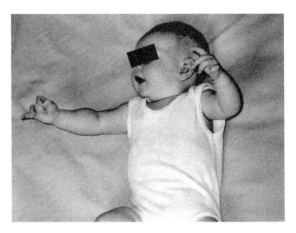

Figure 1

Asymmetrical Tonic Neck Reflex (ATNR) at two months.

movements are triggered by a stationary stimulus for which no following eye movement is needed (Fig. 2). If the baby tries to follow a moving stimulus with his eyes, the arm movements cease. There are still no voluntary hand movements during this period. The grasping reflex shifts from the ulnar palmar side of the hand to the radial palmar side of the hand.

1–2 months

In this period the baby is learning to control eye and head movements, which are prerequisites for eye–hand coordination. The movements of the arm are at first random, unrelated to stimuli. The movements of the arms and head are linked because of the Asymmetrical Tonic Neck Reflex (ATNR). Turning of the head, whether active or passive causes an increase of extensor tone in the arm on the face side and as a result it will extend. Simultaneously the arm on the skull side will flex due to an increase of flexor tone (Fig. 1).

This reflex prevents a baby from incidentally turning from the supine position to the prone position. By the mechanism of this reflex the baby also learns to look at and to reach for an object. The more voluntary this looking and reaching becomes, the more this reflex gets integrated. At the end of the second month arm

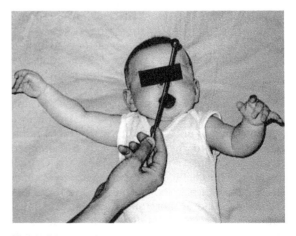

Figure 2

Arm movements triggered by a stationary stimulus.

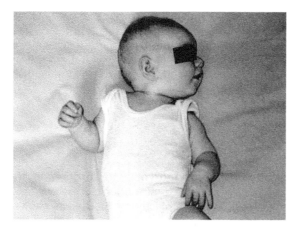

Figure 3

Beginning of the integration of the ATNR: weak reaction.

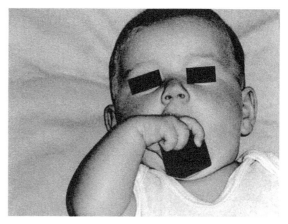

Figure 4

Wrist flexion during grip in a four-month-old baby.

Three months

About this time the baby starts looking at its own hands. By now it is able to follow, with head and eyes, the uncoordinated movements of arm and hands. From now on the motor cortex starts to play an increasing role. The rapid development of voluntary arm movements enables the baby to look better at its hands and much more important, to put them in its mouth in order to really learn something about them.

If an object is held at approximately 45° to the lateral side of the baby, it shows a unilateral approach with elbow, wrist, and fingers in a flexed position. The ATNR is starting to integrate; responses are weak or delayed (Fig. 3).

Four months

Around this time the grasping reflex is disappearing and voluntary prehension is beginning. The sight of an object causes approaching movements in both digits and the entire upper extremity. Still lying supine with firm support of head and trunk, the baby now exercises the stability and coordination of his shoulder girdle, which is a prerequisite for eye–hand coordination. The approach is uncoordinated. When the object is found the grasp is mostly ulnar, an object that is offered on the radial side of the hand cannot be grasped. Although the thumb is no longer held closely into the palm of the hand, there is no thumb involvement in the grasp. Release of objects mostly happens by accident, due to the still strong effect of the grasping reflex. During grip the wrist is flexed (Fig. 4).

Most objects are put in the mouth for strong tactile information. The baby is now making symmetrical movements. Therefore it will reach and grasp with both hands simultaneously. This accounts for the fact that a baby will release an object it is holding in one hand, while grasping something with the other hand. It is an example of symmetrical movement. The baby opens both hands in order to grasp something with one hand. This phenomenon will be present until almost 30 months but with decreasing intensity and frequency.

Another remarkable fact is that the baby cannot cross the midline of its body. It will grasp with its nearest hand. An object that is offered on the right side of the body will be grasped with the right hand. When offering it on the left side it will be grasped with the left hand. This phenomenon will be present until almost the seventh year. It is not until then that a child is able to incorporate this crossing of the body's midline into all his actions. Both phenomena serve the same purpose; it is through these mechanisms that both hands can develop the same basic skills.

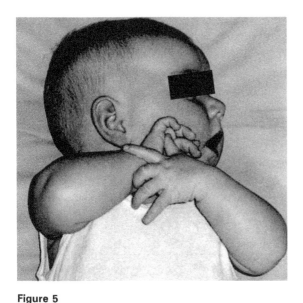

Figure 5

Integration of ATNR: dissociated movements of head and arms.

The ATNR integrates further and by now the changes in arm tone do not result in the characteristic arm movements any more (Fig. 5). From now on head and hands can develop apart from each other. The hands are now able to meet each other in the midline of the body.

Five months

Since the hands are able to function in the body's midline the first, rather clumsy transfers of objects will take place (Fig. 6). Objects need to be substantial, small objects like pellets are visualized but mostly without an attempt to grasp.

As the hands meet in the body's midline strong proprioceptive information about them is supplied. When brought in the prone position the baby will now learn to shift its weight laterally to the other arm and to the chest in order to reach for an object (Fig. 7). By doing so it exercises the

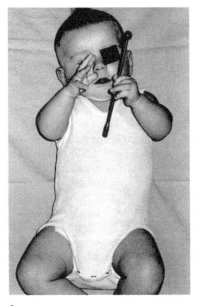

a

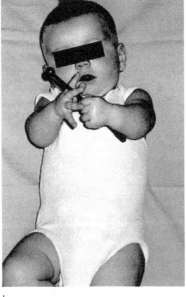

b

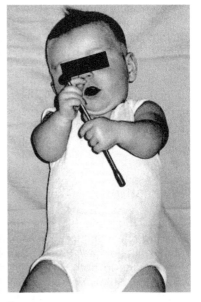

c

Figure 6 (a–c)

First transfer of an object in a five-month-old baby.

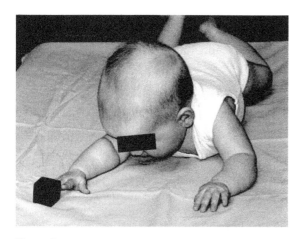

Figure 7

Beginning of weight shifting while reaching in the prone position.

coordination of movements of one shoulder as well as the stability of the other shoulder.

Six months

Now the child approaches an object with intent once it is seen. Ulnar grasping is slowly turning into radial grasping. Grasping is done with full finger extension. The thumb is used incidentally. Small objects are therefore still too difficult to grasp. In the supported sitting position the child reaches out with the unilateral arm once an object is seen (Fig. 8). Around this time the ATNR is almost completely integrated and the child is now able to learn to turn to the prone position.

7–9 months

Approach of an object is still performed with excessive extension of the digits, which will moderate with maturation. Grasping on the radial side of the hand is slowly turning into digital pinching because the thumb is used more and more frequently. Small objects are picked up clumsily. During grasping the wrist is held straight (Fig. 9).

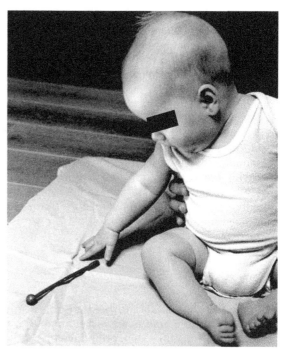

Figure 8

Unilateral approach with excessive finger extension in supported sitting.

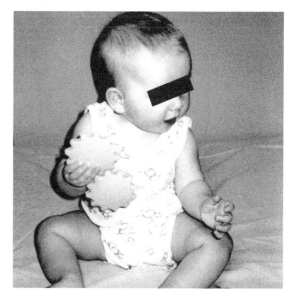

Figure 9

Straight wrist and supination while grasping/holding at eight months.

Release of grip is still difficult but is sometimes possible thus indicating the beginning of cortical control of finger extension, which takes place only after reaching and grasping have been perfected. The forearm will be more frequently supinated. Until this moment the child was reaching and grasping mainly from the lying position. With the capacity for free sitting the child now needs to place the hand in the correct position and this need is provided through the beginning of voluntary pronation and supination. So with the capacity for free sitting the child reaches a developmental phase in which the intentional, coordinated movements of arm and hand can mature.

10 months

By now the child is able to hold an object in a tripod pinch. Little objects are picked up in a two-point grip (Fig. 10). This grip develops from thumb to lateral side of the index finger into thumb opposite the top of the index finger.

The index finger develops the capacity for poking and this indicates that the grasping reflex is fully fractionated by now. The poking of the index finger allows the discovery of the third dimension. Holding an object is now frequently

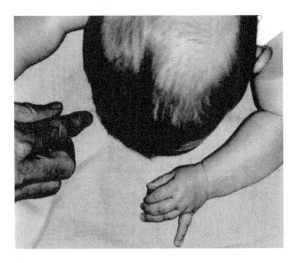

Figure 10

First two-point grip at 10 months.

done with the wrist in extension, which indicates the beginning of coordination between extensor and flexor apparatus.

One year

Around this period the child learns to open its hands more in relation to the object it wants to grasp. Pronation of the forearm is still the favourite position for grasping but supination is more and more coming under cortical control. Extension of the wrist while holding an object is improving and this makes the various grips more stable. Coordination is still poor and sometimes the release of an object can cause a problem.

15 months

At approximately this time the child is able to walk around and from now on it will learn to carry objects. It can grasp and hold more objects at the same time with one hand. This requires more effort, which shows in associated movements of the other hand and sometimes of the mouth. Prewriting skills are establishing. A pencil is grasped proximally and held in a fisted hand. The shoulder is stabilized while the arm moves as a unit, the forearm is slightly supinated and the wrist is slightly flexed. The child scribbles, at first in imitation and later on more spontaneously.

2–3 years

During the second year of life motor patterns are generally asymmetrical. This means that the child cannot make the same movement simultaneously with both hands. Although the child uses both hands in activities, only one hand is performing, while the other hand is used for fixation. When an object is placed on the child's right side it will grasp and perform with its right hand; when the object is placed on the left side it will grasp and perform with its left hand. It still cannot cross the midline of its body and there is not yet a dominant hand.

Prewriting skills develop. A pencil is still grasped proximally but is now held with all fingers and the thumb. The shoulder is freer in movement, the elbow is stabilized, while the forearm functions as a unit. The forearm is now held slightly pronated and the wrist is held straight. The child imitates horizontal and vertical strokes and attempts to copy circles. In this second year of life the child learns to perform activities in which both hands function together.

3–4 years

In this period the child learns to make symmetrical voluntary movements. These movements are mainly symmetrical in the dorso-ventral direction like pushing or throwing a ball with both hands. Manual skills that require manipulation and coordination become more and more complex. The child now frequently uses one hand in particular but it still cannot cross the midline of its body. It will grasp with the nearest hand or it will rotate the trunk and grasp with the favourite hand in order to avoid crossing the midline. This is an important fact and examiners who are not familiar with it can easily get the impression that the child is not using one of his hands.

Prewriting skills are still developing. The pencil is still grasped proximally and held in a gross tripod or four-finger grip. Shoulder and elbow have free movement but now the wrist is stabilized while the hand functions as a unit. The forearm is held slightly supinated and the wrist is held straight. The child learns to copy crosses and circles and traces diamonds, squares, and triangles.

4–5 years

Symmetrical movements are very strong during this period of life. Both hands can now work together to make the same movement. It is not yet possible to make different movements simultaneously with both hands. At the end of the fifth year the child is learning to cross the midline of its body. This is the beginning of lateralization, the conscious choice between the right and the left side of the body. It is not until the seventh year that a child can incorporate this crossing into all his actions.

At the end of the period the prewriting skills have developed to a normal distal grasping of a pencil, which is held in a tripod pinch with precise opposition of the volar pads of thumb, index finger and middle finger. The two ulnar fingers are flexed. Shoulder, elbow, and wrist are free in movement and now the metacarpophalangeal (MCP) joints are stabilized during proximal interphalangeal (PIP) movements. At the end of this period the child is able to copy triangles, squares and diamonds.

Six years

At this age the child can make different movements simultaneously with both hands. Social influences like shaking hands, school influences like learning to write and activities of daily living like eating with a knife and fork are pressuring the child to choose a dominant hand. Mostly there is a dominant hand by the end of the sixth year. It is not until the age of 12–14 that all fine finger manipulation skills are fully developed.

Summary and conclusions

The period from birth to approximately 15 months is the one in which the biological maturation of prehension takes place (Erhardt et al 1981). During the first two months of life the motor cortex is only marginally involved in movements. Movements are dominated by reflexes and reactions originating from the lower parts of the brain (i.e., brain stem and spinal cord). From approximately three months the motor cortex becomes involved, starting with the capacity for visual control of involuntary hand movements (Table 1). At the same time the mouthing of the hand starts, and strong sensory stimuli are reaching the brain. The essential components for prehension are functional by approximately the age of 15 months. Reflexes and reactions are well integrated at that time, and voluntary patterns of approach, grasp,

Table 1 Maturation of prehension

Activity	0	1	2	3	4	5	6	7	8	9	10	11	12	15
								(months)						
Uterine flexion posture	⊠	⊠												
Tactile grasping reflex														
: ulnar palmar side	⊠	⊠												
: radial palmar side			⊠	⊠	▫	▫	▫	▫	▫	▫				
Assym. Tonic Neck Reflex	⊠	⊠	⊠	◑	▫	▫								
Eyes follow movements				⊠	⊠	⊠	⊠	⊠	⊠	⊠	⊠	⊠	⊠	⊠
Voluntary prehension														
: ulnar grasp, wrist flexed					⊠	⊠	◑	◑	◑	◑	▫			
: no thumb involvement					⊠	⊠	◑	▫						
: symmetrical movements in both hands					⊠	⊠	◑							
: no active release					⊠	⊠	⊠	◑	◑	▫				
: radial grasp							⊠	⊠	⊠					
: thumb used incidentally							⊠	◑	▫					
: full finger extension							⊠	⊠	⊠	◑	▫			
: digital pinching								⊠	⊠	⊠	⊠	⊠	⊠	⊠
: thumb used frequently								⊠	⊠	⊠	⊠	⊠	⊠	⊠
: wrist straight								⊠	⊠	⊠	◑	▫		
: start of active release								▫	◑	⊠	⊠	⊠	⊠	⊠
: tripod pinch											⊠	⊠	⊠	⊠
: two-point grip											⊠	⊠	⊠	⊠
: wrist in extension											⊠	⊠	⊠	⊠
: poking of index finger											⊠	⊠	⊠	⊠
Hands in midline; transfer of objects						⊠	⊠	⊠	⊠	⊠	⊠	⊠	⊠	⊠
Active approach							⊠	⊠	⊠	⊠	⊠	⊠	⊠	⊠
Voluntary pro- and supination								⊠	⊠	⊠	⊠	⊠	⊠	⊠
Maturity of prehension														⊠
Start of refinement/skills														⊠

Key: ▫-◑-⊠ = appearing-developing-fully present
      ⊠-◑-▫ = fully present-diminishing-disappearing
      ⊠ = present

manipulation and release have been perfected. From now on the child will refine its movements and increase its skills, and prehension will become perfected through experience.

References

Ayres AJ (1973) *Sensory Integration and Learning Disorders* (Western Psychological Services: Los Angelos).

Ayres AJ (1974) Ontogenetic principles in the development of arm and hand functions. In: *The Development of Sensory Integrative Theory and Practice. A Collection of the Works of A. Jean Ayres*, (Kendall/Hunt, Dubuque IA).

Bower TGR (1979) *Human Development* (WH Freeman: San Francisco).

Erhardt RP (1994a) *Developmental Hand Dysfunction: Theory, Assessment and Treatment*, 2nd edn (Therapy Skill Builders: San Antonio, Texas).

Erhardt RP (1994b) *Erhardt Developmental Prehension Assessment (EDPA) revised*, (Therapy Skill Builders: San Antonio, Texas).

Erhardt RP, Beatty PA, Hertsgaard DM (1981) A developmental prehension assessment for handicapped children, *Am J Occup Ther* **35**:237–42.

Gesell A, Armatruda CS (1969) *Developmental Diagnosis*, 2nd edn (Harper and Row: New York).

Gilfoyle EM, Grady AP, Moore JC (1981) *Children Adapt* (Charles B. Slack: Thorofare, NJ).

5

Psychological behaviour of the child with a congenital difference of the upper limb

Eileen Bradbury

When children are born, they become part of a hereditary line, taking their place in the family, with generations going before and generations to come. Parents' hopes for the future are invested in their children, whether the parent is a single mother or part of a wide extended family and social network.

When children are born with physical anomalies, that hope is compromised. Those who witness the birth of a child with a hand difference will observe the responses of the parents and family members—responses that include sadness, disappointment, pity, loss, anger, and guilt (Solnit and Stark 1962). The range and intensity of the emotions will vary from parent to parent but they will be different from those emotions greeting the birth of the average child with no such imperfections (Varni and Setoguchi 1993). Through different societies, this is a universally observed phenomenon.

Children grow up and become adults. The role of the family and institutions such as school and church is to raise them to adulthood so that they can take their place in society. This development is mediated through the formality of social rules taught by parents, teachers and others, and informally through family life and contact with other children. The families of children with hand anomalies have a special task; they have to raise children who look different from others. The particular social meaning of the anomaly varies between and within societies, but it always carries some social meaning. And in addition to the normal tasks of development, such children face the additional tasks of adjusting to their physical difference, managing social encounters,

developing self-esteem and coping with functional limitations. They are also involved in making decisions about reconstructive surgery that change their appearance at an age when other children may only have to decide which television programme to watch.

This chapter examines the problems facing parents and children, and describes clinical approaches to these problems. There will be particular emphasis on clinical interactions within children's hand surgery service; running the clinic, facilitating decision-making and helping the child and parent cope with surgery and its outcome.

The social meaning of congenital anomalies

From the earliest writings to the present day, those born with congenital anomalies have been viewed as flawed, a visible sign of punishment from the gods (Shaw 1981). The world's literature includes many tales of people whose visible difference marks them out as being dispossessed and punished, isolated people living on the margins of society. Fairy stories passed down by folk mythology document a belief in the goodness of beauty and the evil of ugliness and deformity. In the story of Beauty and the Beast, the Beast is ugly, animalistic, deformed, and isolated. The Beauty is pure, good, and innocent. The love of the Beauty transforms the Beast and makes him physically perfect, taking away the stigmata of an animal-like deformity (Bettelheim

1976). In many films and plays, deformity is the shorthand for evil—those who are affected are different and disadvantaged. It is rare to find a positive role model in any story, play, or film for individuals who have a visible congenital difference.

Those born with congenital anomalies share this common culture—they understand its impact. It is generally more difficult for a child to explain being born with a different hand than to explain that the hand is the result of trauma. We are all at risk of injury, and there may be something heroic in surviving such injury. However, these children commonly say that it is embarrassing to have to admit to being born with a visible difference—it implies a central deficiency, a weakness, a fundamental flaw (Bradbury 1996).

Add into this the particular importance of hands. They play a crucial role in human communication, in representing function, strength, and power, and in touch and intimacy. Our hands are in front of us all the time; they cannot be hidden unless we keep them in pockets or otherwise covered. A hand that is deficient may not function well, may be clumsy and inefficient, and may look unattractive. The individual may not want to expose this hand to the curiosity and critical judgement of others.

Hands have a particular meaning for children in their development. They use their hands continually in gesture. McGrew documented over 100 bodily movements characteristically used by children, including a repertoire of 29 distinct hand gestures (McGrew 1972). In addition to hand gestures, children's hands are exposed to others in play and in the classroom. It is difficult for the child to avoid the hand being noticed by others, and indeed the act of concealing draws attention to the hand and increases the self-consciousness and sense of difference experienced by the child.

Early responses to the birth

Attachment between mothers and babies does not begin at birth but as the child moves within the mother. By the time the baby is born it has been incorporated into the mother's hopes for the future. For all parents there will be some discrepancy between the fantasized baby and the actual child. Winnicott described how all parents harboured a secret fear about their ability to produce the perfect child: 'It is as if human beings find it very difficult to believe that they are good enough to create within themselves something that is quite good' (Winnicott 1965). Thus when the child is born and has no obvious deficiency, there is a sense of relief. It is interesting how often parents recount that the first thing they do is to count the fingers and toes as though this is the talisman of perfection.

For parents who have had a child with an imperfect hand, there is no such reassurance. Instead there is the need to adjust to a child with a compromised future. Those parents who project their own needs onto their children may experience the fear that this child will never carry forward the parents' aspirations. Those with low self-esteem may see in their child the external embodiment of their sense of internal imperfection. For all there is disappointment, sadness for the child and for themselves, and the need to grieve the loss of the anticipated fantasized baby (Bradbury and Hewison 1993). That grief often includes anger that can be directed at the professionals involved.

The surgeon needs to understand that the angry parent with the baby is not angry with the surgeon, but with the anomaly and all that it implies. The parents need clear information about what is known and what could be done. They do not need false reassurance, wild hopes or inappropriate complex technical discussions. Nor do they need to hear any judgemental comments about themselves—they feel badly enough about themselves already as they search for cause and meaning. Parents recall very clearly, for the rest of their lives, all that the surgeon says at such a sensitive and vulnerable time. One parent reported to the author how a surgeon picked up the baby's arm, dropped it saying, 'well, this is no good, is it' and walked out. Another recalls a surgeon making a joke about the hand. When the surgeon is self-indulgent in this first encounter, he or she may never regain the trust of the parent.

The first encounters on the ward and in clinic provide an invaluable opportunity to meet together, form a working relationship, develop mutual trust, work out a treatment plan, and thus reassure the parents that their child is in safe hands. The parents are part of the team and the hostile or distressed parent is not going to function effectively in that team and may sabotage the surgeon's efforts. Parents appreciate an open approach, honesty, relevant information, and a feeling that their needs are being heard and met.

The psychological impact of the hand for the developing child and for the surgeon

As children with hand differences grow up, they can become self-conscious about their hands. The first significant questions come when the child is between two and four years old, when they tend to ask 'why'. This word is commonly used by all children, often to the exasperation of parents who grow tired of having to explain everything to the curious youngster. For the parents of these children, the question carries a particular significance. They may have been dreading this question since the birth, especially if they feel guilty and have not adjusted to the hand. If the child asks such a question and the parent becomes upset, the child quickly learns to ask no more. Children need the protection of their parents and do not want that parent to show an inability to protect. They may also feel that the hand is too serious and distressing to be mentioned again. For these children, the risk to their psychosocial well-being is that they will hide their hands in shame and avoid talking about them.

From the early days after birth, parents need advice on what reactions to expect from their children and how to handle such questions. They need to be told that it is normal for the child to ask 'why' and indeed for the child to say that it is not fair and to be upset or angry. When children are able to make social comparisons with other children then they will notice differences and focus on them. This is normal. They need reassurance that the parents understand how they feel, that they can talk about their feelings and that they are loved for who they are. They should not be told that everything is going to be fine because the surgeon can make the hand 'better'. Although parents may say such things to calm the child, they will later have to

let the child down, and the surgeon may find that a good technical result is rejected by the child who had been led to expect that the hand would be normal after surgery. It is easy to collude and reassure the child that all will be well. The author has heard parents telling children that the doctor will fix the hand. To the child, that can only mean normalizing the hand, taking away the problem.

It should be noted that surgeons may also raise the same false hopes with the distressed child, and that everyday comments such as 'we will sort it out for you', and 'we will make it better' are likely to be misinterpreted by the child who wants to hear that the anomaly will disappear and who does not have the adults' perspective on what is possible.

As the child grows and develops, there are certain times of particular difficulty. Any transition can be problematic, such as a move to a new school where new people will be met and new questions may be asked. As children grow from infancy into childhood, towards social friendships and affiliations, then the need for acceptance is particularly acute and is often based on attractiveness and 'fitting-in'. Children with physical differences are often teased and bullied at this age. Such experiences are common in childhood—a study of some six-year-olds found that 54.7% of English children reported having been frequently bullied at school with name-calling as the most common type of bullying (Wolke et al 2001). Many cross-cultural studies have found name-calling to be the most common type of bullying in 8–12 year olds across Europe (see for example, Baldry 1998). Boys are generally found to be more at risk than girls.

Children who are easy targets for name-calling because of their obvious difference are more at risk, especially if they have low self-esteem resulting from feelings of shame absorbed from their parents. The social pressures at school may lead the child and the parents to seek surgery to resolve the problem. This can be of benefit to the child who finds it easier to explain surgical scars than congenital anomalies. It can also benefit those children who feel that they are being listened to and helped. However, the child who has become a chronic victim is unlikely to gain in confidence from surgery, as the playground interactions have become habitual. In fact, if surgery removes the child's understanding of the reasons for being bullied, but the bullying continues, then the child may feel a greater sense of despair. The excuse for being bullied has now been minimized and the child has to face up to the bleak possibility that it may be personality rather than an external anomaly that is at fault. This has been found in children having surgery to correct prominent ears (Bradbury et al 1992).

Children who are chronic victims would benefit from psychological help in coping with bullying. Successful coping strategies and the development of positive self-belief will strengthen the child's persona, build self-esteem and self-confidence and encourage the child to develop internal means of resolving difficulties rather than external solutions (Olweus 1993). Surgery may be effective within this context as a way of validating the child's efforts and improving the hand, thus reducing stress. However, it is interesting to observe how often children will be happy to postpone surgery when the immediate threat from other children has been lifted. Thus a multi-disciplinary approach is effective in these circumstances.

The next significant developmental stage comes at the transition from childhood into adolescence. This is a time of emotional instability and rapidly changing body image (Smith and Cowie 1983). The young person moves away from the family, relies much more on friendships, and moves into a world dominated by fierce competition, feelings of loneliness, obsessive concerns about appearance, short-term gratification, and sexual adventure. Adolescents are narcissistic and believe that they are constantly under the spotlight and the centre of everyone's attention. Those with hand differences may feel particularly self-conscious in adolescence where the hand signifies lack of competitiveness and unattractiveness. Physical intimacy can be difficult for the self-conscious adolescent to contemplate, and potential partners may reject them because they carry a stigma, thus reducing their status in the eyes of others. Such problems can be cloaked in silence, defensiveness, and/or aggression, and these adolescents are not always easy to reach and help. Such adolescents are often found to be going through their own grieving process, for the loss of the perfect hand they never had. Thus they may well exhibit the range of grieving emotions: anger, denial, and distress. They will generally benefit from the opportunity to talk to someone neutral, away from family and school.

In clinic, these adolescents have a particular need to discuss surgical issues without too much pressure. For some, that will mean talking to the surgeon whilst parents take a back seat. For others, it may mean talking to the surgeon alone, without an audience. Those who are timid and self-effacing with dominant parents may need to find an independent voice and an advocate in clinic.

Development does not abruptly end in adolescence but continues throughout life. The young person faces new challenges entering the world of work where more demands may be made away from the protecting environment of home and school. Many report being teased by workmates. Having children of their own may cause them to focus once more on the hand as their own children ask questions. It is a time when they may seek further reconstructive surgery, having come through the defensive posture of adolescence. All that has gone before in their lives will profoundly affect their ability to cope and their ability to integrate into the working world and form satisfactory relationships.

A recent (as yet unpublished) research study involving the author looked at adults with a different congenital anomaly—cleft lip and palate. Of those assessed, one-third felt that the cleft had not fundamentally affected them as human beings. These were mainly people whose parents had rapidly adjusted to the condition and had supported them throughout. A further third reported that they had been profoundly affected and had suffered low self-esteem and self-confidence as a result. The final third reported that they too had been profoundly affected—they were more sensitive to others and were stronger people through having coped. This last group had developed effective coping strategies for dealing with others and felt in control of their lives.

Thus a congenital anomaly does not inevitably cause major problems; those with well-adjusted parents and those who have developed effective coping strategies can survive remarkably well. Some children are more resilient than others (Fonagy et al 1994). Early intervention to support parents and help them adjust and later intervention helping children develop effective coping strategies are useful forms of clinical intervention (Bradbury 1996). It is important for the surgeon to recognize developmental issues and integrate that knowledge into a multi-disciplinary clinical approach.

Meeting psychological need in the children's hand surgery service

Organizing a psychological service

The aims of surgical reconstruction to children's hands will always be affected by the psychological and social experience of children and their families. This is true even when the reconstruction is entirely to improve function. Hand anomalies always carry meaning for the child and any change to the hand will have psychological implications. The child is a moving target, growing, and changing, and this meaning changes as the child moves through infancy, childhood, and adolescence.

An effective surgical service needs to take account of that meaning. Failure to understand and take account of the whole child in the family and social context can compromise surgical decision-making and diminish satisfaction with outcome. In addition, an integrated service with a team of clinicians working together provides the child and family with the opportunity to treat the child's condition in the most effective way (Lansdown et al 1997). There are three levels at which psychological intervention should be organized:

• *Increasing psychological awareness for the whole team.* Every member of the team interacting with the child and family should have knowledge of psychological issues and how they may impact on the child and family. They should be aware of potential problems, be sensitive to signs of distress and difficulty, understand questions that need to be raised and feel comfortable in responding to psychological and social issues raised during treatment. Those who are used to dealing in practical treatments may become uncomfortable when faced with a weeping mother or withdrawn child. However, if these difficulties are addressed in a relaxed and appropriate way through the normal interactions of clinic

and treatment, then the service will improve and the needs of the child are more likely to be met. Such a general increase in psychological awareness and competence will reduce the need for a more specialist intervention for the average patient.

• *Identifying a team member to take responsibility for counselling.* In every child's surgery team there will be someone who could be identified as the person responsible for offering counselling. This may be the nurse in the outpatient clinic who is interested in counselling, or the occupational therapist who has had training in psychological therapies. Further training in counselling skills may be needed, and the funding of this should be seen as part of the normal costs of running the service. Once that person has been identified and accepts the role, then clinical time needs to be allocated, even if it means increasing the levels of staffing to take account of this. It is not satisfactory to ask the nurse to take responsibility for counselling the distressed family whilst also having to run a busy outpatient clinic single-handed. The effective intervention of such a team member in a general counselling role will enable other team members to do their work more effectively as they gain valuable information about the child and family, and will provide support to the child and family through difficult times.

• *Appointing a specialist psychologist to the team.* There are some children and families who need specialist psychological intervention, for example, mothers suffering from post-natal depression, children with serious anxiety disorders or suffering depression, or children with major social problems that lead to isolation or rejection by their peers. In addition, there will be children who consistently hide their hands and cannot adjust to them, children who have phobias about needles and surgery, and children who have difficulty making decisions about treatment. The team psychologist should have experience of working with children and families and be able to develop specialist skills in this service. He or she would take responsibility for the education of team members in psychological and social issues, support and supervise the team member responsible for counselling, liase with outside agencies such

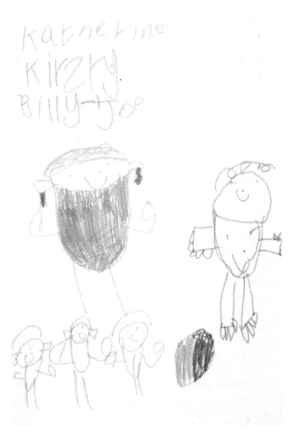

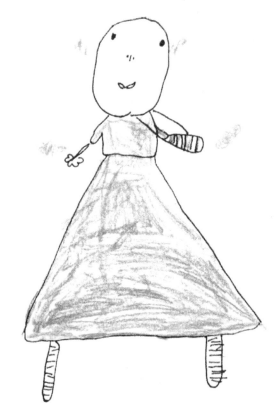

Figure 1

Overpowered by the bully (left); teacher (right) cannot help, nor can friends.

Figure 2

After toe to hand surgery.

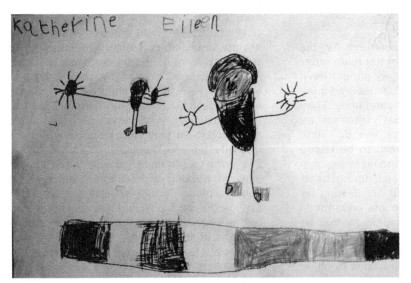

Figure 3

Working with the psychologist!

as schools and local psychological services and assess and treat those children and families with special psychological needs. It should be noted at this point that having a counsellor as a team member and a team psychologist does not absolve other team members from their responsibility in understanding and coping with day-to-day psychological issues that arise during normal clinical interactions. Each layer of this service would be dependent on the other to work effectively.

Decision-making about surgery for children and families

Many decisions taken by surgeons treating those with congenital hand problems are driven by psychological and social needs, even when the gains are primarily functional. This is not life-saving surgery, and there are children who do not have surgery, and yet who grow up to be happy and healthy members of society. Surgeons are often aware of pressure from parents for surgery which might not always be in the interests of the child, and also that some children avoid surgery which would be of great benefit to them. The role of the child and family in such decision-making is complex and difficult, but needs to be addressed.

Making decisions about quite trivial matters can be difficult. Decisions about whether or not to have reconstructive surgery can be extremely difficult for parents and children and they often revert to asking the surgeon what he or she would do. However, being involved in the decision-making process can be of immense benefit to them. The process requires them to evaluate the impact of the hand, consider what they want to achieve, understand what can be achieved, and commit to the surgical intervention. Thus they are more likely to be satisfied with outcome.

The decision is difficult because it is unfamiliar, it is often taken at times of stress, it is based on technical information which may be difficult to understand, and the outcome cannot be guaranteed. In addition, there are secondary factors that will impact on the decision, such as the ability of parents to tolerate their child undergoing surgery and the fears of the child in relation to the surgical process. There is also the issue of possible hidden agendas on the part of parents, children, and the surgeon. Parents may want the surgery to absolve them of the guilt they feel about the hand, children may want a normal hand, and the surgeon may want to use the opportunity to try out new techniques. The whole process is multi-layered and complex and time needs to be given to it to ensure that an effective decision is made which is in the best interests of the child (Bradbury et al 1994b).

Who makes the decision, parent or child? For the child up to the age of about five or six years old, the parents will have to make the decision and will need to ensure that the child has given assent and is not distressed at the prospect of surgery. Thus the parents of children older than babies but too young to make decisions should explain to the child what is to happen in a language the child can understand, and help the child cope with fears about the process of surgery. In order to do this, the parents need to have the relevant information themselves and feel reassured that they are doing the right thing for their child. An uncertain or frightened parent can convey negative feelings to the child. Parents may need support to carry out their role with the child (Alderson 1990).

The older the child and the greater the uncertainty about benefits and outcome, then the more likely it is that the child will be involved in the decision. Alderson found that young children could play an effective part in decision-making if they understood what was involved. In these circumstances, it is the responsibility of the surgeon and the parent to explain the relevant issues to the child in comprehensible language (Alderson 1993). Experts on child development such as Donaldson (Donaldson 1987) have shown that young children can make informed decisions if the adult has communicated the issues effectively. The child who has participated in the decision-making process will benefit psychologically as the outcome is anticipated, uncertainties are tolerated, and the child does not have unrealistic expectations.

Adolescents pose a particular problem. They tend to be defensive and unwilling to discuss psychological and social problems, particularly in a busy clinic where they feel under the spotlight and self-conscious. They may be experiencing denial, they may be hostile to adults, they may be resentful of having to be there in the first place, or they may just be very shy. They do need the opportunity of having one-to-one discussions with the counsellor or the psychologist, away from professionals and family. For them, such discussions about making a decision can bring forward a lot of other issues and lead to a resolution of hidden problems.

In order to facilitate the decision-making process, the family need information and the opportunity to discuss this. A clinical room full of personnel may be a reasonable environment to hear and discuss technical information, but some may want the opportunity to return to discuss the issue with the surgeon, or with the team counsellor or psychologist. This is particularly likely when there are other problems associated with the hand, and also when the decision is a particularly difficult one, such as deciding on toe-to-hand transfer (Bradbury et al 1994a).

Verbal information is enhanced if it is backed up by other types of information; written information, photographs and videos of other children and possibly contact with other parents and children who have made similar decisions. Thus a resource bank should be built of such material, and with contact details of other families willing to be approached.

Not every decision results in surgery, and the process should not be designed to persuade parents and children to proceed, but to enable them to make the best decision for the child at that time. Saying 'no' can be extremely difficult for the child or family. They may feel grateful for all that has been done and is being offered, they may feel that the surgeon really wants to do this surgery and they cannot let him or her down, they may feel that they seem hostile. Above all, the decision to say 'no' requires a psychological leap—because the child and family then have to adjust to the hand as it is. There is no further 'magic', no surgical solution, and thus they can no longer postpone that adjustment. Because this can be such a difficult task, some people continue to have operations to postpone the day when they have to accept the hand.

Helping children and families cope with surgery and its outcome

If the decision-making process is carried out effectively to the satisfaction of all those involved, then there will be less need to support children and families through surgery and its outcome because they have already invested in this and are prepared for what is likely to happen. They are also willing participants.

However, some parents and some children do need particular support. Parents who have not yet adjusted to the hand or who have their own unhappy experiences of surgery may become very distressed prior to surgery. This will affect the child. The support they need is the opportunity to talk through their concerns, to resolve the underlying issues and therefore to feel able to cope with surgery. Generally the team psychologist should carry out this work since it is likely that there will be complex psychological issues to deal with.

Some children become very frightened prior to surgery (Peterson 1989). Those who have had previous surgical experience may have been upset by unfamiliar sights and smells, being restricted, having injections, losing consciousness and/or by post-operative pain. For them, the journey to the operating theatre will be a nightmare, and they are likely to struggle and resist, to the distress of all those involved. A child who has gone through this experience will be more reluctant to agree to surgery in the future.

There are simple and effective approaches to this problem. The child needs to desensitize to the experience. The best way of doing this is to expose the child to the feared stimulus in a reassuring way. Showing pictures of the anaesthetic room and the operating theatre and reading them children's stories about hospital, and by helping them develop coping strategies when they feel frightened such as distraction, can do this. The most effective approach is to take the child into the anaesthetic room before surgery, let the child see what is fearful and previously only glimpsed, help them acclimatize to the smell of the theatre by breathing in and out together, and generally make it an interesting place for the child.

It is important for the team to have a strategy for dealing with parents and children's fears. The fearful parent or child may refuse surgery because of their fear and thus miss the opportunity to gain all the benefits that surgery can offer.

Surgery to improve hands with congenital anomalies may be complex technically, but it is also complex from a psychological and social perspective. The surgeon needs to understand the impact of the hand and the impact of surgery for the child and family, and find ways of organizing a multi-disciplinary service that takes into account the psychological issues. This will benefit the surgeon, the parents and family and above all, it will benefit the child.

References

Alderson P (1990) *Choosing for Children: Parents' Consent to Surgery* (Oxford University Press: Oxford).

Alderson P (1993) *Children's Consent to Surgery* (Open University Press: Buckingham).

Baldry AC (1998) Bullying among Italian middle school students, *Sch Psychol Int* **19**:361–74.

Bettelheim B (1976) *The Uses of Enchantment* (Penguin: London).

Bradbury ET, Hewison J, Timmons M (1992) Psychological and social outcome of prominent ear correction in children, *Br J Plast Surg* **45**:97–100.

Bradbury ET, Kay SPJ, Hewison J (1994a) The psychological impact of microvascular free toe transfer for children and their parents, *J Hand Surg* **19B**:689–95.

Bradbury ET, Kay SPJ, Tighe C, Hewison J (1994b) Decision-making by parents and children in paediatric hand surgery, *Br J Plast Surg* **47**:324–30.

Bradbury ET, Hewison J (1993) Early parental adjustment to visible congenital disfigurement, *Child Care Health Dev* **20**:251–66.

Bradbury ET (1996) *Counselling People with Visible Disfigurement* (British Psychological Society: Leicester).

Donaldson M (1987) *Children's Minds* (Fontana Press: London).

Fonagy et al (1994) The Emmanuel Miller Memorial Lecture 1992. The theory and practice of resilience, *J Child Psychol Psychiatry* **35**:231–57.

Lansdown R, Rumsey N, Bradbury E, Carr T, Partridge J (1997) *Visibly Different: Coping With Disfigurement* (Butterworth-Heinemann: Oxford).

McGrew WC (1972) *An Ethological Study of Children's Behaviour* (Academic Press: New York).

Olweus D (1993) *Bullying at School* (Blackwell Scientific Publications: Oxford).

Peterson L (1989) Coping by children undergoing stressful medical procedures: some conceptual, methodological, and therapeutic issues, *J Consult Clin Psychol* **57**:380–87.

Shaw WC (1981) Folklore surrounding facial deformity and the origins of facial prejudice, *Br J Plast Surg* **34**:237–46.

Smith PK, Cowie H (1983) *Understanding Children's Development*, 2nd edn (Blackwell Scientific Publications: Oxford).

Solnit A, Stark MH (1962) Mourning and the birth of a defective child, *Psychoanal Study Child* **16**:9–24.

Varni JW, Setoguchi Y (1993) Effects of parental adjustment on the adaptation of children with congenital or acquired limb deficiencies, *J Dev Behav Pediatr* **14**:13–20.

Winnicott D (1965) *The Maturational Process and the Facilitating Environment* (Hogarth: London).

Wolke D, Woods S, Stanford K, Schulz H (2001) Bullying and victimisation of primary school children in England and Germany: prevalence and school factors, *Br J Psychol* **92(4)**:673–96.

6

First approach to a child with a congenital difference of the upper limb

Luc De Smet

The confrontation of (healthy) parents with their newborn child with a hand anomaly (or malformation or difference) is usually a great shock. The deformity is obvious and visible for them, their family, and others. The first expert advice is crucial and of utmost importance—based on his (or her) explanation they will be able to cope with the child and its hand problem, to help their child in its development, and its adaptation to the environment and support it through the (surgical) treatments and rehabilitation.

Who has to be this expert?

Congenital hand malformations are not very frequent and the hand surgeon is supposed not only to be a surgeon, but also a geneticist, a dysmorphologist, a rehabilitation expert, a psychologist, and a social worker, ready to answer all the questions of the parents, to provide the necessary information and to execute a perfect reconstruction.

Only a few departments have the luxury of an organized multi-disciplinary outpatient clinic, where different interested and motivated experts are gathered around one patient. Mostly however, the lonely hand surgeon is confronted with anxious, disappointed parents and their child. It is this first approach that will influence how these parents will react and accept any treatment—they're not only just interested in what surgery can do, more often than not all they want are some answers to some basic questions.

Basic information

The basic facts on congenital hand anomalies are well known. Their incidence is about 1/200 to 1/675 births. The aetiology is not clear in two-thirds of them (Table 1). Probably a single mutation is present in most cases, but environmental influences cannot be excluded, as well as (accidental) vascular disruptions. Bilateral malformations, and associated foot malformations are indications for a syndromic diagnosis. The presence of more than three other so-called minor anomalies is an obvious reason to suggest a syndrome diagnosis—thumb anomalies for example, are present in about 60% of syndromic cases (cardial, Holt Oram Syndrome, blood dyscrasia, Fanconi Syndrome and VACTERL associations). In Western European Caucasians, syndactyly is the most frequent major hand anomaly. Other populations and races do not always follow the same pattern. An operative treatment for congenital hand anomalies is necessary in two out of three hands.

Table 1 Congenital malformations of the hand

Aetiology	
• Genetic	
– Chromosomes	10%
– Single gene	5%
• Syndrome	
– Environment	5%
– Multifactorial	20%
• Unknown	

Table 2 Basic questions

- Why? Guilt!
- Can it recur?
- Is it associated with other problems?
- What to do about it?
- When?
- How will it look like?

Parents, however, have more fundamental questions (Table 2):

- Why did it happen to them? They feel guilty and want an extensive explanation of the aetiology.
- They want to know if there is a possibility of the problem reoccurring, its probability, and whether their child will transmit the malformation to their offspring?
- Is the hand anomaly isolated or associated with other problems? In other words a syndrome diagnosis has to be postulated.
- What to do, when, and by whom? They want a clear programme, including all practical considerations such as duration of hospitalization, and financial costs.
- How will the hand(s) look after the operation? How will it function? Will the child be able to use its hand(s) normally; will the child be able to perform a job and practise sport or music?

It is obvious that not all aspects can be dealt with in one visit. The surgeon has to answer all questions of which he is sure. There is no place for guessing or speculations. It is better to be safe rather than sorry and postpone some answers or transmit these questions to other experts. The Internet has proved to be a useful tool providing a gateway by which both surgeon and parents alike can access pertinent information. Such demands for information mean that any hand surgeons dealing with congenital malformations need to have basic knowledge of genetics, dysmorphology, teratology, psychological aspects, social provisions, orthotics and prosthetics, and of course the more specific features of congenital hand problems—areas that are constantly evolving and require continuous dedicated research and study. For the hand surgeon, regular conferences, and (in Europe) the presence of several 'congenital clubs', which meet on different occasions, are valuable.

When is the first consultation?

There has been a shift in the timing of the first visit. In the past, the parents would get to see a surgeon a few weeks after the birth of their child. Nowadays hand surgeons are called soon after the birth, even when the neonate has a lot of other problems—a situation that renders it difficult to discuss the hand problem with an exhausted mother in bed, a disappointed father and the rest of the family circulating in a restricted area.

More often, however, the surgeon is requested when the gynaecologist observes a hand malformation on foetal ultrasound (for instance at 20 weeks gestation). How good all these imaging techniques are remains to be seen since the shadowy images hardly provide a decent impression on the real aspect of the hands (although there is a strong positive correlation of the detected malformation on ultrasound in relation to the diagnosed difference at birth). It is likely that in the near future, molecular screening will be used to predict hand anomalies, since more and more genes involved in normal and abnormal hand development are being discovered. Perhaps the time will come when the hand surgeon will be able to discuss a hand problem with the future parents based purely on the DNA analysis—but until then, some recommendations regarding present day practices need to be made.

Psychological considerations

The parents of any child born with a visible malformation need time to adjust. Every parent expects to give birth to a perfect child. The obvious visible testimony of a congenital problem is a shock for them. They may feel guilty; they may feel disappointed—a narcissistic trauma—and have a feeling of loss of control. They will need to mourn for the loss of the 'perfect' child—a process that takes time and sometimes requires additional support. The grandparents, especially the mother's parents, play an important role in this mourning process. Once the parents have come to terms with their child's situation, they can take part in the medico-surgical management of the hand malformation.

It becomes clear that parents have accepted the situation once they start taking pictures of their child and increasing its exposure to family and friends. There are several crucially important periods in the child's life when he or she is confronted with the hand malformation. Apart from the adjustment period for the parents, the first one for the child itself will be at the age of five or six years, when the conscious confrontation with other children can cause problems. Naturally during the turbulent years of puberty, all misadventures will be blamed on the hand problem, but a very real problem period, and potentially a more frightening one, is the time when the child makes plans for his future professional career, where the choices to be made are either influenced or limited by the hand problem. Fortunately these problem periods can be anticipated and the child can be prepared in advance. However, the coping capacities of the parents will also be transmitted to the child and in cases where the parents have still not accepted the problem, this will negatively influence the child's acceptance of its own handicap.

The surgeon has to be careful in his predictions: realistic expectations are mandatory. As much information as possible has to be provided but perhaps not all in the same (first) session. A correct forum is required. The place and timing for adequate information and explication has to be created so that everybody feels comfortable. Last but by no means least, and especially in older children, one has to be aware that the child has ownership of his own body. This means that one has to convince him or her to collaborate in the treatment and rehabilitation.

Record keeping

General information for each child with a congenital hand malformation has to be stored. The cause, problems, and duration of the pregnancy, the birth, the birth weight and length (and head circumference) are elementary data.

The psychomotor development of the child from birth gives the surgeon an idea of the general and mental development. Details on the family are required—the parents' age and health status, and possible consanguinity. Also medication, trauma, and exposures during pregnancy

are important features. The hands (and of course the whole upper limb), and feet, should now be inspected, palpated and described. A young child can be examined in the arms or whilst sitting on the lap of its mother (or father). Older children are observed when playing or eating, and from the age of three or older, specific tasks can usually be requested. An examination is not complete if the general physical, neurological, and orthopaedic features are not examined. Important features for a syndrome diagnosis are posture, head circumference, facial dysmorphism, genital development, and mental evolution.

Medical imaging has, at the first visit, only a limited value. Plain radiographs only give an illusion of the real bones. Incomplete ossification and overlap of fingers often disturbs the radiographs. Ultrasound does little to provide more detail. More sophisticated imaging techniques require general anaesthesia and should be planned carefully and the possible benefit judged against the inconveniences. Photographs are a powerful tool for case documentation—a picture does tells more than a thousand words—but taking pictures can give the wrong impression to the parents. It is a violation of their privacy and it would be courteous to ask permission before doing so. It should be remembered that taking pictures is a tool, not a purpose—one should not surprise them by behaving like the paparazzi—taking photographs at the end of the visit, just before saying goodbye, has proved to be good time.

Once the basic data (Table 3) has been collected and a view of the skeleton constituted, time has to be made for extensive explanations (see basic questions) on cause, pathogenic associations, and syndromes. All areas should be covered thoroughly, and repetitively if necessary, since false expectations are a serious threat to the parents' confidence in their surgeon's

Table 3 Basic data

- General information
- Pregnancy
- Psychomotor development
- Family history
- Detailed description of the hand
- Complete examination
- Medical imaging
- Photographs

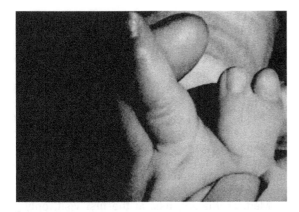

a

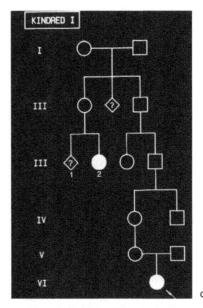

c

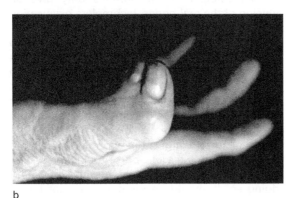

b

Figure 1

Index-patient (a) with unilateral radial polydactylism. No associated dysmorphologic features were present and both parents were normal. It was considered a non-hereditary (spontaneous) deformity, until an old ancestor with a similar deformity (b) was discovered. The family relationship was obvious although the genetic mechanism was not resolved (c).

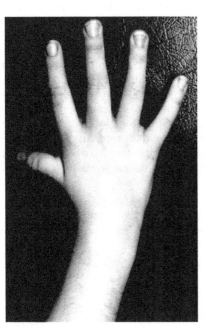

a

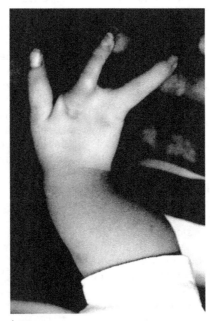

b

Figure 2

(a) The first child of a diabetic mother with radial hypoplasia (thumb hypoplasia Blauth type IIIB). The origin was explained as teratogenic and the mother was informed that with good diabetic control, the recurrence rate was low. She subsequently had a miscarriage (despite scrupulous diabetic care) and the next child (b) had an ulnar ray aplasia.

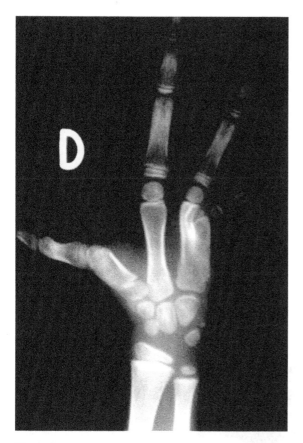

Figure 3

A radiograph showing a unilateral hand malformation with occult polydactyly (delta metacarpal of the first ray), missing index and ulnar regression (teratologische Reie), and absence or late ossification of the lunate. The pathogenic explanation of such a hand development has not yet been made and so classification not possible.

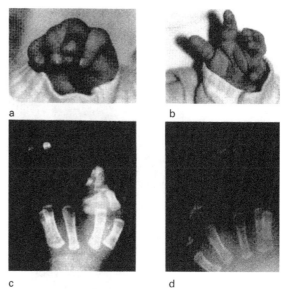

Figure 4

Central polydactyly showing complex syndactyly with rearrangement of metacarpals and metatarsals, inherited as an autosomal dominant trait. Skin fibroblast investigations showed a balanced translocation (t [12,22] [p11.2, q13.3]) present in all family members. This finding formed the basis relating to the discovery of a breakpoint in a gene. (The pathogenesis of which is still under investigation).

competence. The line between coincidental associations or as a result of some syndrome-related cause is not always obvious. Genetic mechanisms and the teratology can be very complex (Figs 1–5). Management does not only involve treatment and treatment does not only involve surgery. The child and its parents should, at any time, have the freedom of choice.

If in doubt, additional help in the form of a geneticist, pediatrician, psychologist, and social worker should be considered to facilitate the provision of all the necessary information. A follow-up visit can be planned, not necessarily immediately, but over the long term and not too close to each other. In the meantime, the parents should be encouraged to write down their questions and observations—not only does this provide important information and help for the surgeon, it is a good base for further cooperation. Try to be as realistic as possible, and predict the adaptations of the child to his hands and to calculate the growth potentials of such a hand.

Although the diagnosis is usually obvious, classification of the malformation into the IFSSH (International Federation of Societies for Surgery of the Hand, Table 4) classification is useful for

Table 4 IFFSH classification

- Failure of formation
- Failure of differentiation
- Duplication
- Overgrowth
- Hypoplasia
- Amniotic band syndrome
- Generalized disorders

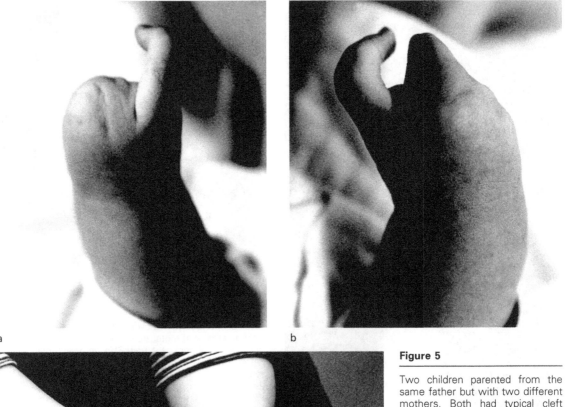

a

b

c

Figure 5

Two children parented from the same father but with two different mothers. Both had typical cleft hands (a,b) and feet (c). The father had perfectly normal hands and feet. The genetic explanation of this pedigree was thought to be gonadal mosaicism (a mutation in the precursor cells of the spermatozoids giving rise to a population of abnormal cells responsible for the hand malformations).

data collection and scientific processing. This classification is now considered as descriptive rather than aetiological or pathogenic, and has been proven to be reliable and easy in use (there is, however, a constant debate between splitters and lumpers).

The first visit forms the basis of a long treatment process for a child with a congenital hand difference. Beside the more specific hand problems, genetic, syndromic, and psychological aspects should be addressed. All the relevant information must be collated and summarized and then related back to the parents. At all times the parents (and/or the child) should be encouraged to participate in the treatment and its management—agreeing on a diagnostic/therapeutic schedule and regular follow-up appointments.

Bibliography

Bradbury E, Kay S, Tighe C, Hewison J (1994) Decision making by parents and children in paediatric hand surgery, *Br J Plast Surg* **47**:324–30.

Bradbury E (1998) Psychological issues for children and their parents. In: Buck-Gramcko D, ed, *Congenital Malformations of the Hand and Forearm* (Churchill Livingstone: London) 49–56.

Buck-Gramcko D (1998) Teratologic sequences. In: Buck-Gramcko D, ed, *Congenital Malformation of the Hand and Forearm* (Churchill Livingstone: London) 17–20.

De Smet L, Matton G, Monstrey S, Cambier E, Fabry G (1997) Application of the IFSSH (3) classification for congenital anomalies of the hand: results and problems, *Acta Orthop Belg* **63**:182–88.

Dobyns J (1990) Helping parents to decide what is best for their child, *Hand Clin* **4**:551–54.

Flatt A (1994) *The Care of Congenital Hand Anomalies*, 2nd edn (Quality Med Publ Inc: St. Louis) 1–2.

Goldberg M., Bartoshesky L (1985) Congenital hand anomaly: aetiology and associated malformations, *Hand Clin* **1**:405–15.

Lister G (1993). *The Hand: Diagnosis and Indications*, 3rd edn (Churchill Livingstone: Edinburgh) 450–512.

Luijsterburg A, Van Huizum A, Impelmans B, Hoogeveen E, Vermeij-Keers C, Hovius S (2000) Classification of congenital anomalies of the upper limb, *J Hand Surg* **25B**:3–7.

Swanson A, De Groot-Swanson G, Tada K (1983) A classification for congenital malformations, *J Hand Surg* **8**:693–702.

7
Syndactyly

David M Evans with Bruno C Coessens and Rolf Habenicht

Since the first publications in the early nineteenth century on surgical techniques for the release of congenital syndactyly, this condition has received constant interest in the medical literature. On Medline, over the last five years, there have been more than 500 publications on syndactyly, many of which focus on new or modified surgical techniques. This clearly indicates that the quest for an optimal treatment is still ongoing.

Syndactyly results from of a failure of digital rays to separate from one another during the fifth to eighth week of intrauterine life by programmed cell death (Entin 1976). This condition is therefore classified with arthrogryposis, camptodactyly, trigger thumb, and other malformations in group II (failure of differentiation or separation of parts) of the International Federation of Societies for Surgery of the Hand (IFSSH) classification (Swanson 1976). Acrosyndactyly occurring in amniotic band syndrome, in which digital rays are fused only distally with a proximal skin-lined fistula, is a different entity of unknown mechanism that is classified in group IV of the IFSSH classification along with intrauterine amputations, and is not included in this chapter.

Syndactyly is, with polydactyly, one of the most common congenital malformations of the hand, and the most common in western countries. It is encountered in one out of 2000 live births (Kelikian 1974, Lamb et al 1982, Leung et al 1982). Half of the cases are bilateral, boys are more commonly affected and it occurs more frequently in Caucasians. It accounts for between 9% and 50% of hand malformations in surgical treatment (Leung et al 1982, Luijsterburg et al 2000, Percival and Sykes 1989). The true incidence is difficult to evaluate because of variations among racial groups, different patient referral patterns and the lack of uniform classification for complex cases. Indeed, frequent association of syndactyly with short fingers (symbrachydactyly), polydactyly, oligodactyly or cleft hands may raise a problem for classification (Luijsterburg et al 2000). In syndactyly without associated malformation, the third web is the most commonly affected (57%), followed by the fourth (27%), the second (14%) and the first (3%) (Flatt 1994, Posch et al 1981). The low frequency of first web involvement is explained by the fact that the thumb–index web separates at a different and earlier stage.

Genetic origin is well demonstrated in the pathogenesis of isolated syndactyly. Inheritance is autosomal dominant (Tentamy and McKussick, 1978, Winter and Tickle, 1993). However the genes are of reduced penetrance and variable expression, meaning that the abnormality is rarely found in each generation. Syndactyly also occurs as a part of 48 different syndromes (Engber 1979, Goldberg and Bartoshesky 1985). The most common syndromes associated with syndactyly are craniosynostoses (of which Apert's syndrome is the best-known), Poland, Fanconi, Moebius, and Pierre Robin syndromes. Identification of a syndrome is of prime importance for the treatment of associated anomalies. Indeed, in these cases, syndactyly is often the least important but the most easily treated pathology affecting the child. An excellent index of syndromes associated with syndactyly and other hand malformations is provided in Flatt's textbook (1994).

Of surgical interest, clinical and radiological evaluation allow for classification of syndactyly into four groups. If the web extends to the tip of the digit, the syndactyly is termed 'complete'; in contrast with 'incomplete' for a syndactyly that does not involve the full length of the finger. If radiological evaluation shows bone fusion, the syndactyly is called 'complex'. If the web is formed by skin and connective tissue only, the syndactyly is classified as 'simple'. The degree of complexity may vary from bone fusion at the end of the distal phalanx to complex skeletal anomalies. Some authors further classify complex cases introducing the notion of 'complicated' syndactylies for cases involving more than side-to-side bone fusion.

The optimal age for correction remains controversial (Netscher and Scheker 1990). Patterns of hand function usually develop before 24 months of age (Hajnis 1968, 1969), so there is a consensus that complex cases in which function is impaired should be treated relatively early. This particularly applies in Apert's syndrome. When webbed fingers are of different growth potential, early correction will prevent flexion contracture and lateral deviation of the longer finger, which would otherwise increase with age. Therefore thumb–index and ring–little finger syndactylies should be operated on early (between 6 and 12 months). Some associated anomalies may present problems that delay surgery from the anaesthetic point of view. It goes without saying that the expertise of the surgeon and anaesthetist are paramount.

Surgical options

The goals of surgery should be the separation of independent digits creating a normally formed web, ideally in one operative stage avoiding impairment of function, scar contracture, web creep, and operative complications. The newly created web should look as closely as possible like a normal one. Although some minor variations exist, the anatomy of normal webs is quite constant. The dorsal aspect of the commissure slopes from proximal and dorsal to distal and palmar to form an angle of 45° with the palmar aspect. The apex of the commissure is longitudinally located at the middle of the proximal phalanx. Active abduction of the long fingers (more than 35° for each web) is allowed by transverse redundancy of the skin.

The history of skin release in syndactyly goes back to the early nineteenth century when surgeons used glass setons or ligatures to separate the fingers, leaving large raw areas to secondary epithelialization, which often led to severe recurrences (Davis and German 1930). Recurrence of syndactyly is in fact a scar contracture. In its mildest form it presents as tension on the suture line. Growth leads to deformities of the fingers with different degrees of severity (Toledo and Ger 1979). Unilateral scar contracture leads to bone distortion with rotation of the longitudinal axis during growth. Scar contracture leads to distal migration of the web, called web creep. Upton (1990) has pointed out that a 1.0 mm loss of tissue in an infant becomes a 1.0 cm deficit in the adult. Current techniques for separation of syndactylized digits include three major steps: the commissure reconstruction, the digital incisions, and methods to overcome skin shortage.

Separation of syndactyly has been the subject of many publications during the last two centuries. The main landmarks have been the use of commissural flaps to cover the web and the design of digital zigzag incisions. The need for skin and drawbacks of skin grafts remain a challenging problem. During the last decade, new dorsal flaps have been designed to introduce new skin and to allow primary closure without skin grafts (Niranjan and De Carpentier 1990).

Case reports with discussion

The following cases of syndactyly highlight different technical aspects of separation.

Case 1 (Bruno C Coessens)

A case of complete simple syndactyly is shown, in which separation was carried out without the use of skin grafts. In this technique a dorsal V–Y island flap is used to form the commissure (Fig. 1a) (Sherif 1998). The base of the flap is placed at the level of the metacarpal heads. The tips of the zigzag incisions reach the mid-axial line of each finger, and a curved incision on the palmar side receives the dorsal commissure flap (Figs 1a and b). Figures 1c and d show the skin markings on the hand, and the final outcome in a case of simple syndactyly is shown in Figures 1e and f.

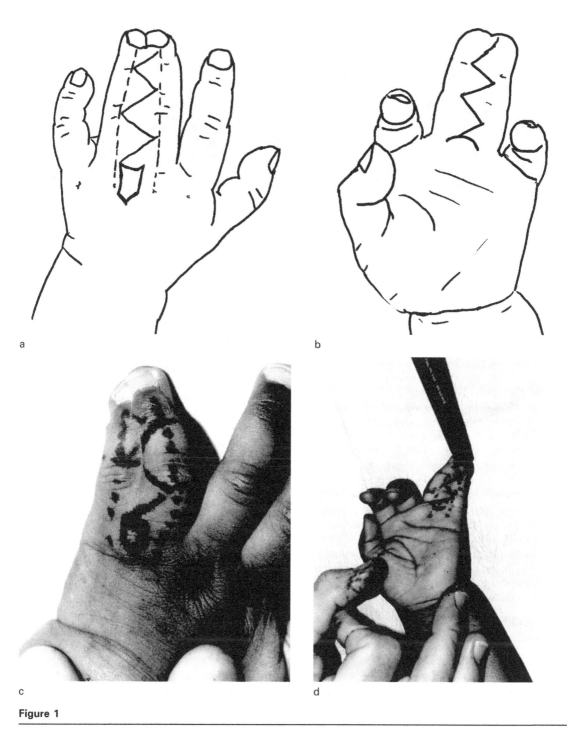

Figure 1

(a, b) Design for separation of simple syndactyly with complete skin closure, using dorsal V–Y island flap for the commissure and wide zigzag flaps reaching the axial line of each digit. (c, d) The skin markings in a clinical case.

continued

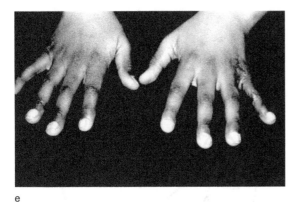

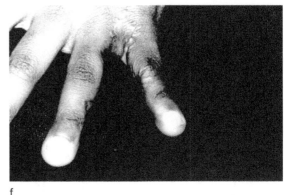

e

f

Figure 1 continued

(e, f) The result of separation using this technique, with no skin grafts. The commissure is well formed. There is still some scar hypertrophy.

Discussion

The shape and position of the web in the results shown are close to normal. One hopes that the position of the web will remain unchanged throughout growth. There is slight hollowing of the shape of the ring finger near the base as a result of fat excision; it would also be interesting to know if that will persist through growth. The preoperative photographs show well the effect of syndactyly of unequal length fingers on growth. There is also fusion of the nails and possibly of the distal phalanges, and this is not evident in the postoperative photographs, which would appear to be a different case with incomplete syndactyly. It would be interesting to discuss further the technique of tip separation when they are closely fused, and also whether complete resolution of the axial growth disturbance can be expected with further growth.

Case 2 (David M Evans)

This girl presented with a first ray cleft and is shown aged four, the thumb position having been previously corrected (Figs 2a and b). There is persistent tight syndactyly between the two radial fingers. At the time of correction of the thumb, the fingers had been explored at the base and she was found to have a common flexor tendon sheath shared between the two fingers extending right across the breadth of the syndactilized digits, and it was initially felt that separation was not feasible. This was strongly requested however, and separation was therefore undertaken by splitting the tendons longitudinally between the two fingers (Fig. 2c) and preserving all the sheath for coverage of the tendons in the middle finger, and enough skin to completely cover the ulnar side of the radial (index) finger after reconstruction of two pulleys using a strip of extensor retinaculum passed around the phalanges. A full thickness skin graft was applied to the large raw area of the tendon sheath on the middle finger (Fig. 2d). The result is shown five years later (Figs 2e and f) and this patient is now fully grown and an accomplished cellist and pianist, and is a medical student. No further surgery was necessary for these two fingers.

The principle of taking sufficient skin to cover one finger completely after syndactyly separation, with the use of a larger single skin graft on the remaining finger, has since been applied in other cases. There are significant advantages in terms of the amount of scarring and the fact that one finger is completely clothed in normal skin. The skin graft in this case was taken from the groin, but a transverse ellipse from the cubital fossa is now used; there is much less of a problem with hair growth later, and the donor site is very convenient and the scar not a problem.

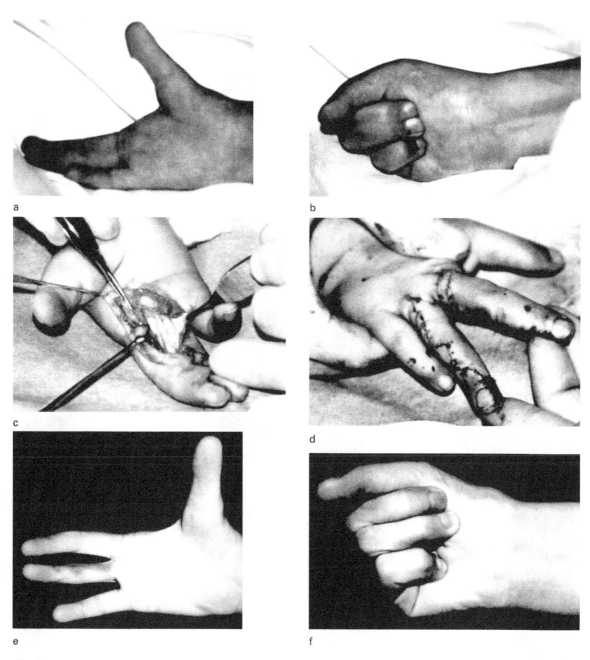

a

b

c

d

e

f

Figure 2

(a, b) Syndactyly associated with cleft hand (first cleft). The thumb has been repositioned. Function is good, and separation strongly requested although it was known that there was a common flexor sheath. (c) The common flexor sheath containing tendons side by side is shown. (d) Separation has been completed, using all available sheath to cover the tendons on the middle finger, with one larger full thickness graft, and complete skin closure on the radial finger which was favoured with the incision design so that this was possible. Two pulleys have been reconstructed beneath this skin closure. (e, f) The result after five years, with no web creep and good function. Figure 2 has been reproduced from *Recent Advances in Plastic Surgery*, Number 5, 1996, edited by Jackson and Sommerlad, Figure 7.4, chapter by D M Evans, by kind permission of the publishers, Churchill Livingstone.

Discussion

There are cases, especially those complicated by the presence of other anomalies such as this one, where there might be good reason to leave two syndactylized digits joined, although this case shows that adequate reconstruction of the tendon anomaly can result in good function. There are advantages in using one large graft as opposed to multiple small ones. Of course, when it proves impossible to close completely a syndactyly separation designed to be graftless, additional skin grafts have to be placed wherever they are necessary.

Case 3 (Rolf Habenicht)

Another method of creating enough skin to resurface tightly syndactylized fingers is soft-tissue distraction. This provides more skin in the pulp region and at metacarpal and phalangeal levels. Such a case is shown in Figures 3a, b and c. Only

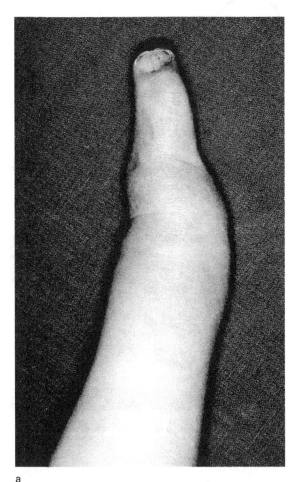

a

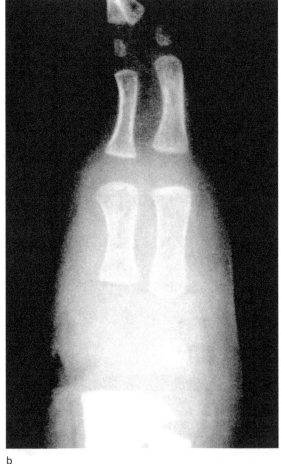

b

Figure 3

(a, b, c) Oligosyndactyly, showing two closely joined digits with fusion of distal phalanges and nails. (d) Fine pins passed through all phalanges and metacarpals of the two digits, avoiding growth plates. (e, f) The modular distraction device in place.

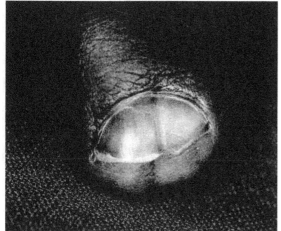

c

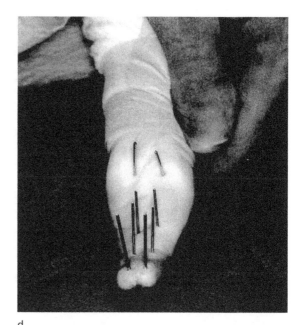

d

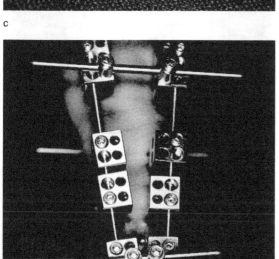

e

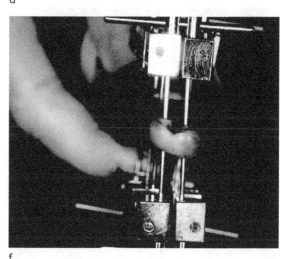

f

continued

two digits are present, they are tightly syndactyl-ized, and the distal phalanges and nails are fused. For cross soft-tissue distraction we use very small and light modular distraction devices, which can be adapted to any individual case. Prior to implantation of the device, fused bones and nails have to be separated, cutting the nail in the middle, and using a percutaneous small osteotome for the distal phalanges. Fine wires are inserted (Fig. 3d), transfixing all bones of the two digits (avoiding growth plates), to avoid joint deviations during distraction. The distraction device is shown in Figures 3e and f.

Distraction starts on the second postoperative day with a speed of between 0.25 and 0.5 mm per day, depending on local circulation and pain

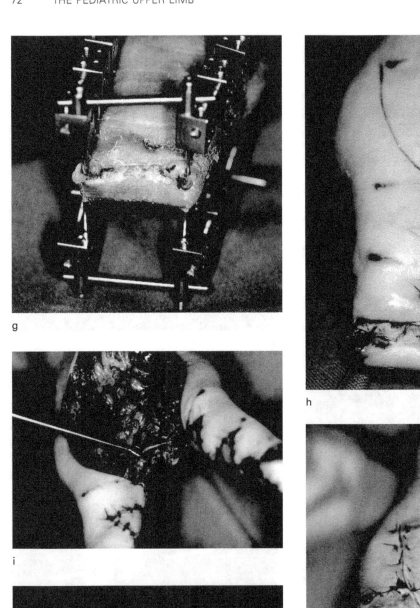

g

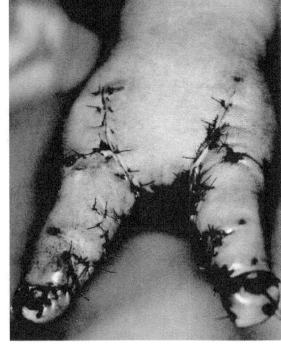

h

i

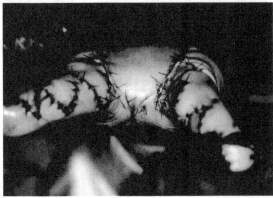

j   k

(g) After distraction. (h, i, j and k) Surgical separation after removal of the device. (l, m, n, o and p) The result of separation.

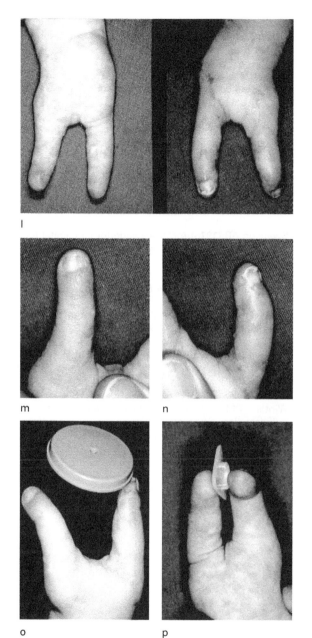

l

m   n

o   p

of distraction at the metacarpal level to form a wide deep new web (Fig. 3h). Distraction takes about 2 weeks and is followed by a consolidation period of 2 to 3 weeks. Then the device is removed and the syndactyly separated by standard techniques (Figs 3h–k). In cases of oligosyndactyly we have achieved closure without skin grafts, and in other cases pulp skin has always been closed directly and proximal areas have needed skin grafts less than with conventional techniques. The result in the case shown can be seen in Figures 3l–p.

Complications include infection, which can be minimized by good pin care and case selection, and we have never had to remove a device in 30 cases. Callus formation may occur in the distal phalanx, especially in Apert's syndrome, and can in fact be used to broaden the phalanx. Blood supply in distracted regions is excellent, and this has contributed to good primary healing and lack of scar contracture with growth. Nail growth resumed normally within 3 months of separation.

Discussion

This technique has clear benefits in tight oligosyndactyly and in Apert's syndrome, and it will be interesting to see how far its use can be extended in other situations, for example in multiple neighbouring syndactylies. Can more than one ray be distracted with one apparatus? Tissue expansion has been tried but abandoned, however horizontal skin stretching by skeletal distraction may prove very useful. One wonders why it is ever necessary to use skin grafts since in theory the distraction could continue until enough skin is available for complete closure.

References

Davis JS, German WJ (1930) Syndactylism. Coherence of the fingers and toes, *Arch Surg* **21**:32.

Engber WD (1979) Syndactyly with Larsen's syndrome, *J Hand Surg* **4**:187–8.

Entin MA (1976) Syndactyly of the upper limb: morphogenesis, classification and management, *Clin Plast Surg* **3**:129–40.

after distraction. If problems arise, speed can be reduced, stopped for one or two days, or distraction temporarily reversed. The amount of distraction depends on the individual requirements, but is normally between 13 and 17 mm (Fig. 3g). In cases of oligosyndactyly we increase the amount

Flatt AE (1994) *The Care of Congenital Upper Limb Anomalies*, 2nd edn (Quality Medical Publishing Inc: St Louis).

Goldberg MJ, Bartoshesky LE (1985) Congenital hand anomaly: aetiology and associated malformations, *Hand Clin* **1**:405–15.

Hajnis K (1968) Growth of the fingers and periods suited for operation on their congenital defects, *Acta Chir Plast* **10**:267–84.

Hajnis K (1969) The dynamics of hand growth since the birth till 18 years of age, *Panminerva Med* **11**:123–32.

Kelikian H (1974) *Congenital Deformities of the Hand and Forearm* (WB Saunders: Philadelphia).

Lamb DW, Wynne-Davies R, Soto L (1982) An estimate of the population frequency of congenital malformations of the upper limb, *J Hand Surg* **7**:557–62.

Leung PC, Chan KM, Cheng JYC (1982) Congenital anomalies of the upper limb among the Chinese population in Hong Kong, *J Hand Surg* **7A**:563–5.

Luijsterburg AJM, van Huizum MA, Impelmans BE, Hoogeveen E, Vermeij-Keers C, Hovius SE (2000) Classification of congenital anomalies of the upper limb, *J Hand Surg* **25B**:3–7.

Netscher DT, Scheker LR (1990) Timing and decision-making in the treatment of congenital upper extremity deformities, *Clin Plast Surg* **17**:113–31.

Niranjan NS, De Carpentier J (1990) A new technique for the correction of syndactyly without skin graft, *Eur J Plast Surg* **13**:101.

Percival NJ, Sykes PJ (1989) Syndactyly: a review of the factors which influence surgical treatment, *J Hand Surg* **14B**:196–200.

Posch JL, Dela Cruz-Saddul FA, Posch JL Jr (1981) Congenital syndactylism of the fingers in 262 cases, *Orthop Rev* **10**:23.

Sherif MM (1998) V-Y dorsal metacarpal flap: a new technique for the correction of syndactyly without skin graft, *Plast Recon Surg* **101**:1861.

Swanson AB (1976) A classification for congenital limb malformations, *J Hand Surg* **1**:8–22.

Tentamy SA, McKussick VA (1978) The genetics of hand malformations, *Birth Defects Orig Artic Ser* **14**:1.

Toledo LC, Ger E (1979) Evaluation of the operative treatment of syndactyly, *J Hand Surg* **4**:556–64.

Upton J (1990) Syndactyly. In: May JW, Littler JW, eds, *Plastic Surgery*, Vol. 8. (WB Saunders: Philadelphia) 5279.

Winter RM, Tickle C (1993) Syndactylies and polydactylies: embryological overview and suggested classification, *Eur J Hum Genet* **1**:96–104.

8

Thumb polydactyly

Alain Gilbert with Michael A Tonkin and Steven ER Hovius

An excess of digits on the human hand has always been a source of philosophical discussions. In the past, many have followed the mythical theory of atavism, expressed and developed by Darwin (1896). He felt that extra digits were 'the result of reversion to a remote ancestor'.

In several civilizations, polydactylism was considered part of social organization or as proof of heredity; for example in a family from the Arabic tribe of Hyamites (Devay 1862), all the children had six fingers and a pentadactyl child was considered as adulterine. In the Ukrainian village of Jetnick, as cited by Sysak (1928), the Jetnicki family had five fingers but all the Siomak family members had seven fingers on each hand, and any intermarriages between the two groups resulted in six-fingered children. In contrast, in some African tribes, a six-fingered child was considered as a bad omen and immediately put to death.

Although polydactylism is considered as essentially sporadic, all these examples demonstrate a condition known as endemic polydactylism, many of which have been in Europe, for example in the villages of Izeaux (Devay 1862) and Colombes (Benard 1916) in the French mountains of Isere, or from the village of Cervera de Butigo, close to Madrid in Spain (De Linares 1930). One of the longest family histories concerns the descendants of Scipo Africanus (185–129 BC) who allegedly had six fingers and six toes. Manoilof (1931) said he could trace the family of a patient living in Russia, going back over 2000 years and 80 generations, with the same anomaly—a family that still bears the same name. Closer to home, there is the Maltese family of Kalleray as described by Morand (1773) with three generations of polydactylism documented.

In most cases, polydactylism should be considered as a result of a mutation. In other cases and in some syndromic syndromes such as Ellis-Van Creveld, Laurence-Moon-Bardet, recessive polydactylism will be part of the features.

Incidence

Most studies concern the overall types of polydactylism (pre- and postaxial). In 1885, Tapie found five polydactyl babies in 2200 births. In 1958, Shapiro recorded 80 polydactylies in 30,388 births but only two were from Whites and 78 from Blacks. This very large racial difference in the incidence of polydactylism was confirmed by Frazier (1960) who, in a study of 200 cases, reported 179 being Black and only 21 being White. Mellin (1963) stated that the incidence of polydactyly was 10.68 per 1000 births in Blacks but 1.56 per 1000 births in Whites, with a medium range for the Orientals. Handforth (1950) confirmed that in Chinese people the rate of polydactyly was 2.5 per 1000—95% of which were thumb duplications; coincidently, in Blacks the same percentage applies to fifth finger duplications.

Classification

There are three types of polydactyly:

- Postaxial, on the side of the little finger
- Central, in one of the central digits, mainly the fourth
- Preaxial, on the side of the thumb.

We shall deal only with the last group. Some authors include the duplication of the index finger in preaxial polydactyly (type III in

Temtamy and McKusick [1985] or polysyn-dactyly-type IV). In this chapter only thumb polydactylism will be discussed.

The most commonly used classification is the Wassel classification (1969). This classification is extremely useful and easy to use. However, it is sometimes difficult to include some cases and the grade VII comprises a very wide group. Several authors have proposed their own classi-fication, for example before Wassel, Millesi had proposed a classification of five types (1967), Tada (1983) had proposed a classification of six types with a rudimentary grade called VII and Ikuta (1998) had added his own subclassification, dividing the cases into 'balanced' (if the two thumbs are of equal size) or 'unbalanced' (if the two thumbs were different size). The Wassel classification gives insufficient information in types IV and VII and some authors have proposed more detailed stages in types IV and VII, and expanding the descriptions of the differ-ent types (Wood 1978). In the literature, most of the authors have used Wassel's classification and in all publications, grade IV is the most common (Table 1).

Age for treatment

In order to avoid severe desaxations with growth, it seems obvious that there is some necessity to treat as early as possible. But treat-ing at too early a stage may be technically demanding since in some instances this small digit requires two osteotomies, flexor tendon relocation, and joint reconstruction etc. The treat-ment has to be a compromise and we feel that the optimum time is between 12–14 months of age.

Problems of treatment

Difficulties arise in grades I or II when the two thumbs are small and 'balanced' (equivalent in size). In instances like these it is tempting to use the Bilhaut-Cloquet technique and fuse the distal phalanges, but the problem comes in the restora-tion of nail growth, and avoiding the central groove.

In grade IV, one of the thumbs (usually the radial thumb) will be excised and the metapha-langeal (MP) joint reconstructed. At this level the problem is more complex (Fig. 1) owing to:

- Deformity of the MP joint.
- Deviation of the proximal phalanx.
- Lateral insertion of the flexor tendon.

Usually, the radial thumb is excised with conser-vation of the ulnar finger (Fig. 2). Most of the thenar muscles are inserted on the radial thumb, and so preserved for future reinsertion. The extensor tendon is sutured onto the other finger and the flexor tendon is sectioned at the level of its division.

The MP joint is roof-shaped and each thumb base is an adaptation. When one of the thumbs is excised, the new joint is oblique and needs to be remodelled. A triangular piece of the metacarpal head and neck is excised, and a new horizontal joint created. A piece of the metacarpal head is also excised for cosmetic reasons. The osteotomy is fixed with a pin and the radial ligament is reconstructed. Stability is enhanced by reattachment of the thenar muscles.

Excision of the extra thumb is not sufficient, since the new thumb has a radial clinodactyly, due to deviation of the proximal phalanx and lateral insertion of the flexor tendon. By a lateral

Table 1 Anatomical findings in the literature

	Nb	Grade I	Grade II	Grade III	Grade IV	Grade V	Grade VI	Grade VII
Wassel (1969)	70	2%	15%	6%	10%	10%	49%	20%
Cheng (1984)	95	6%	17%	9%	46%	12%	3%	6%
Tada (1983)	156	5%	16%	9%	44%	14%	3%	9%
Light (1991)	50	6%	12%	10%	44%	4%	6%	18%
Gilbert (1995)	103	6%	27%	7%	38%	5%	2%	15%
Ikuta (1998)	267	5.3%	20.1%	4.6%	31.9%	3.9%	8.2%	13.8%

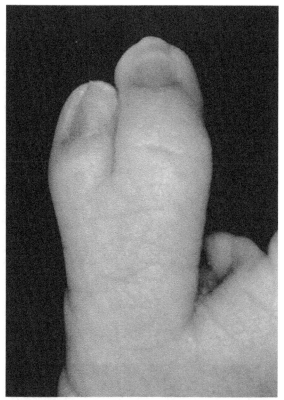

a

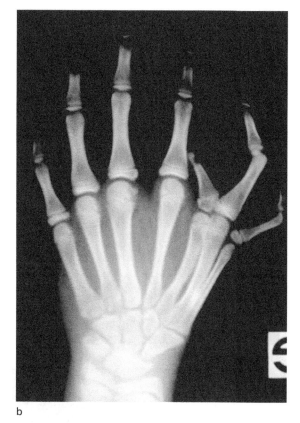

b

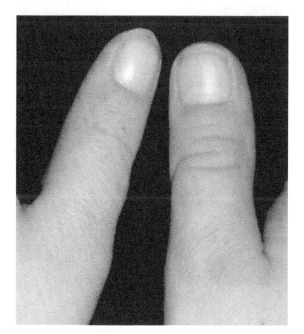

c

Figure 1

Radial polydactyly case with 3 thumbs (a,b). (c) Post-operative result

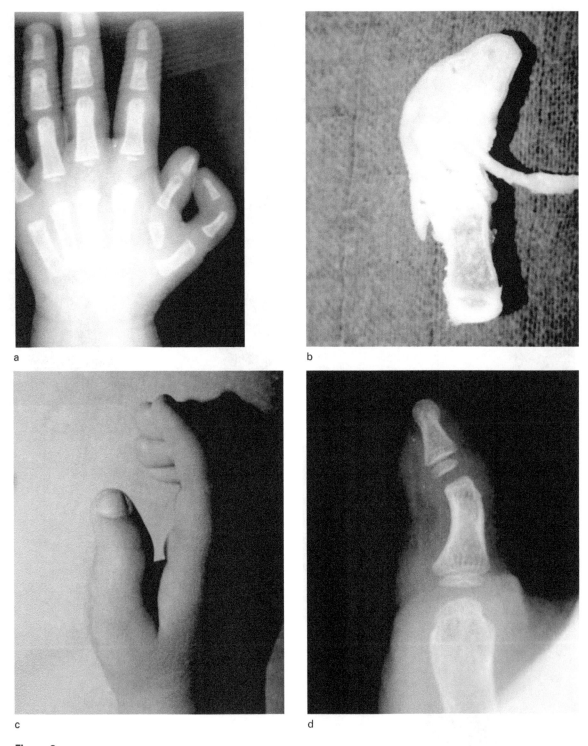

Figure 2

Radial polydactylyl (a); radial thumb resected (b); (c and d) postoperative result of ulnar thumb with slight clinodactyly

incision, osteotomy of the phalanx allows correction of the deviation.

Relocation of the flexor tendon is mandatory in order to avoid recurrence of the deviation. Some authors have advocated sectioning and reinsertion of the flexor tendon, but this carries risks of severe adhesions. We prefer to detach the lateral insertion of the tendon and, folding it on itself, to suture it to the medial part. The treatment is then complete and the skin flaps can be finally adapted and sutured and the pins can be taken out after five or six weeks. The ideal age for this operation is between 12 and 18 months. Understanding the factors involved in the deformity will facilitate a good initial treatment with secondary surgery and if the initial procedures are incomplete, determine the complications and future treatment.

Residual deformity is difficult to treat but there have been some good results. In 1996, Hung and colleagues specifically studied the duplication at a metacarpophalangeal level. They described a classification according to the aspect of both thumbs: convergent, divergent, hypoplastic, from grade A to D. They reviewed the treatment of 21 cases with a long follow-up and found 75% of patients had a good range of movement; there was stability in all but one of the patients and in 85% of the cases, the patients were satisfied.

The relationship between polydactyly and the triphalangeal thumb is still being debated. More than 50% of cases with triphalangeal thumbs are part of a polydactyly. In 1978, Wood devised a new subclassification of Wassel's classification, comprising types A to D—the most common being type C. These patients often needed several procedures: in our own series for example, there were 78 procedures split between just 23 patients. The authors note that the best results are often obtained when the triphalangeal thumb rather than the biphalangeal thumb is removed, (even if it is more rudimentary).

Results of treatment

In the literature there are several large series showing that the results of treatment are usually good, with a few exceptions. In 1969, Wassel reviewed the results of treatment of 22 thumbs. He showed that almost all had some deviation.

This was especially obvious in grades II, IV, and VII. In grade IV, the MP joint mobility was limited.

In 1983, Tada and colleagues published a review of a large number of cases (237 patients and 261 hands). The results were evaluated in 94 hands. The end results were good in 75.5%, fair in 20.2% and poor in 4.3%. In another group, 36 hands with residual deformities were followed-up after operation and it was found that in 13 cases there was no improvement (i.e. only 63.9% in this group had good results). They recommended that surgery should be done at about six months for grades I–VI and at three months for grade VII. In these cases, the grade IV patients were initially treated with the complete procedure involving joint shaving, osteotomy, and tendon relocation. The results were in the same range (75%) as the global series. The grade VII types cannot be compared to any other series since the authors eliminated the triphalangeal thumbs, replacing them with a floating thumb.

Our own series of 106 patients operated between 1976 and 1995 was presented at the International Symposium on Congenital Anomalies in Milan in 1996 (Gilbert and Harguindeguy 1996). We were able to review 76 patients (81 thumbs) with an average follow-up of 36 months. Only 9% of the patients had any bilateral involvement and the average age at operation was 13.5 months. We used a clinical grading system comprising three stages: 0–3, poor results; 3–6, average results and 6–8, good results. The average result in this series was 6.55. We tried to evaluate the results according to several factors:

- Age at operation: patients under age two had a 17% rate of re-operation. Between 2–4 years, the re-operation rate had reduced to 1%, with no re-operations in patients aged four and over. The results were 6.88 for the patients operated on before two years of age, 6.0 for those between 2–4 years old and 6.37 for patients over the age of four.
- Type of anomaly: the number of re-operations is at its highest (47%) in grade VII, with 29% in grade V, and 10% in grade IV. The results also varied with the type: 8 in grade I; 6.68 in grade II; 6.87 in grade III; 6.15 in grade IV; 6.95 in grade VI and 6.0 in grade VII.

The conclusions of this study are that grade VII carries the highest rate of re-operation with the poorest end results, and overall, that the patients operated on before their second birthday had the most re-operations but the end results were better than in patients who were operated on later in life.

Radial polydactyly—distal duplication

Michael A Tonkin

Reconstructive surgery for thumb duplication aims to achieve a thumb of appropriate size, stability, and motion with minimal deformity and scarring. The methods of surgical reconstruction include:

- The removal of one thumb and reconstruction of the other.
- The removal of equal parts from both thumbs with a combination of the retained parts (Bilhaut-Cloquet).
- A combination of asymmetric parts from both thumbs (modified Bilhaut-Cloquet).

For Wassell types I and II thumb duplication (distal duplication), the choice of surgical reconstruction is determined by clinical and radiological assessment. In general, if the thumb to be retained is greater than 70% of the width of the normal opposite thumb and is stable, supplementation of tissue from the removed digit is unnecessary. When the nail is joined, the nail fold will require reconstruction minimally. It may be necessary to reconstruct a collateral ligament, usually the radial collateral ligament, of the interphalangeal joint. Marked deviation of the retained thumb may necessitate an osteotomy at the neck of the proximal phalanx with or without realignment of eccentric flexor and extensor tendon insertions.

If the retained thumb is inadequate in size, the alternatives include the Bilhaut-Cloquet or a modified Bilhaut-Cloquet procedure. The latter aims to avoid a nail ridge by using the nail and nail bed of the retained thumb and supplementing tissue, bone, pulp bulk, and skin as necessary, from the other. Most consider this preferable to the classical Bilhaut-Cloquet procedure with its complication of a nail ridge. However, with atten-tion to technical detail, the nail ridge can be minimized such that the classical Bilhaut-Cloquet procedure remains useful if alternative reconstructions are likely to result in a small or deviated and unstable thumb. Optimal results are achieved by utilizing the following technique:

- The width of the opposite thumbnail is measured.
- The nail or nails of the duplicated thumb are removed.
- Equal parts of both thumbs are removed in a V-shape such that the addition of the two remaining parts results in a width equal to the opposite thumb. A beaver blade is used to divide the bone of the distal phalanges.
- Because the proximal phalanx is too broad, it is difficult to appose the adjacent surfaces of the distal phalanges unless more than half of the width of each distal phalanx is retained. This results in an obviously broad thumb. Therefore, a triangle of bone and cartilage is excised from both sides of the proximal phalangeal head to decrease its bulk and to provide adequate length in the collateral ligaments to allow bone apposition. The collateral ligaments remain attached to the bases of the distal phalanges and in continuity with the periosteum of the proximal phalanx.
- The nail beds are elevated minimally from the dorsal aspects of the distal two-thirds of the distal phalanges beyond the physes.
- The physes, not necessarily the articular surfaces, are apposed. It is more important to match the physes to prevent partial physeal fusion, than to match the joint surfaces. These can be fashioned with a beaver blade to create a congruous joint surface, and will mould if the surgery is done early in life.
- A 0.028 Kirschner wire (K-wire) is used to drill adjacent holes in both distal phalanges in two places. Two 28-guage interosseous wire sutures achieve the osteosynthesis. The wire sutures are tightened on the palmar surface of the bone.
- The nail bed is repaired with interrupted 8-0 vicryl sutures. The dorsal nail bed should also be sutured. The distal ends of the extensor tendons and flexor tendons are co-apted longitudinally with 6-0 vicryl on the dorsal and palmar aspects. The skin is sutured with 6-0 vicryl.

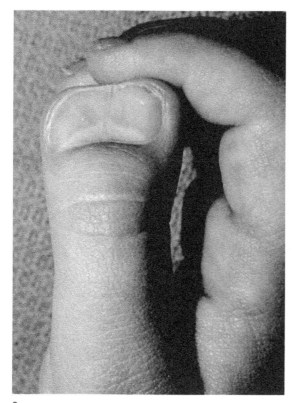

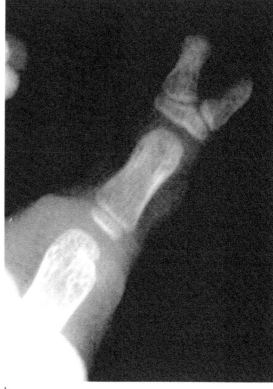

a

b

Figure 3

(a,b) Type I Wassell thumb duplication.

- The more appropriate of the nails is trimmed to fit beneath the nail fold to prevent nail bed-skin adhesion.
- A fine K-wire maintains the joint in extension for 3–4 weeks.

Nine such procedures have been reviewed at an average follow-up of two years. The average parental satisfaction score on a questionnaire was 94 (range 88–100). The operated thumbs were used normally and the procedures not seen to affect the child's preference for hand use.

Appearance was considered satisfactory in all but one case. Length, circumference, shape and nail width were uniformly good. Angulation of 5° and a sharp nail ridge occurred on the dominant hand of one patient. Interestingly, the appearance

and stability of this, the most unsatisfactory case, was considered superior to the opposite thumb that had been treated by ablation and reconstruction resulting in a smaller and less stable thumb.

All interphalangeal joints were stable on clinical examination with a range of flexion from 10–70°. Metacarpophalangeal joint ranges of motion were as present preoperatively. Interphalangeal joint incongruency and physeal bridging occurred in one thumb.

The preoperative appearance, operative technique, and final result are fully illustrated for one case (Figs 3–9). Pre- and postoperative illustrations are available for other cases.

The most appropriate reconstructive procedure for Wassell type I and II thumb duplication will be determined by the individual presentation.

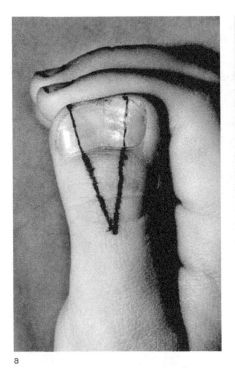

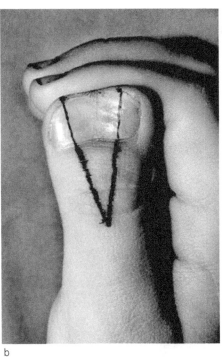

Figure 4

(a,b) Excision of central aspect of thumb duplication.

a

b

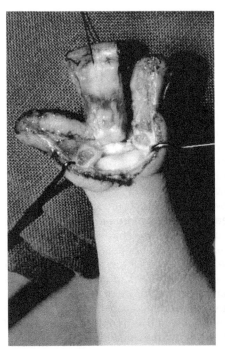

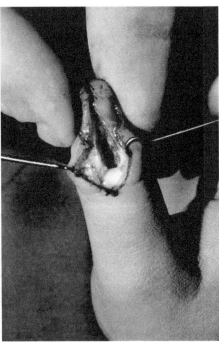

Figure 5

(a,b) Difficulty in apposition of retained thumbs.

a

b

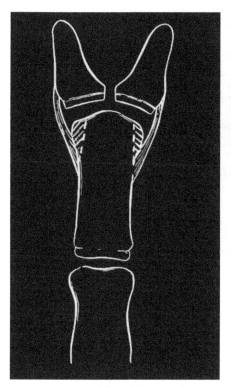

a

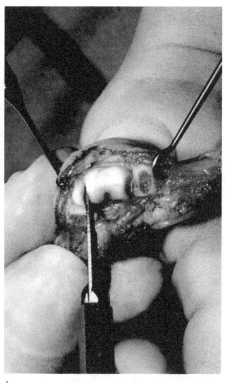

b

Figure 6

(a,b) Excision of lateral aspects of proximal phalangeal head with maintenance of capsulo-periosteal flaps.

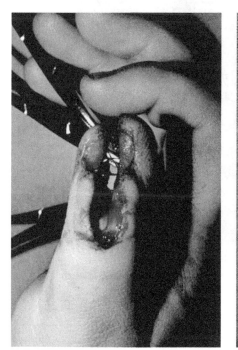

a

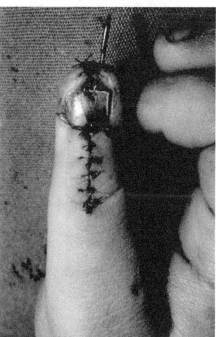

b

Figure 7

(a,b) Bone apposition and nail and skin repair.

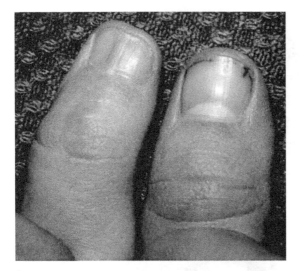

a

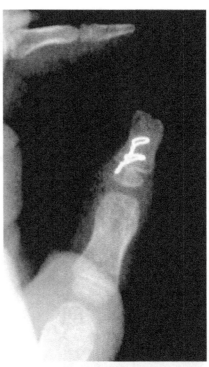

a

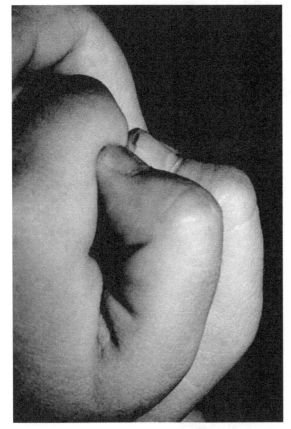

b

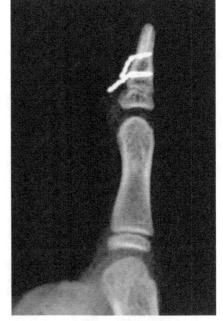

b

Figure 8

(a,b) Postoperative results.

Figure 9

(a,b) Postoperative x-rays.

The classical Bilhaut-Cloquet procedure remains applicable for selected cases when the two thumbs are of equal size and shape. It is then possible to achieve a stable thumb of normal size with satisfactory motion and appearance.

The triphalangeal thumb

Steven ER Hovius

A triphalangeal thumb is a thumb consisting of three 'phalanges'. The middle 'phalanx' can vary from a very small delta-shaped sized bone to a fully developed phalanx as in a normal finger. The incidence is reported to be 1:2500 live births (Lapidus 1943), which has been questioned as being low by Buck-Gramcko. However, he also included a long epiphysis of the distal phalanx with or without slight deviation. The unilateral cases with a short triangular middle phalanx are mostly sporadic; the other types mostly have a positive inheritance (Buck-Gramcko 1998).

The hand can look like a five-fingered hand, or the hand can present itself with one or two extra thumbs, either biphalangeal or triphalangeal. Our series comprise large pedigrees with triphalangeal thumbs demonstrating the whole variety as described above, often associated with an extra thumb and a varying degree of thenar hypoplasia to nearly complete absence of thenar muscles. Genetic analysis revealed the locus to be on the long arm of chromosome 7, more precisely 7q36 (Heutink 1994).

Triphalangeal thumbs can be associated with polydactyly, syndactyly, a typical cleft hand, radial dysplasia, synpolydactyly, ear and toe anomalies and systemic diseases like cardiovascular and gastrointestinal anomalies, blood dyscrasias and noxious agents like thalidomide (Upton 2000).

Many classifications have been provided (Buck-Gramcko 1998, Temtamy 1978). Buck-Gramcko has provided the so-called teratologic sequence in six types from a rudimentary middle phalanx to a fully developed triphalangeal thumb associated with radial polydactyly (type VI) in which treatment options can vary from doing nothing, excision, closing wedge osteotomies, metacarpal osteotomies, tendon transfers, intrinsic tightening, web deepening, pollicization and combinations of the above techniques. As this is a case illustration

and not an extensive paper on triphalangeal thumbs, I will confine myself to an example of type VI of the teratological sequence of Buck-Gramcko's classification. This is, as a matter of fact, the largest group of triphalangeal thumbs.

In our series of this type the ulnar thumb is nearly always the most developed one and nearly always triphalangeal. The radial thumb or thumbs can either be tri- or biphalangeal or more rudimentary (a few cases had three thumbs). The goal is to form one thumb out of two instead of merely amputating one.

In the illustrated case the following procedures were undertaken in a one-stage operation. No further operations were performed. The operative procedure in both hands consisted of the following:

- Reduction osteotomy of mostly the distal and middle part of the middle phalanx and a short part of the distal phalanx via a dorsal incision, resulting in an arthrodesis of the DIP joint.
- Longitudinal removal of a part of the ulnar nail and ulnar distal phalanx with reconstruction of the ulnar nail wall.
- Extirpation of the radial ray with isolation of the rudimentary extensor tendon, flexor tendon, and radial collateral ligament tissues.
- Rotation, shortening, and abduction osteotomy of the ulnar first metacarpal at mid-shaft level (two growth plates are often present).
- Reconstruction of the radial collateral ligament with the rudimentary radial collateral ligament tissues covered with the rudimentary extensor tendon to strengthen the new radial collateral ligament.
- Shortening of the intrinsics at the lateral slip level. The intrinsic muscles are already freed at the metacarpal level when performing the reduction osteotomy.
- Skin alignment.

In this case a double distal phalanx was present and therefore the thumb was reduced longitudinally.

Reduction osteotomies at the DIP level are nowadays conducted via a Y-V incision instead of transverse and longitudinal incisions. If necessary fist web deepening or radial transposition of the ulnar ray are performed. Sometimes volar plate plasty and opponens plasty are performed later on. The length of the thumb is of continuous concern, especially in the presence of two growth plates. The reduction is started at the DIP level, as shortening is limited at this site, followed by reduction at the metacarpal level.

The length of the thumb should be proximal to the PIP joint of the index finger. Although advocated by various authors, I seldom perform a formal pollicization in these cases. See Figures 10–19; all figures are of the same patient.

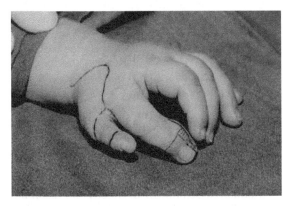

Figure 10

Type VI triphalangeal thumb with polydactyly: dorsal view.

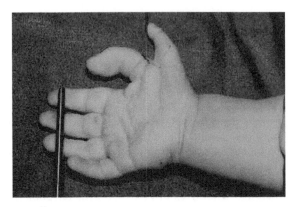

Figure 11

Type VI triphalangeal thumb with polydactyly: palmar view.

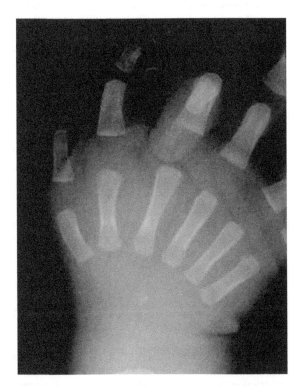

Figure 12

X-ray: note partial presence of a third thumb (middle and distal phalanx).

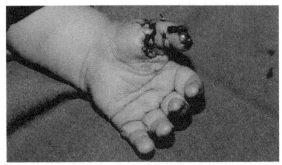

Figure 13

Direct post-operative view: palmar view.

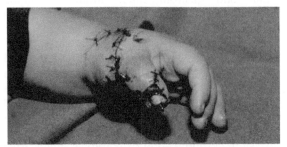

Figure 14

Direct post-operative view: dorsal view.

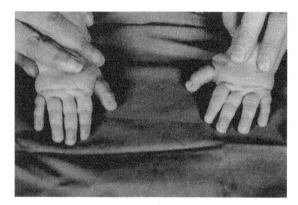

Figure 15

Both hands respectively 1 and 1.5 years postoperatively.

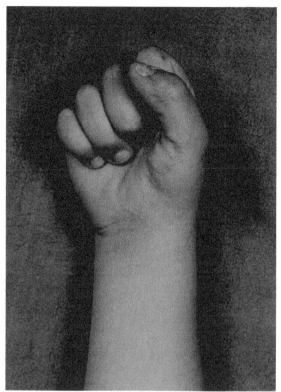

Figure 16

Right hand 6.5 years postoperatively.

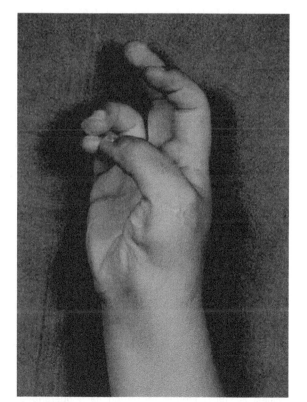

Figure 17

Same as Figure 16 with flexion of thumb.

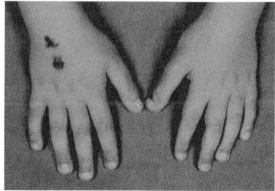

Figure 18

Both hands 6.0 and 6.5 years postoperatively.

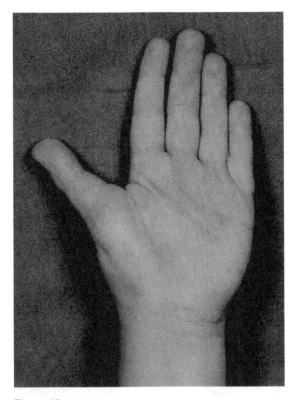

Figure 19

Left hand 6 years postoperatively: palmar view.

References

Bilhaut M (1890) Guérison d'un pouce bifide par un nouveau procédé opératoire, *Congrès Français de Chir* 4/576.

Blauth W, Olason AT (1988) Classification of polydactyly of the hands and feet, *Arch Orthop Traum Surg* **107**:334–44.

Buck-Gramcko D (1998) *Congenital malformations of the hand and forearm* (Churchill Livingstone: London) 403–25.

Buck-Gramcko D, Behrens P (1989) Classification for polydactyly hand and foot, *Handchir Mikrochir Plast Chir* **21**:195–204.

Cheng JCY, Chan KM, Ma GFY et al (1984) Polydactyly of the thumb: a surgical plan based on 95 cases, *J Hand Surg* **9A**:155–64.

Dobyns JH (1988) Duplicate thumbs (pre-axial polydactyly) In: Green DP, ed, *Operative hand surgery*, 2nd edn, (Churchill Livingstone: New York).

Dobyns JH, Lipscomb PR, Cooney WP (1985) Management of thumb duplication, *Clin Orthop* **195**:26–44.

Egawa T (1966) Surgical treatment of polydactyly of the thumb, *Jpn J Plast Reconstr Surg* **9**:97–101.

Goffin D, Gilbert A, Leclercq C (1990) Thumb duplication: surgical treatment and analysis of sequels, *Ann Hand Upper Limb Surg* **9**:119–28.

Heutink P et al (1994) The gene for triphalangeal thumb maps to the sub-telomeric region of chromosome 7q, *Nature Genet* 287–92.

Hung L, Cheng JC, Bundoc R, Leung P (1996) Thumb duplication at the metacarpophalangeal joint, management, and a new classification, *Clin Orthop Rel Res* **323**:31–41.

Kawabata H, Tada K, Masada K et al (1990) Revision of residual deformities after operations for duplication of the thumb, *J Bone Joint Surg* **72A**:988–98.

Kelikian H, Doumanian A (1957) Congenital anomalies of the hand, *J Bone Joint Surg* **39A**:1002.

Lapidus PW et al (1943) Triphalangeal thumb, *Surg Gyaecol Obstet* **77**:178–86.

Light TR (1991) Duplication du pouce: pathologie et traitement. *Monographies du Groupe d'Etude de la Main: Les Malformations Congénitales du Membre Supérieur* (Expansion Scientifique Française, Paris).

Light TR (1992) Treatment of pre-axial polydactyly, *Hand Clin* **8**:161–75.

Manoiloff EO (1931) A rare case of hereditary hexadactylism, *Am J Phys Anthropol* **15**:503.

Manske PR (1989) Treatment of duplicated thumb using a ligamentous/periosteal flap, *J Hand Surg* **14A**:728–33.

Marks TW, Bayne LG (1978) Polydactyly of the thumb: abnormal anatomy and treatment, *J Hand Surg* **3A**:107–16.

Millesi H (1967) Fingerverformung nach operationen wegen polydaktylie, *Klin Med Wien* **22**:266–72.

Miura T (1977) An appropriate treatment for postoperative z-formed deformity of the duplicated thumb, *J Hand Surg* **2A**:380–6.

Miura T (1982) Duplicated thumb, *Plast Reconstr Surg* **69**:470–5.

Tada K, Yonenobu K, Ysuyuguchi Y et al (1983) Duplication of the thumb. A retrospective review of 237 cases, *J Bone Joint Surg* **65A**:584–98.

Temtamy S, McKusick V (1978) *The genetics of hand malformations*, (Alan R. Liss Inc: New York) 364–82.

Townsend DJ, Lipp EB, Chun K et al (1994) Thumb duplication, 66 years' experience: a review of surgical complications, *J Hand Surg* **19A**:973–6.

Tuch BA, Lipp EB, Larsen IJ, Gordon LH (1977) A review of supernumerary thumb and its surgical management *Clin Orthop* **125**:159–67.

Upton J (2000) In: Gupta A, Kay SPJ, Scheker LR, eds, *The growing hand. Diagnosis and management of the upper extremity in children* (Harcourt Publishers Ltd: London) 255–69.

Wassel HD (1969) The results of surgery for polydactyly of the thumb: a review, *Clin Orthop* **64**:175–93.

Wood VE (1978) Polydactyly and the triphalangeal thumb, *J Hand Surg* **3A**:436–44.

9
Symbrachydactyly

Steven ER Hovius and Teun JM Luijsterburg with Guy Foucher,
Chantal MAM van der Horst and Simon PJ Kay

Symbrachydactyly is an intriguing conglomerate of congenital differences of the upper limb. Literally translated, symbrachydactyly comprises of syndactylous fingers combined with short fingers. Besides clean-cut definitions such as isolated polydactyly, most congenital differences have some form of symbrachydactyly. Therefore, it cannot be considered to be 'a' congenital difference or entity.

Confusion starts with the nomenclature. German, Japanese, and English speaking authors interpret the term symbrachydactyly differently (Buck-Gramcko 1985 and 1999). German and Japanese authors use the term symbrachydactyly for congenital differences ranging from brachydactyly with syndactyly up to absent fingers with only nubbins left (Blauth and Gekeler 1971 and 1973, Buck-Gramcko 1985 and 1999, Miura et al 1994, Ogino 1996, Yamauchi and Tanabu 1999). English speaking authors did not use the term symbrachydactyly before 1993. Cleft hands were classified into typical and atypical cleft hands (Barsky 1964). After the IFSSH meeting in 1992, consensus was established that atypical cleft hand should be called symbrachydactyly (Flatt 1994, Manske 1993). However, the English definition of symbrachydactyly covers only part of the German symbrachydactyly (Buck-Gramcko 1985). As a result of this confusion, literature concerning treatment strategies is not consistent. Similar differences are called symbrachydactyly, ring constriction syndrome, transverse defects, and Poland's syndrome. Clinical studies are difficult to compare. Therefore, it seems more appropriate to discuss a congenital difference by its soft tissue and bony appearance.

Furthermore, pathoembryology is not well understood. Symbrachydactyly is said to stem from the middle phalanges in the mid-hand, and to progress proximally and predominantly to the ulnar side (Buck-Gramcko 1999). However, the cleft hand type of symbrachydactyly cannot easily be explained in this way, as the cartilaginous models of the middle phalanges are the last to be ossified during development (see Chapter 3). Therefore, disturbances of distal or proximal phalanges have already taken place. Keeping this in mind, it is difficult to imagine the pathogenesis in a hand with a thumb syndactylous with a hypoplastic index finger, absent middle and ring fingers, and a relatively normal little finger, all with different disturbances in ossification of the various phalanges (see case 1). Furthermore, the supposed tight link to syndactyly does not seem to be related to disturbances in ossification of the middle phalanges. Moreover, a significant number of the symbrachydactylies do not display syndactyly at all. Finally, to our knowledge no experimental data seem to be available to confirm or refute any assumption, except for one study (Imagawa 1980).

Despite this confusing situation, the term symbrachydactyly will be used following the German interpretation, thereby enabling discussion of clinical manifestations and treatment strategies.

Clinical manifestations

Because of the numerous manifestations any attempt to group patients is somewhat arbitrary. Four distinct morphological types are distinguished that may be useful for decisions in treatment strategies (Blauth and Gekeler 1971 and 1973, Buck-Gramcko 1985 and 1999). Gradually

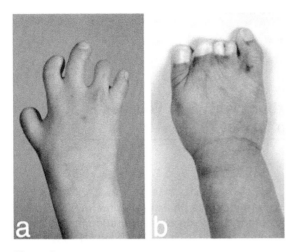

Figure 1

Short finger type.

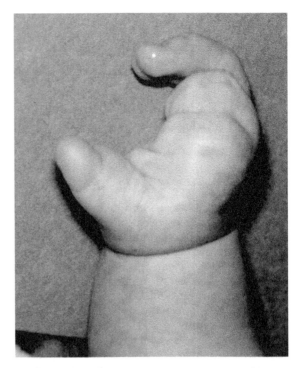

Figure 2

Cleft hand type.

ranging from a relatively mild form to more severe differences, patients may demonstrate short finger type, cleft hand type, monodactylous type, or peromelic type. This teratological sequence of reduction was first recognized by Müller in 1937 (Blauth and Gekeler 1971 and 1973, Buck-Gramcko 1999). A supposedly consistent finding in all types is the presence of distal phalanges with (rudimentary) nails (Blauth and Gekeler 1971 and 1973, Buck-Gramcko 1999).

- Short finger type. Patients exhibit complete or incomplete (soft tissue) syndactyly of the digits. The middle phalanges are hypoplastic, malformed or absent. The long finger is usually most severely affected, followed by the index finger, the ring finger, the little finger, and the thumb. The interphalangeal joints may be dysplastic, and may be (sub)luxated. Often a clinodactyly exists. The thumb is relatively normal, but occasionally with an adduction contracture without opposition. Also, the thumb can be situated more in the plane of the hand (Fig. 1).
- Cleft hand type. One, two or all mid-hand rays are absent. There may be a small or larger gap in the mid-hand. Often the preserved digits have a distinct shape, and syndactyly is

observed between the remaining ulnar digits. Carpals may be hypoplastic, malformed, or synostotic (Fig. 2).
- Monodactylous type. Gradually the fingers are reduced, leaving only bud-like fingers and a marked reduced thumb. The finger buds contain cartilage or bony pieces, and malformed nails. Carpals are malformed or synostotic and a malformed radius or ulna may be present (Fig. 3).
- Peromelic or adactylous type. If the fingers are absent as well as the thumb, the most severe form emerges. An amputation-like appearance of the hand shows finger buds with nail remnants. Carpal synostosis is observed (Fig. 4).

Yamauchi and Tanabu (1999) have provided another classification based on the radiographic pattern of bone reduction leading to seven types:

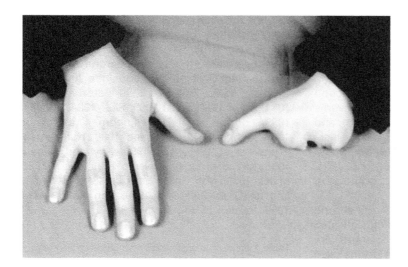

Figure 3

Monodactylous type.

- Triphalangia type. No phalanges are missing, though some may be hypoplastic or malformed (often middle phalanges).
- Diphalangia type. One phalanx is missing in one or more rays (usually the middle).
- Monophalangia type. One or more rays display only one phalanx.
- Aphalangia type. Two phalanges are absent in one or more digits.
- Ametacarpia type. One or more rays are absent.
- Acarpia type. No rays are observed and carpal bones are partially or completely absent.
- Forearm amputation type. Absence of the distal portion of the forearm, often with rudimentary digits on the stump.

According to Buck-Gramcko (1999) this division is not always consistent. Classification is impossible if one digit has two phalanges, another digit has one phalanx, and a third digit is missing.

A few patients display bilateral symbrachydactyly (Blauth and Gekeler 1971 and 1973, Buck-Gramcko 1999). An associated finding may be an absent or malformed ipsilateral pectoralis major and minor muscle (the sternocostal portion), i.e. Poland's syndrome (Castilla et al 1979, Buck-Gramcko 1999, Gausewitz et al 1984, Glicenstein and Haddad 1999). Seldom, the lower limbs are involved or craniofacial aberrations are observed, such as in Hanhart's syndrome (Herrmann et al 1976).

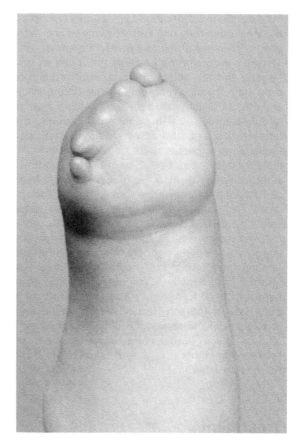

Figure 4

Peromelic type.

Differential diagnosis

Because of the wide spectrum of the four morphological types and their transitional forms, symbrachydactyly may resemble other congenital differences. These include ring constriction syndrome, cleft hand, and 'true' transverse reduction defects (Barsky 1964, Blauth and Gekeler 1971 and 1973, Büchler 2000, Buck-Gramcko 1988 and 1999, Miura 1976, Miura and Suzuki 1984, Miura et al 1986, 1992 and 1994, Ogino 1996, Ogino and Saitou 1987, Ogino et al 1981).

Symbrachydactyly usually involves the second and third rays, and digits are increasingly affected to the ulnar side. The middle phalanges are always affected, and more severe forms also include more proximal structures. Subsequently, the distal phalanges and (rudimentary) nails are mostly present at the distal border. The proximal bones and the border digits are usually hypoplastic. Most often only one limb is involved and there is no occurrence among relatives. In contrast, ring constriction syndrome involves the index to ring fingers, and the defect progresses from distal to proximal. The distal border of this difference is smooth or displays soft tissue swelling due to lymphoedema, and the proximal tissues are normal. One or both limbs may be affected, and there is no inheritance. If ring constrictions or lymphoedema are absent, the diagnosis shifts to symbrachydactyly in our experience. Cleft hand consists of a central wedge shaped defect, and the digits are gradually more affected on the radial side. The distal border is smooth, and the proximal tissues as well as the border digits are not hypoplastic. Moreover, there is a frequent strong familial inheritance and mostly more than one affected limb. Finally, some confusion may exist between 'true' transverse reduction defects and peromelic symbrachydactyly. 'True' transverse reduction defects display no finger buds, have a smooth distal border, and show no aberrant proximal structures. It is mostly unilateral, and there is no inheritance.

Treatment

Variability in clinical manifestations has led to various treatment strategies, which should be tailored for each individual, thereby challenging the capabilities of the reconstructive surgeon. Many reconstructive options and their results have been reported in the literature (Table 1) (Blauth and Gekeler 1973, Büchler 2000, Buck-Gramcko 1985, 1988 and 1999, Eaton and Lister 1991, Entin 1981, Ezaki 1999, Flatt 1994, Foucher 1999, Foucher et al 2001, Friedman and Wood 1997, Gilbert 1982, 1989 and 1998, Hulsbergen-Kruger et al 1998, Kay 1999, Kay and Wiberg 1996, Kay et al 1996, Leclercq 1999, Lister 1988, Malek 1999, Neff 1981, Seitz Jr 1998, Swanson and de Groot-Swanson 1999, Van Holder et al 1999, Yamauchi and Tanabu 1999).

Table 1 Various reconstructive techniques, which may be combined if necessary

Syndactyly release
Widening and deepening of the first web
Rotation osteotomy of phalanges and/or metacarpals
Fusion of unstable joints
Tendon transfers
Local flaps and skin grafts
Removal of non-functional digits
Create an opposing post against which the other ray(s) oppose:
1. Double or asynchronous or synchronous one or two single toe transfers
2. Lengthening and/or stabilization using a proximal toe phalanx transfer and/or distraction lengthening and/or iliac crest bone graft or bone grafts from phalanges/metacarpals to be removed
3. Unfolding a dorsal pedicle
Krukenberg procedure

Deciding which treatment strategy could be proposed is also dependent on cultural and social philosophies of both parents/patient and surgeon. The congenital difference often presents itself in 'aesthetic balance'. One should be careful not to disturb this balance for instance by placing a 'long finger' on top of the hand. However, a clear functional benefit may prevail, which can alter the 'aesthetic balance'. Furthermore, anatomical aberrations may greatly restrict or enhance reconstructive possibilities. For instance, if thenar and hypothenar activity is absent, the value of distraction, toe to finger/thumb transfer, or bone graft may be limited. However, if thenar or hypothenar activity is observed, creating an ulnar or radial post may improve hand function. These posts are usually less mobile, even if a toe to finger/thumb transfer is performed.

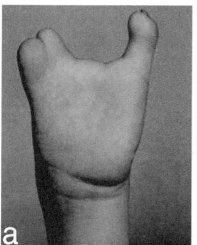
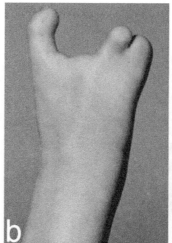
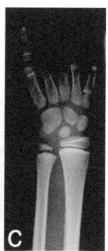

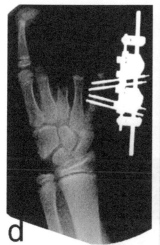
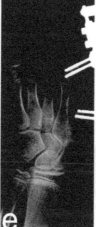
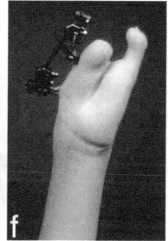

Figure 5

Case 1.
Preoperative dorsal (a) and ventral (b) photographs as well as the x-ray (c) of the left hand. (d) Peroperative x-ray of the distraction of the first metacarpal. (e, f) Satisfactory distraction was obtained after four months. (g–i) After removal of the second ray, and filling the gap of the distracted first metacarpal with the second metacarpal as a bone graft, 'pinch' and 'grip' was enabled.

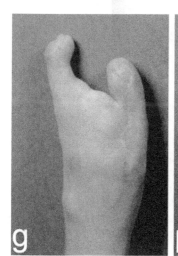
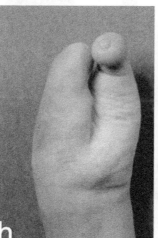
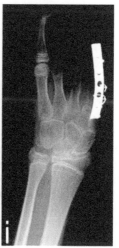

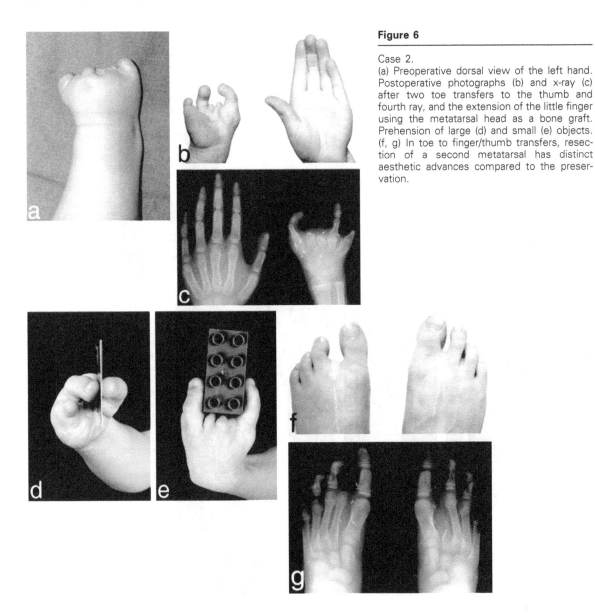

Figure 6

Case 2.
(a) Preoperative dorsal view of the left hand. Postoperative photographs (b) and x-ray (c) after two toe transfers to the thumb and fourth ray, and the extension of the little finger using the metatarsal head as a bone graft. Prehension of large (d) and small (e) objects. (f, g) In toe to finger/thumb transfers, resection of a second metatarsal has distinct aesthetic advances compared to the preservation.

Progression in 'grip' and 'pinch' mostly originate from carpometacarpal joints and less from other joints. The latter remain restricted in their motion, and can be stiff or unstable. Removal of digital stumps without any function may create a web providing space for grip and pinch.

In addition to the surgical reflections, psychosocial factors, such as motivation and compliance of the parents and patient, are of paramount importance for success in any operation. Furthermore, especially when performing more advanced surgery like a vascularized toe transfer, one should bear in mind his/her own surgical capabilities and preferences, including meticulous technique and microreconstructive skills. Moreover, all pre-, per-, and postoperative personnel have to be sufficiently trained to cope with all aspects of pediatric hand surgery. Extensive collaboration with specialists in pediatric rehabilitation medicine and hand therapy pre- and postoperatively will provide optimal conditions to obtain the desired outcome.

To illustrate the aforementioned criteria, four cases will be discussed. Treatment strategy for each case will be outlined, and the decision process discussed.

Case 1

An 11-year-old male patient was referred to our outpatient clinic with congenital differences in both hands, severe cleft feet, and craniofacial aberrations. The same differences of the limbs were present in a fourth degree relative. Both shoulders and elbow regions were symmetrical, as were the pectoralis muscles. The left hand showed symbrachydactyly of the cleft type (Figs 5a–c). Physical examination showed impaired wrist mobility. Thenar activity was not observed, but hypothenar muscles did contract. The little finger had a mobile metacarpophalangeal joint, and showed radial clinodactyly and campto-dactyly of the interphalangeal joint. The motion of other metacarpophalangeal joints was limited. The right hand demonstrated symbrachydactyly of the short finger type (see Fig. 1a).

The function of the left hand could be greatly improved if a radial digit could reach the little finger, thereby creating some 'grip' and 'pinch'. To achieve this, several strategies were considered. First, one or two toe-to-finger/thumb transfers were not possible because of the severe cleft feet. Second, desyndactylization of the thumb and index finger could create a two finger post. However, no thenar activity was observed and joint motion was limited. Therefore, the only option left was the creation of a first web and lengthening of the thumb. The first web was created by the removal of the second ray. At the same time distraction osteotomy of the first metacarpal was performed (Fig. 5d). In addition, the nail of the second digit was transferred to the first. Following satisfactory distraction of 2.5 cm (Figs 5e and f), the thumb was lengthened using the

second metacarpal as bone graft to fill the gap created by distraction. An AO plate was used to fix the bone graft. After the procedure 'pinch' and 'grip' were possible (Figs 5g–i).

Case 2

This case was kindly provided by SPJ Kay from St James's University Hospital, Leeds, UK. The male patient exhibited symbrachydactyly of the peromelic type (Fig. 6a), without any opportunity for prehension. The choice was to perform two asynchronous toe to finger/thumb transfers. In the first stage a second toe was transferred to the thumb, and in the second stage a toe was transferred to the fourth ray. Furthermore, a bone graft from the discarded metatarsal head was used to augment the fifth ray (Figs 6b and c). Postoperatively, the patient could grasp small and large objects (Figs 6d and e) and became bimanual. Clearly the aesthetic benefit is demonstrated by resection of the second metatarsal in the right foot compared to the preserved second metatarsal of the left foot (Figs 6f and g).

Case 3

A one-year-old male patient was referred to our outpatient clinic with a cleft hand type symbrachydactyly of the left hand (Fig. 7a). Thenar activity was observed, but no hypo-thenar contractions. The thumb was very hypoplastic with a carpometacarpal and rudimentary metacarpophalangeal joint. The little finger was severely malformed and very short. To provide hand function for this child 'pinch' and 'grip' should be created. Distraction of one or both rays was not an option due to severe hypoplasia. A non-vascularized phalangeal toe transfer could have been performed but would not have given satisfactory results in terms of adequate movement. Therefore, a second toe transfer to the little finger was chosen (Fig. 7b), and in the second stage the other second toe was transferred to the thumb. Unfortunately, the toe-to-thumb transfer failed, and therefore a groin flap was subsequently used to cover the defect. Finally, an iliac crest bone graft was used to augment the thumb. Evaluation after four

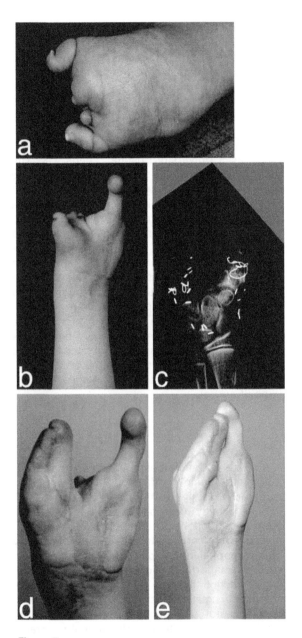

Figure 7

Case 3.
(a) Preoperative dorsal view of the left hand showing symbrachydactyly of the cleft hand type (rudimentary). (b) Postoperative view of the left hand after transfer of the left second toe to the little finger. (c) X-ray of the left hand after the toe transfer and the creation of a radial post (bone graft with groin flap) at a 4-yr follow-up. Palmar view of the left hand in open (d) and closed (e) situation 4 years postoperatively.

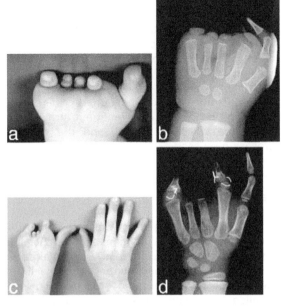

Figure 8

Case 4.
(a, b) Symbrachydactyly of the monodactylous type of the left hand. The thumb was normal as well as the hypothenar. (c, d) Dorsal view of the left hand after two vascularized proximal phalangeal toe transfers to the second and fourth digits at 2 years postoperatively.

years demonstrated a very functional left hand for both small and large objects, with integration of the created 'pinch' and 'grip' (Figs 7c–e). This case shows clearly that even after a failed toe transfer a functional radial post can be created.

Case 4

This patient was kindly provided by CMAM van der Horst, from the University Hospital Amsterdam, the Netherlands. The left hand demonstrated symbrachydactyly of the monodactylous type with a relatively normal thumb and hypothenar (Figs 8a and b). At two years and two and a half years of age respectively a non-vascularized proximal phalangeal toe transfer was performed to nubbins of the second and fourth digits. Evaluation two years postoperatively showed adequate bone growth (Figs 8c and d), and useful outcome.

Finger and thumb instability in symbrachydactyly

Guy Foucher

Symbrachydactyly frequently demonstrates unstable joints. The instabilities are induced by two mechanisms. Firstly, hypoplasia or absence of the middle phalanx (brachymesodactyly) may lead to a flail digit or thumb. Secondly, incompetent ligaments may cause a true joint instability with a moderately hypoplastic metacarpophalangeal joint. These two types of joint instability should be managed differently, and growth potential should be considered in the choice of treatment strategy.

With respect to the first mechanism, we have proposed to divide monodactylous hands into type IIIA with a normal thumb (or a thumb with symphalangism) and type IIIB with brachymesophalangy of the thumb (Foucher et al 2000). In type II with didactylous hands, brachymesophalangy occurs infrequently. In type IIIB, the treatment consists of reconstructing finger(s) and stabilizing the thumb to create a 'pinch'. To balance length and growth potential, the technique for thumb stabilization has to take into account the technique for finger reconstruction.

A non-vascularized phalanx transfer to a finger 'pocket' could be accompanied by the same kind of transfer to stabilize the thumb. If peroperatively the gain in length is adequate, growth rate will be moderate, but both transfers will be in balance, depending on age at operation (Goldberg and Watson 1982). In contrast, a vascularized toe to finger transfer combined with a non-vascularized phalanx transfer to the thumb, will demonstrate imbalance in growth between both transfers (Foucher et al 2001). The initial 'pinch' between the tip of the thumb and the finger may deteriorate progressively due to growth discrepancy. This discrepancy is caused by limited growth potential of a non-vascularized phalanx transfer in comparison with a vascularized toe transfer. Also, peroperatively, the thumb will gain limited length by the non-vascularized phalanx transfer. If the aforementioned strategy

is used, lengthening of the thumb by one or more distractions may often be necessary to maintain pulp-to-pulp contact. Relatives have to be informed in advance that multiple procedures may be necessary. Instead of this strategy, we favour a vascularized epiphysis transfer to the thumb instead of a non-vascularized phalanx transfer (Foucher 1999). This epiphysis is harvested from the second toe and in our experience, symmetrical growth was observed after ten years of follow-up.

In some cases of type II, that have 'floating' fingers without metacarpal bone and advanced hypoplasia, we prefer an alternative procedure. The ulnar rays are stabilized, and the more radial ray is 'sacrificed'. This technique allows the usually insufficient first web to be deepened. Also, at the same time a vascularized skeleton transfer stabilizes the brachymesophalangy of the thumb. While growth is never normal in such hypoplastic fingers, it exceeds growth of non-vascularized phalanges.

The second mechanism, concerning incompetent ligaments, is frequently observed at the metacarpophalangeal joint of either thumb or ulnar digits. We favour stabilizing the thumb by ligament reconstruction or capsulodesis in young patients with unidirectional laxity. However, recurrence of joint instability is not infrequent, primarily due to the use of the hand for body support. A supportive splint has to be applied in order to change the pattern of weight bearing. At the age of seven to ten years, an arthrodesis is the most secure technique, but when using this technique, care should be taken to preserve the growth plate of the proximal phalanx. In our experience, growth is not disturbed, as has been demonstrated previously (Kowalski and Manske 1988).

In patients with closed growth plates, formal arthrodesis is the preferred procedure. The situation is more complex in ulnar fingers as the sacrifice of the metacarpophalangeal joint in a stiff finger (symphalangism) is functionally not advisable. Capsuloplasty has been quite disappointing in our experience except when the unstable finger is supported by stable ulnar finger(s). In isolated and unstable little fingers, we have performed capsuloplasty or ligament reconstruction. The little finger needs protection by a splint, which should be only removed at night.

References

Barsky AJ (1964) Cleft hand: classification, incidence, and treatment, review of the literature and report of nineteen cases, *J Bone Joint Surg* **46A**:1707–20.

Blauth W, Gekeler J (1971) Morphology and classification of symbrachydactylia, *Handchirurgie* **3**:123–28.

Blauth W, Gekeler J (1973) Symbrachydactylias, *Handchirurgie* **5**:121–74.

Büchler U (2000) Symbrachydactyly. In: Gupta A, Kay SPJ, Scheker LR, eds, *The growing hand. Diagnosis and management of the upper extremity in children*, (Harcourt Publishers Ltd: London) 149–58.

Buck-Gramcko D (1985) Cleft hands: classification and treatment, *Hand Clin* **1**:467–73.

Buck-Gramcko D (1988) Syndactyly. In: Nigst H, Buck-Gramcko D, Millesi H, Lister GD, eds, *Hand surgery*, (Thieme Medical Publishers Inc.: New York) 12.22–12.42.

Buck-Gramcko D (1999) Symbrachydactyly. In: Tubiana R, ed, *The hand*, (WB Saunders Company: Philadelphia) 793–806.

Castilla EE, Paz JE, Orioli IM (1979) Pectoralis major muscle defect and Poland complex, *Am J Med Genet* **4**:263–69.

Eaton CJ, Lister GD (1991) Toe transfer for congenital hand defects, *Microsurgery* **12**:186–95.

Entin M (1981) Reconstruction of congenital aplasia of digits, *Surg Clin North Am* **61**:407–24.

Ezaki M (1999) Syndactyly. In: Green DP, Hotchkiss RN, Pederson WC, eds, *Green's operative hand surgery*, 4th edn, (Churchill Livingstone: Philadelphia) 414–29.

Flatt AE (1994) Cleft hand and central defects. In: Flatt AE, ed, *The care of congenital hand anomalies*, 2nd edn, (Quality Medical Publishing Inc: St Louis) 337–65.

Flatt AE, Wood VE (1970) Multiple dorsal rotation flaps from the hand for thumb web contractures, *Plast Reconstr Surg* **45**:258–62.

Foucher G (1999) Vascularized joint transfer. In: Green DP, Hotchkiss RN, Pederson WC, eds, *Green's operative hand surgery*, 4th edn, (Churchill Livingstone: Philadelphia) 1251–70.

Foucher G, Medina J, Pajardi G et al (2000) Classification and treatment of symbrachydactyly. A series of 117 cases, *Chir Main* **19**:161–68.

Foucher G, Medina J, Navarro R et al (2001) Toe transfer in congenital hand malformations, *J Reconstr Microsurg* **17**:1–7.

Friedman R, Wood VE (1997) The dorsal transposition flap for congenital contractures of the first web space: a 20-year experience, *J Hand Surg* **22A**:664–70.

Gausewitz SH, Meals RA, Setoguchi Y (1984) Severe limb deficiency in Poland's syndrome, *Clin Orthop* **185**:9–13.

Gilbert A (1982) Toe transfers for congenital defects, *J Hand Surg* **7B**:118–24.

Gilbert A (1989) Congenital absence of the thumb and digits, *J Hand Surg* **14B**:6–17.

Gilbert A (1998) Microvascular procedures. In: Buck-Gramcko, ed, *Congenital malformations of the hand and forearm*, (Churchill Livingstone: London) 63–71.

Glicenstein J, Haddad R (1999) Poland's sydnrome. In: Tubiana I, ed, *The hand*, (WB Saunders Company: Philaldelphia) 825–30.

Goldberg NH, Watson HK (1982) Composite toe (phalanx and epiphysis) transfers in the reconstruction of the aphalangic hand, *J Hand Surg* **7A**:454–59.

Herrmann J, Pallister PD, Gilbert EF et al (1976) Studies of malformation syndromes of man XXXXI B: nosologic studies in the Hanhart and the Mobius syndrome, *Eur J Pediatr* **122**:19–55.

Hulsbergen-Kruger S, Preisser P, Partecke BD (1998) Ilizarov distraction-lengthening in congenital anomalies of the upper limb, *J Hand Surg* **23B**:192–95.

Imagawa S (1980) Symbrachydactyly: pathogenesis of 5-fluorouracil induced model in mice, *Hiroshima J Med Sci* **29**:169–81.

Kay SP, Wiberg M (1996) Toe-to-hand transfer in children. Part 1: technical aspects, *J Hand Surg* **21B**:723–34.

Kay SP, Wiberg M, Bellew M et al (1996) Toe-to-hand transfer in children. Part 2: Functional and psychological aspects, *J Hand Surg* **21B**:735–45.

Kay SPJ (1999) Hypoplastic and absent digits. In: Green DP, Hotchkiss RN, Pederson WC, ed, *Green's operative hand surgery*, 4th edn, (Churchill Livingstone: Philadelphia) 368–89.

Kowalski MF, Manske PR (1988) Arthrodesis of digital joints in children, *J Hand Surg* **13A**:874–79.

Leclercq C (1999) Other techniques for congenital syndactyly. In: Tubiana I, ed, *The hand*, (WB Saunders Company: Philaldelphia) 818–24.

Lister G (1988) Microsurgical transfer of the second toe for congenital deficiency of the thumb, *Plast Reconstr Surg* **82**:658–65.

Malek R (1999) Congenital syndactylies. In: Tubiana I, ed, *The hand*, (WB Saunders Company: Philaldelphia) 807–17.

Manske PR (1993) Symbrachydactyly instead of atypical cleft hand [letter], *Plast Reconstr Surg* **91**:196.

Miura T (1976) Syndactyly and split hand, *Hand* **8**:125–30.

Miura T, Suzuki M (1984) Clinical differences between typical and atypical cleft hand, *J Hand Surg* **9B**:311–15.

Miura T, Torii S, Nakamura R (1986) Brachymetacarpia and brachyphalangia, *J Hand Surg* **11A**:829–36.

Miura T, Nakamura R, Suzuki M et al. (1992) Cleft hand, syndactyly and hypoplastic thumb, *J Hand Surg* **17B**:365–70.

Miura T, Nakamura R, Horii E (1994) The position of symbrachydactyly in the classification of congenital hand anomalies, *J Hand Surg* **19B**:350–54.

Neff G (1981) Extension according to Matev in malformations of the hands, *Z Orthop Ihre Grenzgeb* **119**:14–20.

Ogino T (1996) Congenital anomalies of the hand. The Asian perspective, *Clin Orthop* **323**:12–21.

Ogino T, Saitou Y (1987) Congenital constriction band syndrome and transverse deficiency, *J Hand Surg* **12B**:343–48.

Ogino T, Ishii S, Shiono H (1981) Transverse deficiency of the hand in one of monozygotic twins, *Hand* **13**:77–80.

Seitz WH Jr (1998) Distraction treatment of the hand. In: Buck-Gramcko, ed, *Congenital malformations of the hand and forearm*, (Churchill Livingstone: London) 119–28.

Swanson AB, de Groot-Swanson G (1999) The Krukenberg procedure in the juvenile amputee. In: Tubiana R, ed, *The hand*, (WB Saunders Company: Philadelphia) 971–81.

Van Holder C, Giele H, Gilbert A (1999) Double second toe transfer in congenital hand anomalies, *J Hand Surg* **24B**:471–75.

Yamauchi Y, Tanabu S (1999) Symbrachydactyly. In: Buck-Gramcko D, ed, *Congenital malformations of the hand and forearm*, (Churchill Livingstone: New York) 149–58.

10
Camptodactyly

Ulrich Lanz with Guy Foucher, Rolf Habenicht, Susanne Kall and Hans-Martin Schmidt,

Camptodactyly is a congenital condition character-ized by a flexion deformity of the proximal inter-phalangeal (PIP) joint of one or more fingers. The term derives from the Greek words 'καμπτειν' (*kamptein*) meaning bent, and 'δακτυλος' (*daktylos*) for finger. Basically it means bent finger without saying anything about its cause or the clinical appearance. Landouzy introduced the term in 1906.

Clinical appearance

The deformity is usually found in the little finger, but can involve the other fingers, with a decreas-ing frequency towards the index finger. The extension of the PIP joint is restricted, often combined with a hyperextension of the metacar-pophalangeal (MP) joint and/or the distal inter-phalangeal (DIP) joint. Passive extension may be fully possible with an extension lag or may consist of a fixed flexion deformity. A short winging skin between the proximal and the

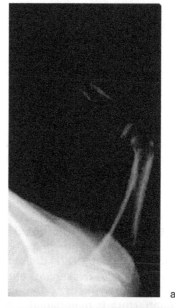

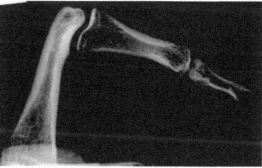

a

b

Figure 2

(a) Roentgenogram of the little finger in a 10-year-old girl. The base of the middle phalanx is widened. (b) Flattening of the head and indentation of the neck of the proximal phalanx, and wide base of the middle phalanx as seen in an adult.

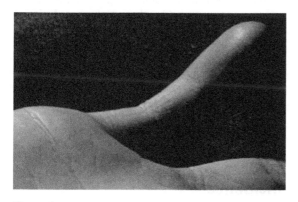

Figure 1

Typical appearance of camptodactyly in a little finger.

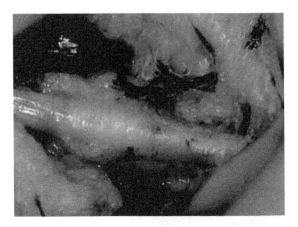

Figure 3

Tight bands (marked with ink) being part of the retinacular ligament system sustaining the flexion contracture of the PIP joint.

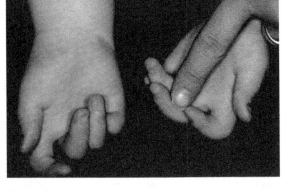

Figure 4

Camptodactyly of multiple fingers on both hands exhibited in Freeman–Sheldon Syndrome.

middle flexion crease of the finger (Fig. 1) is typical, standing in distinct contrast to an acquired flexion contracture of the PIP joint.

Typical x-rays of this condition show the condyle of the proximal phalanx as being dorsally flattened, the neck of the phalanx having an indentation and the base of the middle phalanx being widened (Fig. 2a and b) (Buck-Gramcko 1987, Engber and Flatt 1977). Characteristic changes such as the thickening and shortening of the retinacular ligament system by which the flexion contracture is maintained can be seen intra-operatively (Fig. 3).

Syndromes with camptodactyly

Susanne Kall

Usually camptodactyly occurs as sporadic or as a single autosomal dominant condition in early childhood (type I) or adolescence (type II), but it can also be part of a distinct syndrome (type III) (Temtamy and McKusick 1978). In 1984, Rozin and colleagues reviewed all known camptodactyly syndromes and distinguished three categories: (1) syndromes due to chromosomal anomalies, (2) syndromes with major CNS involvement, and (3) multisystemic disorders. Since 1984 more than 50 additional syndromes associated with camptodactyly have been

reported and are summarized in the Appendix. Camptodactyly is not specific for most of these disorders but accompanies them with varying frequency (Bamshad et al 1996).

The hand surgeon is usually consulted when camptodactyly is presented in the more common, less complex syndromes like distal arthrogryposis type 1 (DA1), Freeman–Sheldon syndrome or in congenital contractural arachnodactyly (Beals and Hecht 1971, Daentl et al 1974, Freeman and Sheldon 1938). Distal arthrogryposis type 1 and Freeman–Sheldon syndrome are frequent causes of inherited multiple congenital contractures including camptodactyly and clubfoot (McKusick 2000) (Fig. 4). Other wider spread syndromes like the cerebro-oculo-facial-skeletal syndrome (COFS syndrome), Pena–Shokeir syndrome II, or the camptodactyly-arthropathy-coxa vara-pericarditis syndrome are usually not seen in the hand surgeon's practice (Jacobs and Downey 1974, Pena and Shokeir 1976). These syndromes often exhibit more serious conditions other than joint contractures—some leading to death in early infancy.

Incidence

The incidence of camptodactyly is thought to be around one per cent of the population (Jones et al 1974, Smith and Kaplan 1968). Most cases are sporadic; a familial occurrence is rare and follows an autosomal dominant pattern of varying penetrance, with a male to female ratio of about 1:3 (Miura et al 1992). Approximately two-thirds of cases are bilateral, however in unilateral cases the right hand appears to be involved slightly more often (Smith and Kaplan 1968).

Pathogenesis

It is commonly accepted that camptodactyly is caused by an imbalance of the flexing and extending forces to the proximal interphalangeal joint of the finger (Engber and Flatt 1977, Hori et al 1987, McCash 1966, Millesi 1974, Miura 1983)—but this seems to be the only point of agreement. Millesi (1968) and Berger and Millesi (1975) believe that a defect in the extensor mechanism is responsible, whereas Koman et al (1990), in their study of 12 children with flexion contractures in one or more fingers (which were already present at birth), found that the central slip was attenuated and the lateral bands subluxed palmarly, concluding that these patients must belong to a distinct subgroup.

Other studies (Frank et al 1997, Jones et al 1974, McFarlane et al 1983, 1992, Wilhelm and Kleinschmidt 1968) have found that abnormal lumbrical muscles are responsible for the imbalance (Figs 5a–f). McFarlane and colleagues (1983, 1992) believe that camptodactyly resembles an intrinsic minus deformity, in addition, they found that the fourth palmar interosseous muscle was abnormal in five of their ten cases (it was missing in two cases, was small in one case, and inserted into the extensor expansion of

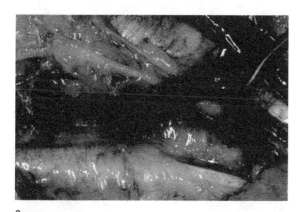

a

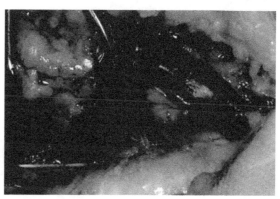

b

Figure 5

Anatomical anomalies found in camptodactyly: (a–c) Complete or partial insertion of the lumbrical muscle into the periosteum of the proximal phalanx.

continued

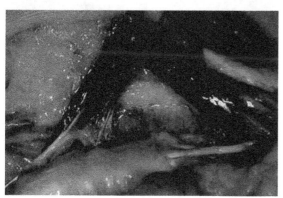

c

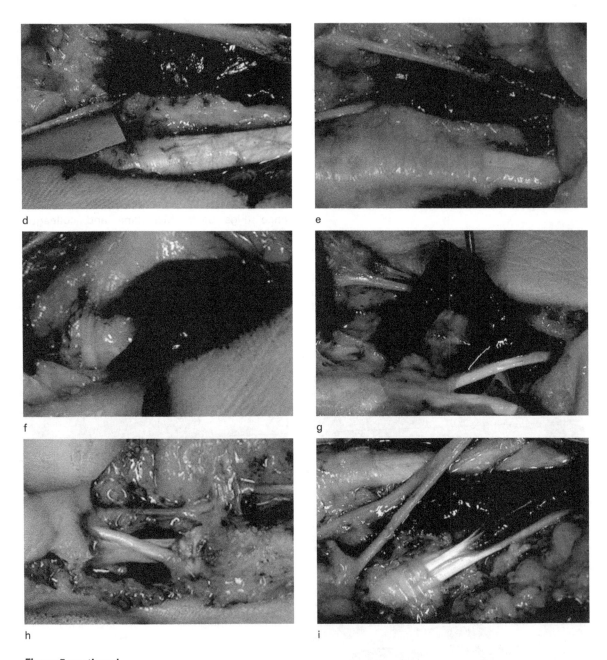

Figure 5 continued

(d and e) Insertion of the lumbrical muscle into the neighbouring finger. (f) Bigastric lumbrical muscle. (g) Bigastric lumbrical, one head inserting into the periosteum of the proximal phalanx, the other joining the FDS tendon. (h) Fibrous band replacing a regular FDS tendon. (i) Lumbrical muscle intercalated into the FDS tendon. (Figures 5a and 5g reproduced from Frank et al (1997) *Handchir Mikrochir Plast Chir* **29**: 284–90 with permission of G. Thieme-Verlag.)

the neighbouring ring finger in two other cases). Wilhelm (2000) saw anomalous insertions of the abductor digiti quinti muscle in 22 of 36 fingers, leading to a tenodesis effect.

The importance of an erroneous insertion of the lumbrical muscles was explained by Rabischong (1962)—these small muscles contain a high number of neuroceptors by which they could act as sensors to coordinate the flexor and extensor muscle system. In contrast Buck-Gramcko (1997) stated that these anatomical variations and abnormalities are a rare occurrence. He considers the rare insertion of the lumbrical muscles into the flexor digitorum superficialis (FDS) tendon as the only anomaly causing the deformity. This variation concerning the lumbrical muscles have also been described elsewhere (Maeda and Matsui 1985, Ogino and Kato 1992, Stedtfeld and Brug 1979) (Figs 5g and i). Maeda and Matsui (1985) observed an abnormal origin in five of six inspected FDS tendons of the small finger—the tendons were hypoplastic, lacked the connection to their muscle belly and originated either from the palmar aponeurosis, the deep surface of the flexor retinaculum or the tendon sheath of the ring finger causing a tenodesis effect (Fig. 5h). McFarlane et al (1992) reported a significant correlation between the independence of the FDS and the severity of flexion contracture of the PIP joint.

Anatomical variability of the structures believed to cause camptodactyly

Hans-Martin Schmidt

This section outlines the anatomy and variations of the third and fourth lumbrical muscles, third palmar interosseus, abductor digiti minimi, and flexor digitorum superficialis muscle.

The third and fourth lumbrical muscles

The human lumbrical muscles originate from the embryonal muscular blastema on the flexor side of the extremities (Čihak 1972, Christ 1990). They are embedded within the loose connective tissue between the palmar aponeurosis, flexor tendons, and deep muscles of the palma manus. The slender muscles arise from the tendons of the flexor digitorum profundus muscle. On the palmar side of the deep transverse metacarpal ligament, within fibrous channels ('lumbrical channels'), they pass distally to the insertions at the fingers. The muscles link up the deep finger flexors and the complex extensor apparatus. As a result the flexor forces are reduced in favour of the increase of the extensor effect.

It has been known for years that the lumbrical muscles belong to the most variable human muscles (Schmidt and Lanz 1992). The variation frequency remarkably increases from the first to the fourth lumbrical muscle, both at the origin and the insertion, with variations normally being found at the third and fourth lumbrical muscle (Mehta and Gardner 1961, Schmidt et al 1963, 1965). In 81% of cases the third lumbrical muscle is bipennate and only 9% unipennate. In the majority of cases the bipennate muscles arise from the ulnar side of the deep flexor tendon of the ring finger and from the radial side of the profundus tendon of the little finger. Unipennate muscles arise from the radial side of the deep flexor tendon and on rare occasions from isolated tendons of the flexor digitorum profundus muscle in the forearm region.

There are a variety of insertion points for the third lumbrical muscle. With a mean length of 59.2 mm (41–77 mm, muscle and tendon) 50% of cases have an insertion point on the radial side of the dorsal aponeurosis of the ring finger (Mehta and Gardner, 1961). In 10% of cases, the insertion point passes to the ulnar side of the middle finger and in 40% of 'double headed' cases the muscle inserts both at the radial and the ulnar side of the middle and the ring finger (Basu and Hasary 1960, Schmidt et al 1963, 1965). Our own investigations revealed additional insertions (with a mean width of 3 mm) at the A1 pulley of the ring finger in 81% of cases as well as insertions at the deep transverse metacarpal ligament (with a mean width of 2.7 mm) in 64% of cases (Ullrich and Schmidt 2001 personal communication). Insertions at the base of the proximal phalanx of the ring finger were observed in 3% of cases and others (Ikebuchi et al 1988, Mehta and Gardner 1961) have described joint insertions both at the dorsal aponeurosis and the proximal phalanx of the ring finger in 17% of cases.

The fourth lumbrical muscle has a mean length of 49.5 mm (36–63 mm) and in 63% of cases is bipennate. The muscle originates from the ulnar side of the deep flexor tendon of the ring finger and the radial side of the tendon of the flexor digitorum profundus muscle of the little finger. In 11% of cases the fourth lumbrical muscle arises solely from the ulnar side of the deep flexor tendon of the ring finger and in 17% of cases from the same tendon in the little finger. Proximal attachments have also been found with the third lumbrical muscle and in 8% of cases, the muscle leaves the carpal tunnel with a small tendon. The fourth lumbrical muscle is rarely absent.

In 85% of cases reviewed in the literature, the insertion of the fourth lumbrical muscle was at the dorsal aponeurosis on the radial side of the fifth finger, with only 3% at the ulnar side of the fourth finger. Eleven per cent exhibited a double-headed insertion at both the ring and the little finger. Additional attachments at the A1 pulley of the little finger (with a mean insertion width of 4 mm) were observed in 86% of cases and at the deep transverse metacarpal ligament (with a mean width of 1.6 mm) in 36% of cases (Ullrich and Schmidt 2001 personal communication). McFarlane and colleagues (1983) reported a common insertion point at both the flexor tendon sheath and the capsule of the metacarpophalangeal joint of the fifth finger and additional insertion points at the dorsal aponeurosis and at the proximal phalanx were described by Mehta and Gardner (1961) in 61% of their cases (although it should be noted that 11% displayed an isolated insertion at the proximal phalanx). On rare occasions, the fourth lumbrical muscle has been reported to insert at the tendon of the superficial flexor muscle of the ring finger (Frank et al 1997, Maeda and Matsui 1985, McFarlane et al 1983, Stedtfeld and Brug 1979).

The third palmar interosseus muscle

As with the other palmar and dorsal interosseus muscles, the third palmar interosseus muscle developed from the short deep flexor (musculus flexores breves profundi) and contrahentes muscles of the hand (Lewis 1965). As a rule, the third palmar interosseus muscle originates from the radial side of the shaft of the fifth metacarpal bone. With a mean length of 23 mm, it passes in a distal direction, dorsal to the deep transverse metacarpal ligament and palmar to the flexion–extension axis of the metacarpophalangeal joint. The muscle inserts with a short but strong tendon into the dorsal aponeurosis. In 6% of the cases reviewed, an additional insertion at the base of the proximal phalanx has been described (Eyler and Markee 1954, Salsbury 1936/37). Accessory tendon separations run to the capsule of the metacarpophalangeal joint of the fifth finger. McFarlane and colleagues (1983) described the complete absence of the third palmar interosseus in two out of ten cases reported and in two cases they found an insertion of the interosseus tendon into the dorsal aponeurosis of the ring finger.

The abductor digiti minimi muscle

This muscle is known to originate from the pisiform bone, the pisohamate ligament and sometimes from the flexor retinaculum. In some cases the muscle arises proximally from the flexor carpi ulnaris muscle or the palmar carpal ligament. The muscle is fusiform shaped and has a mean length of 40 mm. The insertion tendon is divided into three fibre strands, which pass to the ulno–palmar side at the base of the proximal phalanx, to the sesamoid bone (if it exists) and inserts into the dorsal aponeurosis of the little finger. The more ulnar-oriented fibres merge with the digital cord (abductor cord) as described by Littler (1967), Millesi (1959, 1965), Missfelder et al (1990) and Tubiana and Thomine (1967). Any variations in the abductor digiti minimi muscle are normally found in the area of origin (Schmidt and Lanz 1992), and have a strong correlation with Guyon tunnel syndrome.

The flexor digitorum superficialis muscle

As with the lumbrical and palmaris longus muscles, the flexor digitorum superficialis muscle has a variety of origins. The fleshy muscle belly for the little finger is rudimentary. In 20% of cases reviewed it is totally absent (Baker et al 1981, Shrewsbury and Kuczinsky 1974) or has been replaced by tendon fibres from the fourth lumbrical muscle, the flexor retinaculum or from the palmar aponeurosis (Ogino and Kato 1992). Even Curnow (1873) and later Kaplan (1969) and Schmidt (1990) described the crossing of a thin tendon fibre bundle from the flexor digitorum superficialis of the ring finger to the tendon sheath of the little finger as a rare anomaly. Separations out of the fourth lumbrical muscle have been observed by Humphry (1873), Frohse and Fränkel (1908), and Chowdary (1951); from the flexor digitorum profundus muscle by Macalister (1872) and Testut (1884), and from the tendon of the flexor digitorum superficialis muscle of the index finger by Kaplan (1969). Some cases have even reported origins from the tendon sheath of the flexor muscles of the ring finger (Ogino and Kato 1992).

Natural history

There are two separate types of so-called simple camptodactyly: the congenital type which is already present at birth and the juvenile type which appears later in development. According to Engber and Flatt (1977), 84% of their patients developed the deformity within the first year of life, and only 13% after the age of ten. Both types show progression during skeletal growth that appeared to halt after the twentieth year of life (Senrui 1998).

Assuming that the imbalance of forces upon the PIP joint is the central pathogenetic factor involved, the sequence of events outlined here explains the clinical features of camptodactyly although long-time observations are still missing, and one must always keep in mind the fact that any disturbance in mobility of the joints will affect a growing organism. Skin and retinacular ligaments, including the natatory ligaments, Grayson's and Cleland's ligaments, will only grow according to the range of mobility of the adjacent joint and thus produce a fixed flexion deformity. Of special importance is the abductor band of the little finger, which is also involved in the flexion contracture of the PIP joint in Dupuytren's contracture.

A lack of active extension will eventually lead to a fixed flexion contracture. Scharizer (1979) believed that the skeletal changes in the PIP joint were a secondary phenomenon. Hori et al (1987) showed that the bony changes seen on x-rays could remodel after correction of the flexion contracture. This observation seems to prove the secondary nature of the bony changes. Lack of full extension explains the flattening of the head of the proximal phalanx whereas the widening of the base of the middle phalanx may be due to the pull of the palmar plate and the superficialis tendon. A PIP joint held permanently in flexion will exert continuous pressure on the central slip of the extensor mechanism, leading to an attenuation of this structure.

Stages

Back in 1891, Adams produced a camptodactyly staging system: stage I consisted of an extension lag only; stage II had a flexion contracture with shortening of the palmar soft tissue structures; stage III consisted of a fixed flexion contracture (a) without and (b) with visible x-ray changes and stage IV comprised flexion contractures in two or more fingers. We prefer a staging system that includes more therapeutic aspects (Frank et al 1997). In stage I, Frank's system differentiates those cases without (a) and those with (b) moderate skin shortening. Stage II always includes skin webbing with a fixed flexion contracture of less than 50° and stage III is characterized by a flexion contracture of more than 50° with a moderate (a) or severe skin shortening (b).

Therapy

Non-operative treatment should precede any surgical procedure in all but the very advanced cases (McCash 1966). Dynamic and static splints must be adjusted often and be worn for long periods of time (Hori et al 1987, Miura et al 1992). The authors recommend that splints be worn until the growth plates are closed. Flatt (1994) doubts that his patients would tolerate so many years of treatment—the contractures would recur, however, if the splints were discontinued before the twentieth year of life (Hori et al 1987). Nevertheless continuous splinting (24 hours a day) can correct or at least improve a fixed flexion deformity and thus facilitate subsequent operative measures.

Operative treatment deserves careful consideration and caution (Buck-Gramcko 1997) and should only be considered after treatment with splints (where patient compliance can also be assessed). The flexion contracture of the PIP joint should amount to at least 30° (McFarlane et al 1992) or even exceed 60° (Siegert et al 1990) to justify an operation. If a decision to operate is made however, it should be done at an early an age as possible in order to correct the underlying imbalance of forces.

Surgery can be directed towards the different tissues involved. The skin can usually be addressed with a longitudinal incision that can be elongated by a Z-plasty or free skin grafts (Wood 1993). In severe cases of skin shortage a transpositional flap from the dorso–ulnar side of the proximal phalanx, as described by Glicenstein and colleagues (1995), is recommended. Joint contractures can be corrected by arthrolysis, either in its traditional way by sequentially releasing all the contracting structures starting with the retinacular ligaments, the flexor tendon sheath, the check rein ligaments, and if necessary, excising the accessory collateral ligaments or even the palmar plate; or with a total anterior tenoarthrolysis as described by Saffar (1983) in combination with a transpositional flap (Frank et al 1997, Glicenstein et al 1995). Muscular imbalance can be addressed either by repair of the extensor hood with or without resection and/or transposition of the flexor digitorum superficialis (Berger and Millesi 1975, Millesi 1968, Koman et al 1990)—a procedure recommended by Buck-Gramcko (1987) if the lumbrical muscles are incorrectly inserting into this tendon. Wilhelm and Kleinschmidt (1968) and McFarlane and colleagues (1992) pointed out the importance of this malformation of the lumbrical muscles at insertion, which should be corrected eventually in combination with flexor digitorum superficialis (FDS) tendon transposition (Frank et al 1997). McFarlane et al (1992) preferred the use of the FDS IV for transposition due to its more independent function. The FDS IV tendon should be transposed to the

radial lateral band of the fifth finger. Salvage procedures consist of wedged osteotomies of the proximal phalanx aiming at a functionally improved range of PIP joint motion (Engber and Flatt 1977)—the last line of defence being a joint fusion in a good functional position. Wood (1993) mentions the possibility of a soft tissue distraction treatment, which may eventually turn out to be beneficial in severely contracted fingers.

In considering any operative or non-operative treatment one should bear in mind that even severely contracted little fingers impose little or no functional impairment. In treatment any contracture of the PIP joint is critical for the prognosis. All efforts must therefore be directed in maintaining the full passive extension achieved at surgery. It also is of utmost importance that long term splinting follows any surgical treatment.

Results

Results from the treatment of camptodactyly have been reported elsewhere by Berger and Millesi (1975), Frank et al (1997), Hori et al (1987), and Wilhelm (1998). McFarlane et al (1992) believe that an extension deficit of the PIP joint of less than 50° and a full passive extension are prerequisites for a good result. At surgery the FDS tendon should be transected, however the palmar plate should be left untouched, even if a contracture of the joint of 20° or so persists. Engber and Flatt (1977) saw improvements in 20% of their cases after non-operative treatment, and in 35% after operative therapy.

A restricted flexion would not be rare. Siegert et al (1990) reported an 18% success rate after surgical treatment and 66% success rate after non-operative therapy, whereas McFarlane et al (1992) saw full flexion in only 33% of cases treated operatively, with a flexion contracture of 15° in the PIP joint persisting in about 50% of their patients. Our own findings show that flexion contractures of the PIP joint often persist as well as restriction of full flexion, however even in severe cases, it was possible to transfer the arc of motion towards a functionally better extended range.

The general consensus is that the earlier the treatment is initiated, the better the results

(Berger and Millesi 1975), although McFarlane and co-workers (1992) point out that results in very young children can be compromised by lack of compliance.

Treatment strategies

In this section, individual treatment strategies for mild, moderate and severe cases of camptodactyly are described.

Case studies 1 and 2
Guy Foucher

Camptodactyly always remains a challenge for the hand surgeon but for teaching purposes it is possible to separate a simple and a complex case. A simple situation is that of a passively supple joint. This condition can be found in two circumstances: one is a 'late' imbalance that usually occurs in teenage girls; the other involves cases exhibiting an initial stiff camptodactyly, which after a few months of night splinting results in a passive range of mobility, but a lack of active extension persists. Many of these imbalance cases exhibit abnormal flexor superficialis muscles and tendons as well as abnormal lumbrical muscles—a common finding in camptodactyly, and not a rare occurrence in anatomical dissections. However, not all hand surgeons agree to classify these cases as camptodactyly as proposed by Goffin et al (1994).

Case 1: mild case

Our first case exhibited initial stiffness of the PIP joint that was improved passively by a period of splinting. A clinical examination was undertaken and any residual stiffness in flexion demonstrated by the patient was carefully noted—if moderate (less than 30°) surgery would not necessarily offer any improvement. Since wrist extension increases the flexion of the PIP joint a flexor superficialis tenodesis test was then performed, as was a flexor superficialis flexion test (first immobilizing the profundus of all remaining fingers and then fixing the index and

middle fingers only). Between 34–42% of a normal population have no PIP active flexion in the first phase and between 79–96% recover flexion when the fourth finger is liberated—demonstrating not only a connection to the FDS IV but also the presence of an active muscle which could be used surgically (Austin et al 1989, Baker et al 1981). When negative, the test indicates that the FDS V is either absent (i.e. 6% in Furnas 1985) or reduced to a simple fibrous chord as we found in six cases where camptodactyly was operated on. Then a Bouvier (or Beever) test is performed, which involved manually blocking MP joint hyperextension. If full PIP extension was obtained some sort of 'lasso' operation should be considered (as it has been shown to be effective in a reviewed series of 16 cases). If the Bouvier test proves negative, an extensor tenodesis test as proposed by Smith and Breed (1994) for the diagnosis of a boutonnière deformity should be performed; if there is a functioning extensor apparatus at the PIP joint level, extension would be obtained when the wrist and MP joint are flexed. Some resistance could be felt, when opposed. If the manoeuvre is negative some agenesis of the medial band would need to be controlled intra-operatively and more extensive reconstruction performed at this level, however, this would be quite exceptional since the authors have only ever encountered two cases in a series of 89 patients who have undergone surgery.

More often than not, the Bouvier test proves positive with an effective FDS V. Surgery is performed through a Bruner approach at the proximal phalanx level with prolongation into the palm to allow exploration of the flexor tendon and lumbrical muscles, as well as the approach of the extensor hood on the radial side of the metacarpophalangeal joint (MPJ). The flexor superficialis is cut at the proximal phalanx level (combined in case of some persisting lack of passive extension with a Watson check rein operation: extra-articular arthrolysis). The abnormal lumbrical is more frequently found to insert on the lateral aspect of the MP joint or on the flexor superficialis tendon at the entrance of A1 pulley. Careful dissection allows a distal tendon to be prepared using a band from the superficialis. The superficialis tendon is also freed from the profundus since adhesion with the 'tubular' aspect of the superficialis, surrounding the profundus, has been frequently noted and the course of the muscle is checked by traction on the tendon (to confirm preoperative testing). Then both the flexor superficialis and the lumbrical muscles are transferred onto the most palmar fibres on the radial side of the extensor hood (under tension for the superficialis but without tension for the lumbricals to avoid ischaemia). After careful haemostasis and closure of the skin, a dorsal plaster shell is used to maintain the wrist in a neutral position, the MP joint in full flexion, and the IP joints in complete freedom. Active flexion at the IP joint is controlled by day five. The plaster is removed after three weeks and full use of the hand is allowed. If some persistent stiffness of the PIP joint is noticed, night extension splints are recommended for a few more weeks. Following a complete clinical assessment as described above, 14 out of 16 patients that underwent operations have achieved active extension to the same extent (or better in five cases) than preoperative passive extension levels. All these cases have maintained full active flexion. One patient has a recurrence of some claw deformity (30°) and one has lost a few degrees of flexion, touching the palm at 1.5 cm of the distal palmar crease.

Case 2: severe case

This next case is a good example of a complex case; it involved a 6-year-old patient who had undergone two previous operations for trigger finger of the fifth ray. Each operation was said to have aggravated the lack of passive and active extension, which reached 70° at the PIP joint level and flexion was incomplete due to evident flexor tendon bow stringing. Lateral x-rays of the PIP joint of the fifth finger revealed a classic, although mild deformity of the base of the middle phalanx and the head of the proximal one. The camptodactyly was unilateral; there was no familial history and no associated conditions. Since no improvements were obtained following two months of night splinting, surgery was contemplated.

A combined operation as described by Malek (1998) with pulley reconstruction was performed. Malek's approach consisting in cutting a palmar, proximally based rectangular flap, with a distal cut situated at the DIP flexion crease. This flap was then elevated palmar to the neurovascular digital bundles. Fat was preserved on the palmar aspect of the middle phalanx and the dissection only deepened to the flexor sheath level at the PIP joint. The sheath, usually entered transversally to cut the flexor superficialis proximal to the chiasma, was easily opened (the flexors being subcutaneous). Both the A1 and A2 pulleys were entirely absent, having been excised. The chiasma of Camper was elevated from the periosteum and the palmar plate was cut transversally, distal to the retro-tendinous artery. In previous cases, a transection of the check rein ligaments had failed to provided any significant improvements in extension—so a section of the accessory ligament was also necessary, freeing the palmar plate. Full extension was then obtained but bow stringing of the profundus tendon was evident.

A Kirschner wire was used to maintain the extension of the PIP joint for a further two weeks. However in this case adhesion to the pulley reconstruction would be a major complication, so an A2 pulley was reconstructed according to the technique proposed for tenolysis by Foucher et al (1993). An 8 cm long segment of the flexor superficialis tendon was excised and twice passed around the proximal phalanx (and the extensor mechanism) according to Bunnell's technique and then both ends were exteriorized medially through the skin and fixed on a button. The skin flap was put back in its place denuding the entire palmar middle phalanx, which was covered by a full thickness skin graft taken from the groin. The wrist was immobilized in a neutral position and the MP joint in extension. A dynamic extensor spring maintained the IP joints in extension and flexion was not allowed prior to the fifth day to facilitate healing of the graft. Active flexion against the spring was then allowed and passively assisted. The long splint was removed after two weeks and for the next six weeks was replaced by an identical, but shorter, splint that gave the MP joint freedom. After two months a more dynamic splint that improved flexion was used. Two years after the operation the lack of active extension was measured at 10° and flexion was full with no palpable flexor bow stringing. In another case (diagnosed as trigger finger) similar results were obtained and in this instance an extension lack of 20° and a full flexion resulted.

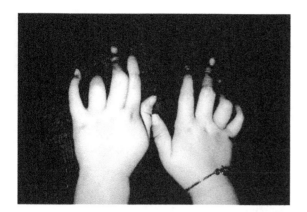

Figure 6

Case 3. Dorsal view of both hands.

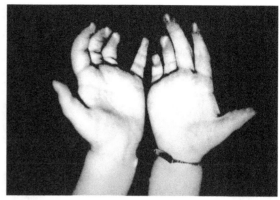

Figure 7

Case 3. Palmar view of both hands.

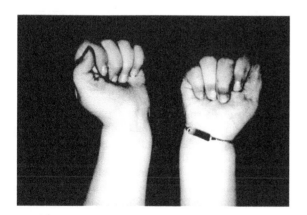

Figure 8

Case 3. Both hands in fist.

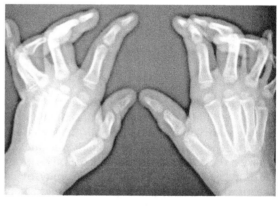

Figure 9

Case 3. X-rays of both hands.

Case studies 3, 4, and 5
Rolf Habenicht

Case 3: presentation of a 3½-year-old girl

A review of the family's medical history revealed that a cousin of the father exhibited a campto-dactyly of the little finger. The girl was the first child of healthy parents. Pregnancy, birth, and development of the child were normal and beside the flexion contracture of the fingers no other malformations were known. Soon after birth, physiotherapy was started to increase finger extension.

During our examination the MP and DIP joint mobility was normal, combined with a hyperextension in the MP joints of the third, fourth, and fifth finger. The PIP mobility of the index finger on both sides was normal. In active motion of the PIP joints of the right hand we found an extension deficit of 25° at the middle finger, 70° at the ring finger and of 45° at the little finger. Passive extension was possible up to 0° in the middle finger but restricted to about 40° in the ring and 15° in the little finger. The left hand presented an active extension deficit of the middle finger of about 30°, of the ring finger of 65° and of the little finger of about 20°. Passive

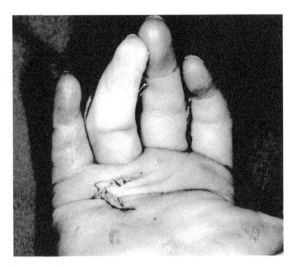

Figure 10

Case 3. Restricted circulation of the ring finger after removal of tourniquet.

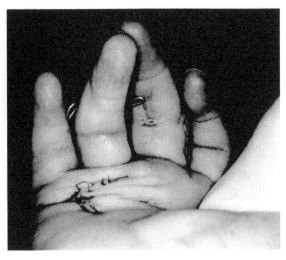

Figure 11

Case 3. Circulation improved after bringing the PIP joint of the finger into a more flexed position.

extension was possible up to 0° in the middle finger and little finger but restricted to about 25° in the ring finger. Flexion of all PIP joints was completely normal and the child was able to make a fist with both hands (Figs 6–8). The x-rays of both hands showed a mild deformity of the heads of the ground phalanges of the middle and ring finger and a slightly broader base of their middle phalanx (Fig. 9).

Due to the almost severe flexion contractures, especially of the ring fingers, an operative treatment was performed when the child was four years old. The operation consisted of an open arthrolysis of the PIP joints of the third to fifth fingers of both hands combined with a flexor digitorium superficialis III/IV transposition to the third to fifth fingers on the right side and an FDS IV transposition to the ring finger of the left hand. Intra-operatively no anomalies of the lumbrical muscles were found. The PIP joints of both ring fingers and of the right middle finger were fixed in extension by percutaneous Kirschner wires. After releasing the tourniquet, the right ring finger showed a circulatory disturbance. The revision did not show any irregularity of the palmar vessels and a duplex-sonograph showed undisturbed blood flow in the palmar

arteries up to the end of the phalanx (Fig. 10). Circulation improved after bringing the PIP joint of the finger into a more flexed position (Fig. 11).

Circulation of the right ring finger remained stable during the first three postoperative days. On the fourth day a necrosis of the distal phalanx developed (Fig.12) and four weeks later an amputation up to the middle of the middle phalanx had to be performed. At this time all corrected PIP joints could be mobilized intra-operatively up to full extension, both ring fingers and the right little finger showing a slightly restricted flexion. Intensive postoperative physiotherapy combined with night splinting followed.

Five years after the operation the result was quite unsatisfactory. All MP joints in both hands presented a free function. On the left hand the PIP joints could be actively extended as follows: index finger up to 10° of flexion, middle finger up to 65°, ring finger up to 40° and little finger up to 80° of flexion. Passively, the PIP joint of the index finger was completely extendable, whereas an extension deficit of about 65° of the middle, 20° of the ring and 55° of the little finger persisted. Flexion was quite normal. On the left hand the PIP mobility of the index and little

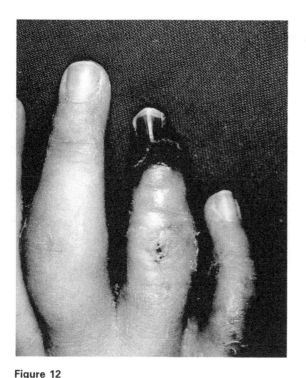

Figure 12

Case 3. Necrosis of the distal phalanx.

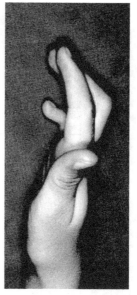
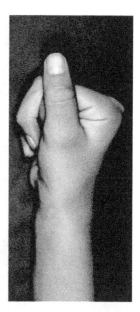

Figures 13 and 14

Case 3. Lateral view of the right hand in extension and flexion.

finger was quite normal, the middle finger showed an active extension deficit of 20° (passive 10°) and free flexion, and the ring finger was completely fixed in 20° of flexion in the PIP joint and showed no active motion in the DIP joint (Figs 13–16).

The disappointing results described above show that the surgical treatment of campto-dactyly, even when performed by quite experienced hand surgeons, might fail simply because of our limited pathological and anatomical knowledge of this complex malformation. Surgical treatment often only improves extension with a loss in flexion and without an increase in the range of motion. Besides surgery, intensive postoperative physiotherapy is of great importance, but is quite difficult to perform in little children, which leads to the difficult dilemma of when is the best time for an operation—very early on in life or at the end of the child's first decade when the patients are able to cooperate?

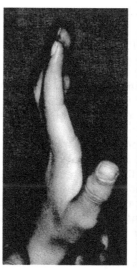
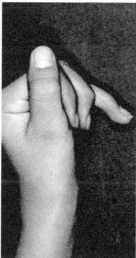

Figures 15 and 16

Case 3. Lateral view of the left hand in extension and flexion.

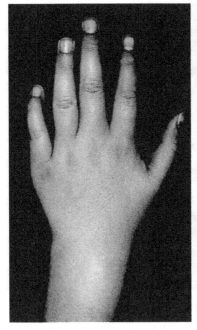

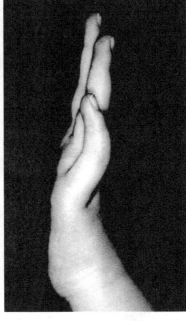

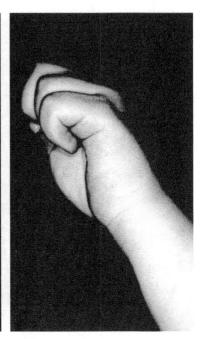

Figure 17

Case 4. Dorsal aspect of the left hand.

Figure 18

Case 4. Lateral view of the left hand.

Figure 19

Case 4. Lateral view of the left hand making a fist.

Case 4: presentation of an 8½-year-old girl

The medical history of the family did not reveal any finger malfunctions. About six months prior to the initial consultation the girl and her parents first observed a malpositioning and malfunction of both little fingers. The girl reported no pain, finger function was not restricted, and she was able to use her hands normally.

During our examination we saw free mobility of the shoulders, elbows and wrists and with the exception of the little fingers, all other digits were normally developed and had free functionality. The little finger of the left hand showed a slight radial deviation in the middle phalanx of about 15° and an ulnar deviation in the distal phalanx of 10° (Fig. 17). The active mobility of the MP joint was 35–0–70° and the restricted active mobility of the PIP joint of 0–30–100° was compensated by hyperextension in the MP joint (Fig. 18). The DIP joint showed a normal mobility of 0–0–60° and the girl was able to make a fist

(Fig. 19). With the MP joint held in flexion the PIP joint could be actively extended up to 15° of extension deficit and passively up to 10° (Fig. 20). The x-ray of the left little finger in lateral view showed a deformity of the head of the ground phalanx and a slightly broader base of the middle phalanx (Fig. 21), however, the clinical and radiological findings of the right little finger were not so pronounced (Fig. 22).

In this case the patient did not complain of any pain. The hand function was completely normal and the girl was able to extend the fingertip of the little finger up to the level of the other fingertips by hyperextension of the MP joint so that the palm was completely open. At this time no surgical treatment is indicated but careful observation during development is recommended in order to detect early any increase in contracture that would make surgery necessary. The girl and her parents were instructed to stretch the corresponding PIP joints as many times a day as possible to improve

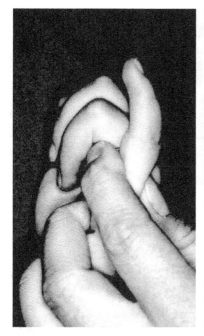

Figure 20

Case 4. Active extension of the left little finger, holding the MP joint in flexion.

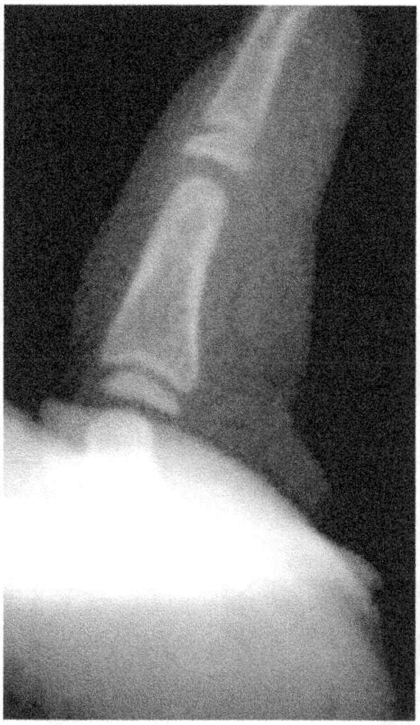

Figure 21

Case 4. X-ray of the left little finger.

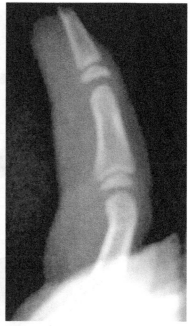

Figure 22

Case 4. X-ray of right little finger.

active and passive extension and to avoid a further increase in contracture.

Case 5: presentation of a 13¾-year-old boy

The boy's history revealed multiple congenital disorders while the history of his family was uneventful. After birth the boy presented an adaptation problem with dysphagia (difficulty in swallowing) and abnormal perspiration. Wrist contractures and functional disorders of the hand were then found, the upper and lower jaws were hypoplastic and the boy presented a severe kyphoscoliosis. Under intensive physiotherapy wrist and hand function were improved considerably, however a weakness in grip strength and a flexion contracture, especially of the middle phalanx of both middle fingers, persisted.

During our examination elbow extension and flexion were slightly restricted with mobility on the right side of 0–20–130° and on the left side of 0–10–120°. Pronation and supination were about 40–0–60° on both sides. Wrist extension and flexion were possible on both sides with 40–0–60°. The CM joint of the thumb showed a restricted radial and palmar abduction of about 25°, the MP joint showed a motion of 0–0–40° on the right and 0–20–40° on the left side, and the DIP joint showed an extension/flexion on the right side of 10–0–80° and on the left of 0–0–80°. Both thumbs showed good opposition. The fingers of both hands showed an almost normal mobility in the MP joint and only a slightly restricted DIP joint mobility. The PIP joints of the index, ring, and little finger could be almost fully extended and showed a normal flexion. The PIP joint of the middle finger showed an active extension deficit of 50° on the left and of 40° on the right hand, which could not be passively compensated. The palmar structures of the middle fingers were quite short (Figs 23–26).

An extensive soft-tissue release by Z-plasty was performed on the palmar side of the middle

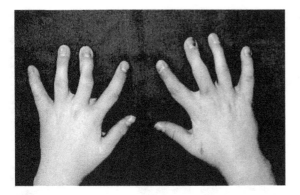

Figure 23

Case 5. Dorsal aspect of both hands.

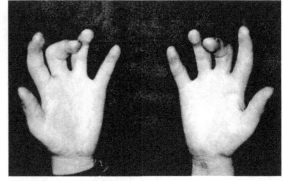

Figure 24

Case 5. Palmar view of the hands.

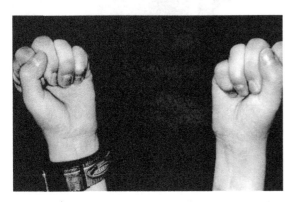

Figure 25

Case 5. Both hands in fist.

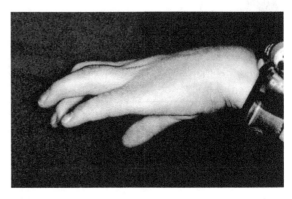

Figure 26

Lateral view of the left hand.

finger of the left hand combined with resection of subcutaneous adhesions and a PIP joint arthrolysis. No lumbrical anomalies were found. After soft tissue release and arthrolysis, a passive full extension of the PIP joint was possible, but due to the remaining tension of the superficial and deep flexor tendons, the digit returned to a flexed position. Therefore, in addition, we performed a fractional lengthening of the superficial and deep flexor tendon of the middle finger at forearm level. After this the PIP joint remained in extension. Forearm and hands were immobilized in splints for three weeks, fixing the middle finger in an almost extended position and afterwards an intensive physio-

therapy regime was started combined with additional long-term nighttime splinting (Fig. 27).

One year after the operation the range of motion of the PIP joint of the left middle finger was almost normal, with an extension/flexion of about 0–50–90° (Figs 28–30). In selected cases, especially in cases of camptodactyly in multiplex congenital arthrogryposis, a fractional lengthening of flexor tendons may help to increase the range of motion. By this method it is possible to increase active and passive mobility of the PIP joint without a loss in flexion. Other techniques also allow an increase in extension but a decrease in flexion. Long term follow-ups are recommended to verify these results.

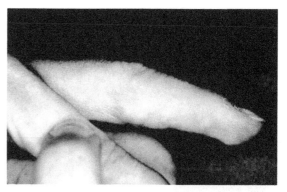

Figure 27

Case 5. Nighttime splint.

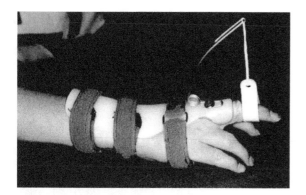

Figure 28

Case 5. Middle finger in extended position in lateral view.

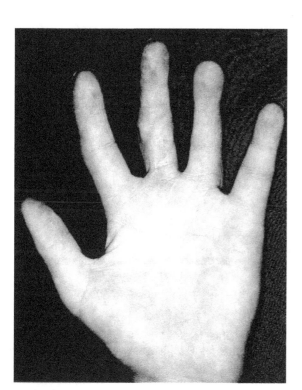

Figure 29

Case 5. Palmar view of the left hand.

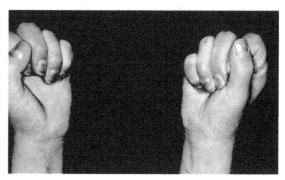

Figure 30

Case 5. Both hands in fist.

Case studies 6, 7, and 8
Ulrich Lanz

Case 6: presentation of a 13-year-old boy

This case details the presentation of a 13-year-old boy with an extension deficit in the PIP joint of both ring fingers of 50° (Figs 31a and b). With full passive extension and full flexion no preoperative splinting was necessary. There were no additional deformities. No lumbricals in the right hand could be identified during surgery (Fig. 31c), but apart from that no other anatomical abnormalities could be detected. Both lateral bands could be identified and complete extension of the PIP joint could be

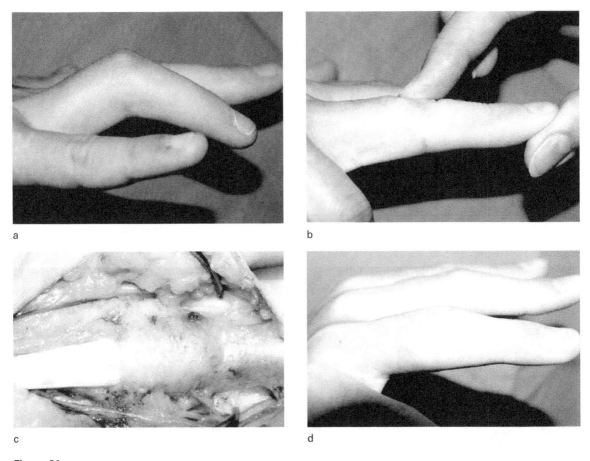

a

b

c

d

Figure 31

Case 6. (a and b) Right hand of an 13-year-old boy with bilateral extension deficit of the PIP joints of his fourth fingers. (c) Intra-operatively there is no lumbrical muscle to the ring finger in the right hand. (d) Three weeks after sectioning of the insertion of the interosseus muscles into the proximal phalanx of the ring finger. PIP extension is almost full.

achieved by pulling on them. The treatment comprised cutting both interossei at their insertion into the proximal phalanx, and directing all their power to the lateral bands of the extensor hood. Three weeks after the operation only a 10° extension deficit remained (Fig. 31d). Splinting is still being continued and a similar surgical approach is planned for the left hand.

Case 7: presentation of a 12-year-old girl

The right hand of a 12-year-old girl showed the little finger as having a fixed flexion contracture of 50° and when flexion was full, active extension

was possible to only 60° (Fig. 32a). The palmar skin over the PIP joint was webbed and splinting could not improve passive extension. At surgery skin was lengthened by a straight incision, followed by a Z-plasty. After a staged arthrolysis, beginning with resection of the tight retinacular skin ligaments, transection of the check rein ligaments and excision of the accessory collateral ligaments, full passive extension of the joint could be achieved. Revision of the lumbrical muscle showed an abnormal insertion of this muscle into the periosteum of the base of the proximal phalanx. No anomalies of the FDS were noted. The lumbrical was detached from its insertion and

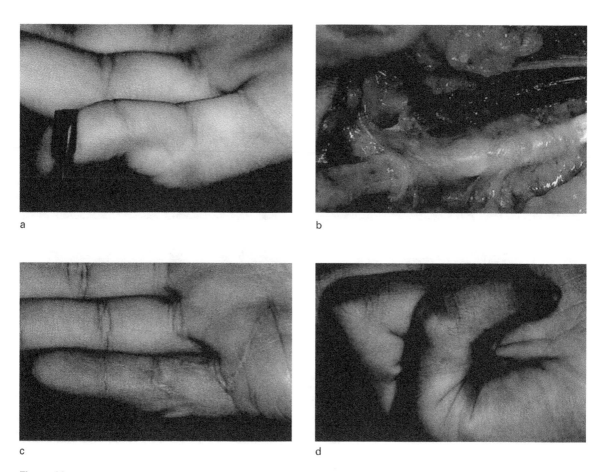

Figure 32

Case 7. Twelve-year-old girl with flexion contracture of the PIP joint of her right little finger. (a) Skin webbing. (b) At surgery after arthrolysis of the PIP joint transposition of the malinserting lumbrical muscle to the lateral band of the extensor mechanism. Z-plasty for skin lengthening. (c and d) Function three months postoperatively.

transferred to the radial lateral band under slight tension (Fig. 32b). Postoperative immobilization took place over a period of three weeks using a plaster splint in an intrinsic plus position. Thereafter physiotherapy was initiated, however between the exercise sessions the PIP joint was still held in extension with a splint. Treatment was continued for three months at which time the extension of the PIP joint was still full with a limitation of flexion to 80° (Figs 32c and d).

Case 8: presentation of a 14-year-old girl

This example highlights the case of a 14-year-old girl with a 65° fixed flexion contracture of the PIP joint of her right little finger. There was severe scarring resulting from previously unsuccessful surgery and marked shortening of the skin between the flexion creases of the proximal phalanx and the middle joint. Splintage showed only little improvement; surgery therefore deemed necessary.

In order to reduce the skin shortage, the midlateral incision was planned to include a transpositional flap from the ulno–dorsal lateral side of the proximal phalanx (Fig. 33a). Full extension could be achieved by total anterior tenoarthrolysis, detaching all soft tissues from

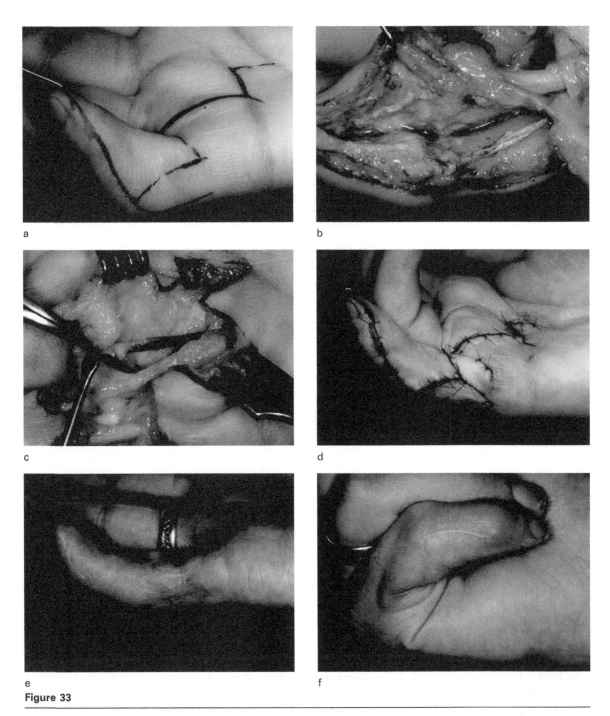

Figure 33

Case 8. (a) Fixed flexion contracture of 65° of the PIP joint in a 14-year-old girl with previous unsuccessful surgery and severe scarring. (b) Total anterior tenoarthrolysis (TATA), temporary transfixation of the PIP joint with a Kirschner wire, and transpositional flap from the dorso–ulnar side of the proximal phalanx. Bigastric lumbrical muscle, one where the belly inserts into the neighbouring finger, the other into the periosteum of the little finger (See Fig. 5f). (c) Transposition of both muscle bellies to the radial lateral band. (d) Skin closure with a transpositional flap. (e and f) Function one year postoperatively. Reproduced from Frank et al (1997) *Handchir Mikrochir Plast Chir* **29**: 284–90, with permission of G. Thieme-Verlag.

the palmar side of the proximal and middle phalanges including palmar skin with both neurovascular bundles, flexor tendon sheath, the palmar plate of the PIP joint and the FDS insertion to the middle phalanx (Fig. 33b). The PIP joint was transfixed in an almost full extension with a Kirschner wire. The lumbrical muscle was found to be bigastric with one belly attaching to the periosteum of the little finger and the other to the ulnar side of the ring finger (see Fig. 5f). No insertion into the extensor mechanism could be detected. Both muscle bellies were detached and transposed to the radial lateral band of the little finger (Fig. 33c). The FDS tendon was very thin. Traction on the tendon showed very little proximal elasticity so that an anomaly in its muscle belly was assumed. The tendon was resected, the skin gap resulting from the PIP extension was covered with the transpositional flap, and the donor defect covered with a split thickness skin graft from the ulnar side of the forearm (Fig. 33d).

Following surgery, a three-week period of immobilization using a plaster splint took place, after which time the Kirschner wire was removed and physiotherapy begun. The PIP joint was kept in extension by a splint for another four months. After a year there was mobility of the PIP joint of 0–20–70° (Figs 33e and f).

Conclusions

No agreement has been reached on the causes of camptodactyly, however, the numerous variations and anomalies of the anatomical structures acting at the PIP joint appear to be the likely cause for the imbalance of forces. These structures include not only the lumbrical muscles and the FDS tendon of the involved fingers, but also the interosseus muscles. But variations and anomalies in the tendons and muscles do not always lead to an apparent camptodactyly—anatomically, they appear to be quite common. Contrary to this, all clinical features of the deformity can be explained as secondary sequelae of an imbalance of forces during the growth period of a child. While mild cases can obviously be treated conservatively with prolonged splinting, more severe cases should be explored as early in life as possible in order to restore the equili-

brium of forces acting on the PIP joint and to prevent secondary deformities. The most important factor affecting the result can be seen in the fixed flexion contracture of this joint—the successful treatment of which is responsible for determining the final outcome.

Appendix

Syndromes associated with camptodactyly

1. Chromosomal
- 10q+ (Gorlin et al 1976)
- trisomy 13 (Zellweger and Simpson 1977)
- trisomy 18 (Zellweger and Simpson 1977)
- triploidy, diploid/triploid mosaics (Gorlin et al 1976)
- partial 11q monosomy (Jacobsen syndrome) (Jacobsen et al 1973)
- 4p+ (Gonzales et al 1977)
- trisomy 8 (Sanchez and Yunis 1974)

2. Major CNS involvement
- Zellweger syndrome (cerebrohepatorenal syndrome) (Bowen et al 1964)
- COFS (cerebrooculofacioskeletal synd., Pena-Shokeir synd. type II) (Pena and Shokeir 1974)
- Marden—Walker synd. (Marden and Walker 1966)
- Neu–Laxova synd. (Neu et al 1971, Laxova et al 1972)
- Pallister W synd. (Pallister et al 1974)
- Lenz microphthalmia synd. (Lenz 1955)
- MacDermont–Winter synd. (MacDermot and Winter 1989)
- Miller–Dieker lissencephaly synd. (Miller 1963, Dieker et al 1969)
- Ritscher–Schinzel synd. (craniocerebellocardiac dysplasia) (Ritscher et al 1987)
- Lin–Gettig synd. (craniosynostosis-mental retardation synd.) (Lin and Gettig 1990)
- distal arthrogryposis with hypopituitarism, mental retardation, and facial anomalies (Chitayat et al 1990)
- Palant cleft palate synd. (Palant et al 1971)
- Fryns synd. (Fryns et al 1979)
- Hennekam lymphangiectasia-lymphedema synd. (Hennekam et al 1989)

- Crisponi synd.(Crisponi 1996)
- Urban–Rogers–Meyer synd. (Urban et al 1979)
- Van Maldergem synd. (cerebrofacioarticular synd.) (van Maldergem et al 1992)
- Juberg–Marsidi synd. (Juberg and Marsidi 1980)
- cleidofacial dysostosis (Kozlowski et al 1970)

3. Multisystemic disorders
- Weaver synd. (Wodniansky 1957)
- Pena–Shokeir synd. type I (COFS II) (Peno and Shokeir 1976)
- Guadalajara camptodactyly synd. type I (facio-thorakoskeletal synd.) (Cantu et al 1980)
- Guadalajara camptodactyly synd. type II (Cantu et al 1981)
- Tel Hashomer camptodactyly synd. (Goodman et al 1972)
- Teebi–Shaltout synd. (Teebi and Shaltout 1989)
- Antley–Bixler synd. (multiple osteodysgenesis w. long bone fractures) (Antley and Bixler 1975)
- Meyer–Schickerwarth synd. (oculodentodigital dysplasia) (Lohmann 1920)
- arthrogryposis multiplex congenita, distal type 1 (DAI) (Daentl et al 1974)
- arthrogryposis multiplex congenita, distal type 2 (DA2, Freeman–Sheldon synd.) (Freeman and Sheldon 1979)
- arthrogryposis multiplex congenita, distal type 2B (DA2B, Freeman–Sheldon variant) (Krakowiak et al 1998)
- arthrogryposis multiplex congenita, distal type 3 (DA3, Gordon Synd.) (Gordon et al 1969)
- arthrogryposis multiplex congenita, distal type 4 (w. scoliosis, DA4) (Hall et al 1982)
- arthrogryposis multiplex congenita, distal type 5 (w. ophthalmoplegia and/or ptosis, DA5) (Hall et al 1982)
- arthrogryposis multiplex congenita, distal type 6 (w. sensorineural deafness, DA6) (Stewart and Bergstrom 1971)
- arthrogryposis multiplex congenita, distal type 8 (w. multiple pterygia, DA8, autosomal dominant multiple pterygium synd.) (Kawira and Bender 1985)
- arthrogryposis multiplex congenita, distal type 9 (w. congenital contractural arachnodactyly, DA9, Beals synd.) (Beals and Hecht 1971)

- Alves synd. (arthrogryposis and ectodermal dysplasia) (Alves et al 1981)
- Kuskokwim disease (arthrogryposis like disorder) (Petajan et al 1969)
- multiple pterygium synd. (many variants) (Matolcey 1936)
- agenesis of corpus callosum synd. (Naiman and Fraser 1955)
- Camera–Maguro–Cohen synd. (Camera et al 1993)
- Silver–Russel synd. (Silver 1964)
- Stuve–Wiedemann synd. (Schwartz–Jampel synd. type II) (Stuve and Wiedemann 1971)
- camptodactyly-arthropathy-coxa vara-pericarditis synd. (Jacobs synd., familial fibrosing serositis) (Jacobs and Downey 1974)
- triphalangeal thumbs and dislocation of patella synd. (Say et al 1976)
- cam ptodactyly-ichtiosis synd. (Baraitser 1982)
- camptodactyly w. fibrous tissue hyperplasia and skeletal dysplasia (Goodman et al 1979)
- facial dysmorphism, cleft palate, hearing loss, and camptodactyly (Courtens et al 1997)
- Liebenberg synd. (Liebenberg 1973)
- Blau synd. (Jabs synd., arthro-cutaneouveal granulomatosis) (Blau 1985, Jabs et al 1985)
- Dincsoy synd. (Dincsoy et al 1995)
- Meier–Gorlin synd. (ear-patella-short stature synd.) (Meier and Rothschild 1959)
- cholestasis w. gallstone, ataxia, and visual disturbance (Schubert et al 1976)
- Borrone dermatocardioskeletal synd. (Borrone et al 1993)
- Goodman synd. (acrocephalopolysyndactyly type IV) (Goodman et al 1979)
- Marfan synd. (McKusick 1972)
- marfanoid craniosynostosis (Shprintzen–Goldberg craniosynostosis synd.) (Shprintzen and Goldberg 1979)
- pseudoaminopterin synd. (Fraser et al 1987)
- progeroid facial appearance w. hand anomalies (Giannotti et al 1997)
- Goltz–Gorlin synd. (Wodniansky 1957)
- mesomelic limb shortening and bowing (Reardon et al 1993)
- familial retroperitoneal fibrosis (Comings et al 1967)
- ODPD synd. (terminal osseous dysplasia and pigmentary defects) (Bloem et al 1974)
- Aase–Smith synd. (Aase and Smith 1968)
- Emery–Nelson synd. (Emery and Nelson 1970)

- Aarskog–Scott synd. (Aarskog 1970)
- frontometaphyseal dysplasia (Gordon et al 1969)
- camptodactyly and absence of fingerprints (Baird 1964)
- OMM synd. (ophthalmomandibulomelic dysplasia) (Pillay 1964)
- Klein–Waardenburg synd. (Waardenburg synd. type III) (Klein 1950)
- German synd. (German et al 1975)
- camptodactyly-taurinuria synd. (Nevin et al 1966)
- camptodactyly w. associated malformations (Pierce 1974)
- camptodactyly-torticollis-scoliosis synd. (Baraitser 1982)
- Karsch–Neubauer synd. (Karsch 1936)
- distal symphalangism w. camptodactyly, (Ohdo et al 1981)
- Fitch synd. (Fitch et al 1976)
- camptodactyly with myopia and fibrosis of the medial rectus of the eye (Kilic et al 1998)
- craniofacial anomalies, ocular findings, pigmented nevi, camptodactyly, and skeletal changes (Gul et al 2000)
- agenesis of corpus callosum, camptodactyly and obesity (Velores and Lesenfants 2000)
- Pointer synd. (Huq et al 1997)
- phocomelia, flexion deformities and absent thumbs (Holmes and Borden 1974)
- growth and mental retardation, microcephaly, preauricular skin tags, cleft palate, camptodactyly and distal limb anomalies (Hall et al 1982)

(w = with, synd. = syndrome)

References

Aarskog D (1970) A familial syndrome of short stature associated with facial dysplasia and genital anomalies, *J Pediat* **77**:856–61.

Aase JM, Smith DW (1968) Dysmorphogenesis of joints, brain and palate: a new dominantly inherited syndrome, *J Pediat* **73**:606–9.

Adams W (1891) On congenital contraction of the fingers and first association with 'hammertoe': pathology and treatment, *Lancet* **2**:107–11, 161–63, 165–68.

Alves AFP, dos Santos PAB, Castelo-Branco-Neto E,

Freire-Maia N (1981) An autosomal recessive ectodermal dysplasia syndrome of hypotrichosis, onychodysplasia, hyperkeratosis, hyphoscoliosis, cataract, and other manifestations, *Am J Med Genet* **15**:213–18.

Antley RM, Bixler D (1975) Trapezoidocephaly, midface hypoplasia and cartilage abnormalities with multiple synostoses and skeletal fractures, *Birth Defects Orig Art Ser* **XI**:397–401.

Austin GJ, Leslie BM, Ruby LK (1989) Variations of the flexor digitorum superficialis of the small finger, *J Hand Surg* **14A**: 262–67.

Baird HW III (1964) Kindred showing congenital asbsence of the dermal ridges (fingerprints) and associated anomalies, *J Pediat* **64**:621–31.

Baker DS, Gaul JS, Williams VK (1981) The little finger superficialis: clinical investigation of its anatomic and functional shortcomings, *J Hand Surg* **6A**:374–78.

Bamshad M, Jorde LB, Carey JC (1996) A revised and extended classification of the distal arthrogryposes, *Am J Med Genet* **65**:277–81.

Baraitser M (1982) A new camptodactyly syndrome, *Am J Med Genet* **19**:40–3.

Basu SS, Hasary S (1960) Variations of the lumbrical muscles of the hand, *Anat Rec* **136**:501–4.

Beals RK, Hecht F (1971) Congenital contractural arachnodactyly: a heritable disorder of connective tissue, *J Bone Joint Surg* **53A**: 987–93.

Berger A, Millesi H (1975) Spätergebnisse der Operativen Behandlung der Kamptodaktylie. *Handchirurgie* **7**:75–79.

Blau EB (1985) Familial granulomatous arthritis, iritis, and rash, *J Pediat* **107**:689–93.

Bloem JJ, Vuzevski VD, Huffstadt AJC (1974) Recurring digital fibroma of infancy, *J Bone Joint Surg* **56B**:746–51.

Borrone C, Di Rocco M, Crovato F, Camera G, Gambini C (1993) New multisystemic disorder involving heart valves, skin, bones, and joints in two brothers, *Am J Med Genet* **46**:228–34.

Bowen P, Lee CSN, Zellweger H, Lindenberg R (1964) A familial syndrome of multiple congenital defects, *Bull Johns Hopkins Hosp* **114**:402–14.

Buck-Gramcko D (1987) Congenital and developmental

conditions. In: Bowers W, ed *The Interphalangeal Joints. The Hand and Upper Extremity* (Churchill Livingstone: London) 199–202.

Buck-Gramcko D (1997) Comment on Operative Therapie der Kamptodaktylie by Frank et al, *Handchir Mikrochir Plast Chir* **29**:293–96.

Camera G, Marugo M, Cohen MM Jr (1993) Another postnatal-onset obesity syndrome, *Am J Med Genet* **47**:820–22.

Cantu JM, Rivera H, Nazara Z, Rojas Q, Hernandez A, Garcia-Cruz D (1980) Guadalajara syndrome camptodactyly: a distinct probably autosomal recessive disorder, *Clin Genet* **18**:153–9.

Cantu JM, Garcia-Cruz D, Ramirez ML, Sole-Pujol MT (1981) Guadalajara syndrome camptodactyly syndrome type II. *Sixth Internal Congress on Human Genetics*, Jerusalem; Abstract: 263.

Chitayat D, Hall JG, Couch RM, Phang MS, Baldwin VJ (1990) Syndrome of mental retardation, facial anomalies, hypopituitarism, and distal arthrogryposis in sibs, *Am J Med Genet* **37**:65–70.

Chowdary DS (1951) A rare anomaly of flexor digitorum sublimis, *J Anat* **85**: 100–1.

Christ B (1990) Entwicklung der Extremitäten. In: *Humanembryologie Hrsg* (K Hinrichsen Springer: Berlin, Heidelberg, New York).

Čihak R (1972) Ontogenesis of the skeleton and intrinsic muscles of the human hand and foot, *Ergebn Anat Entwickl-Gesch* **46**:1–194.

Comings DE, Skubi KB, Van Eyes J, Motulsky AG (1967) Familial multifocal fibrosclerosis: findings suggesting that retroperitoneal fibrosis, mediastinal fibrosis, sclerosing cholangitis, Riedel's thyroiditis, and pseudotumor of theorbit may be different manifestations of a single disease, *Ann Intern Med* **66**:884–92.

Courtens W, Perlmutter N, Dan B, Vamos E (1997) New syndrome or severe expression of Gordon syndrome? A case report, *Clin Dysmorph* **6**:39–44.

Crisponi G (1996) Autosomal recessive disorder with muscle contractions resembling neonatal tetanus, characteristic face, camptodactyly, hyperthemia, and sudden death: a new syndrome?, *Am J Med Genet* **62**:365–71.

Curnow J (1873) Notes of some irregularities in muscles and nerves, *J Anat Physiol* **7**: 304–10.

Daentl DL, Berg BO, Layzer RB, Epstein CJ (1974) A new familial arthrogryposis without weakness, *Neurology* **24**:55–60.

Dieker H, Edwards RH, zu Rhein G, Chou SM, Hartman HA, Opitz JM (1969) The lissencephaly syndrome. In: Bergsma D, ed.: *The Clinical Delineation of Birth Defects: Malformation Syndromes*. New York: National Foundation-March of Dimes, 2nd edn, 53–64.

Dincsoy MY, Salih MAM, Al-Jurayyan N, Al Saadi M, Patel PJ (1995) Multiple congenital malformations in two sibs reminiscent of hydrocephalus and pseudotrisomy 13 syndromes, *Am J Med Genet* **56**:317–21.

Emery AEH, Nelson MM (1970) A familial syndrome of short stature, deformities of the hands and feet, and an unusual facies, *J Med Genet* **7**:379–82.

Engber WD, Flatt AE (1977) Camptodactyly: an analysis of sixty-six patients and twenty-four operations, *J Hand Surg* **2A**:216–24.

Eyler DL, Markee JE (1954) The anatomy and function of the intrinsic musculature of the fingers, *J Bone Joint Surg* **36A**:1–9.

Fitch N, Jequier S, Papageorgiou A (1978) A familial syndrome of cranial, facial, oral and limb anomalies, *Clin Genet* **10**:226–31.

Flatt E (1994) *The Care of Congenital hHand Deformities*, 2nd edn (Quality Medical Publishing Comp: St. Louis).

Foucher G, Lenoble E, Ben Youssef K, Sammut D (1993) A post-operative regime after digital flexor tenolysis: a series of 72 patients, *J Hand Surg* **18B**:35–40.

Frank U, Krimmer H, Hahn P, Lanz U (1997) Operative Therapie der Kamptodaktylie, *Handchir Mikrochir Plast Chir* **29**:284–90.

Fraser FC, Anderson RA, Mulvihill JI, Preus M (1987) An aminopterin-like syndrome without aminopterin (ASSAS), *Clin Genet* **32**:28–34.

Freeman EA, Sheldon JH (1938) Cranio-carpotarsal dystrophy: undescribed congenital malformation, *Arch Dis Child* **13**:277–83.

Frohse F, Fränkel M (1908) Die Muskeln des menschlichen Armes. In: Bardeleben KV, *Handbuch der Anatomie des Menschen* (G. Fischer: Jena).

Fryns JP, Moerman F, Goddeeris P, Bossuyt C, Van Den

Berghe H (1979) A new lethal syndrome with cloudy corneae, diaphragmatic defects, and distal limb deformities, *Hum Genet* **50**:65–70.

Furnas DW (1985) Muscle tendon variations in the flexor compartment of the wrist, *Plast Reconstr Surg* **3**:320–24.

German J, Morillo-Cucci A, Simpson JL, Chaganti RSK (1975) Generalized dysmorphis of a similar type in 2 unrelated babies, *Birth Defects Orig Art Ser* **XI**(2):34–8.

Giannotti A, Digilio MC, Mingarelli R, Marino B, Dallapiccola B (1997) Progeroid syndrome with characteristic facial appearance and hand anomalies in father and son, *Am J Med Genet* **73**:227–9.

Glicenstein J, Haddad R, Guero S (1995) Traitement chirurgical des camptodactylies, *Ann Chir Main* **14**:264–71.

Goffin D, Lenoble E, Marin Braun FM, Foucher G (1994) Camptodactylies: classification et résultats thérapeutiques: a propos d'une série de 50 cas, *Ann Chir Main* **13**:20–5.

Gonzales CH, Sommer A, Meisner F, Elejalde BR, Opitz J (1977) The trisomy 4p syndrome: case report and review, *Am J Med Genet* **1**:137–56.

Goodman RM, Katznelson MB-M, Manor E (1972) Camptodactyly: occurrence in two new genetic syndromes and its relationship to other syndromes, *J Med Genet* **9**:203–12.

Goodman RM, Sternberg M, Shem-Tov Y, Katznelson MB-M, Hertz M, Rotem Y (1979) Acrocephalopolysyndactyly type IV: a new genetic syndrome in 3 sibs, *Clin Genet* **15**:209–14.

Gordon H, Davies D, Berman MM (1969) Camptodactyly, cleft palate and clubfoot: syndrome showing the autosomal-dominant pattern of inheritance, *J Med Genet* **6**:266–74.

Gorlin RJ, Cohen MM Jr (1969) Frontometaphyseal dysplasia: a new syndrome, *Am J Dis Child* **118**:487–94.

Gorlin RJ, Pindborg JJ, Cohen MM Jr (1978) *Syndromes of the Head and Neck.* New York: McGraw-Hill, 2nd edn.

Guion-Almeida ML, Zechi-Ceide RM, Richieri-Costa A (1999) Multiple congenital anomalies syndrome: growth and mental retardation, microcephaly, preauricular skin tags, cleft palate, camptodactyly, and distal limb anomalies. Report of two unrelated Brazilian patients, *Am J Med Genet* **87**:72–7.

Gul D, Oktenli C, Saglam M, Erdem U (2000) Craniofacial anomalies, ocular findings, pigmented nevi, camptodactyly, and skeletal changes: a possible new autosomal recessive disorder, *Clin Dysmorph* **9**:61–2.

Hall JG, Reed SD, Greene G (1982) The distal arthrogryposes: Delineation of new entities—review and nosological discussion, *Am J Med Genet* **11**:185–239.

Hennekam RCM, Geerdink RA, Hamel BCJ, Hennekam FAM, Kraus P, Rammeloo JA, Tillemans AAW (1989) Autosomal recessive intestinal lymphangiectasia and lymphedema, with facial anomalies and mental retardation, *Am J Med Genet* **34**:593–600.

Holmes LB, Borden S (1974) Phocomelia, flexion deformities and absent thumb: a new hereditary upper limb malformation, *J Pediat* **54**:461–5.

Hori M, Nakamura R, Inoue G et al (1987) Non-operative treatment of camptodactyly, *J Hand Surg* **12A**: 1061–65.

Humphry GM (1873) Lectures on the varieties in the muscles of man. Lecture II. The muscles of the upper limb, *BMJ* **2**:51–54.

Huq AH, Braverman RM, Greenberg F, Bacino CA, Rimoin DL, Lachman RS, Levin ML (1997) The Pointer Syndrome: a new syndrome with skeletal abnormalities, camptodactyly, facial anomalies, and feeding difficulties, *Am J Med Genet* **68**:225–30.

Ikebuchi Y, Murakami, Ohtsuka A (1988) The interosseus and lumbrical muscles in the human hand, with special reference to the insertions of the interosseus muscles, *Acta Med Okayama* **42**:327–34.

Jabs DA, Houk JL, Bias WB, Arnett FC (1985) Familial granulomatous synovitis, uveitis, and cranial neuropathies, *Am J Med* **78**:801–4.

Jacobs JC, Downey JA (1974) Juvenile rheumatoid arthritis. In: Downey JA, Low NL, eds, *The Child with Disabling Illness* (WB Saunders: Philadelphia) 5–24.

Jacobsen P, Hauge M, Henningsen K, Hobolth N, Mikkelsen M, Philip J (1973) An (11;21) translocation in four generations with chromosome 11 abnormalities in the offspring: a clinical, cytogenetical, and gene marker study, *Hum Hered* **23**:568–85.

Jaquemain B (1966) Die angebohrene Windmühlenflügelstellung als erbliche Kombinationsmißbildung, *Z Orthop* **102**:146–54.

Jones KG, Marmor L, Lankford LL (1974) An overview on new procedures in surgery of the hand, *Clin Orthop* **99**:154–67.

Juberg RC, Marsidi I (1980) A new form of x-linked mental retardation with growth retardation, deafness, and microgenitalism, *Am J Med Genet* **32**:714–22.

Kaplan EB (1969) Muscular and tendinous variations of the flexor superficialis of the fifth finger of the hand, *Bull Hosp Joint Dis* **30**:59–67.

Karsch J (1936) Erbliche Augenfehlbildung in Verbindung mit Spalthand- und Fuß, *Z Augenheilkd* **89**:274–9.

Kawira EL, Bender HA (1985) An unusual distal arthrogrypsis, *Am J Med Genet* **20**:425–9.

Kilic I, Kilic BA, Ergin H, Aygun MG, Aksit MA (1998) Camptodactyly, myopia, and firosis of the medial rectus of the eye in two sibs born to consanguineous parents: autosomal recessive entity?, *Am J Med Genet* **77**:28–30.

Klein D (1950) Albinisme partiel (leucisme) avec surdi-mutite, blepharophimosis et dysplasie myo-osteo-articulaire, *Helv Paediat Acta* **5**:38–58.

Koman LA, Toby EB, Poehling GG (1990) Congenital flexion deformities of the proximal interphalangeal joint in children: a subgroup of camptodactyly, *J Hand Surg* **15A**: 582–86.

Kozlowski K, Hanicka M, Zygulska-Machowa H (1970) Dysplasia cleido-facialis, *Z Kinderheilk* **108**:331–8.

Krakowiak PA, Bohnsack JF, Carey JC, Bamshad M (1998) Clinical analysis of a variant of Freeman-Sheldon syndrome (DA2B), *Am J Med Genet* **76**:93–8.

Landouzy L (1906) Camptodactylie, stigmate organique precoce de neuro-arthitisme, *Presse Med* **14**: 251–53.

Laxova R, Ohdra PT, Timothy JAD (1972) A further example of a lethal autosomal recesive condition in sibs, *J Ment Defic Res* **16**:139–43.

Lenz W (1955) Recessiv-geschlechtsgebundene Mikrophthalmie mit multiplen Missbildungen, *Z Kinderheilk* **77**:384–90.

Lewis OJ (1965) The evolution of the mm. interossei in the primate hand, *Anat Rec* **153**:275–88.

Liebenberg F (1973) A pedigree with unusual anomalies of the elbows, wrists and hands in five generations, *S Afr Med J* **47**:745–7.

Lin AE, Gettig E (1990) Craniosynostosis, agenesis of the corpus callosum, severe mental retardation, distinctive facies, camptodactyly, and hypogonadism, *Am J Med Genet* **35**:582–5.

Littler JW (1967) Dupuytren's contracture. In: *Maladie de Dupuytren* (GEM Monograph L'Expansion: Paris).

Lohmann W (1920) Beitrag zur Kenntnis des reinen Mikrophthalmus, *Arch Augenheilk* **86**:136–41.

Macalister A (1872) Additional observations on muscular anomalies in human anatomy (third series), with a catalogue of the principal muscular variations hitherto published, *Trans R Ir Acad* **25**:69–117.

MacDermot KD, Winter RM (1989) Two brothers with facial anomalies, microcephaly, hypoplastic genitalia, and a failure of psychomotor development, *Am J Med Genet* **32**:60–2.

Maeda M, Matsui T (1985) Camptodactly caused by an abnormal lumbrical muscle, *J Hand Surg* **10B**: 95–96.

Malek R (1998) Camptodactylies congénitales. In: Tubiana R, *Traité de Chirurgie de la Main*, vol. V (Masson: Paris) 379–93.

Marden PM, Walker WA (1966) A new generalized connective tissue syndrome, *Am J Dis Child* **112**:225–8.

Matolcsy T, Über die chirurgische Behandlung der angeborenen Flughaut, *Langenbeck Arch Klin Chir* **185**:675–81.

McCash CR (1966) Congenital contractures of the hand, *The Second Hand Club* **22**:399–401.

McFarlane RM, Classen DA, Porte AM, Botz JS (1992) The anatomy and treatment of camptodactyly of the small finger, *J Hand Surg* **17A**: 35–44.

McFarlane RM, Curry GI, Evans HB (1983) Anomalies of the intrinsic muscles in camptodactyly, *J Hand Surg* **8**:531–44.

McKusick VA (1972) *Hereditable Disorders of the Connective Tissue*. St Louis: CV Mosby Co. 4th edn.

McKusick V (2000) Arthrogryposis multiplex congenita, distal, type 2B, AMCD2B, http://www.ncbi.nlm.nih.gov/Omim: entry 601680.

Mehta HJ, Gardner WU (1961) A study of lumbrical muscles in the human hand, *Am J Anat* **109**:227–38.

Meier Z, Rothschild M (1959) Ein Fall von Arthrogryposis multiplex congenita kombiniert mit Dysostosis mandibulofacialis (Franceschetti-Syndrom), *Helv Paediat Acta* **14**:213–6.

Miller JQ (1963) Lissencephaly in 2 siblings, *Neurology* **13**:841–50.

Millesi H (1959) Neue Gesichtspunkte in der Pathogenese der Dupuytren'schen Kontraktur, *Bruns Beitr Klein Chir* **198**:1–25.

Millesi H (1965) Zur Pathogenese und Therapie der Dupuytren'schen Kontraktur, *Ergebn Chir Orthop* **47**:51–101.

Millesi H (1968) Zur Pathogenese und operativen Korrektur der Kamptodaktylie, *Chirurgia Plast Reconstr* **5**:55–61.

Missfelder S, Fischer G, Lanz U, Schmidt H-M (1990) Klinische Anatomie des digitalen Bandzuges an der Ulnarseite des Kleinfingers, *Handchir Mikrochir Plast Chir* **22**:88–91.

Miura T (1983) Non-traumatic flexion deformity of the proximal interphalangeal joint: first pathogenesis and treatment, *Hand* **15**:25–34.

Miura T, Nakamura R, Tamura Y (1992) Long-standing extended dynamic splintage and release of an abnormal restraining structure in camptodactyly, *J Hand Surg* **17B**: 665–72.

Naiman J, Fraser FC (1955) Agenesis of the corpus callosum: a report of two cases in siblings, *Arch Neurol Psychiat* **74**:182–5.

Neu RL, Kajii T, Gardner LI, Nagyfy SF, King S (1971) A lethal syndrome of micrpcephaly with multiple congenital anomalies in three siblings, *Pediatrics* **47**:619–12.

Nevin NC, Hurwitz LJ, Neill DW (1966) Familial camptodactyly with taurinuria, *J Med Genet* **3**:265–8.

Ogino T, Kato H (1992) Operative findings in camptodactyly of the little finger, *J Hand Surg* **17B**: 661–64.

Ohdo S, Yamauchi Y, Hayakawa K (1981) Distal symphalangism associated with camptodactyly, *J Med Genet* **18**:456–8.

Palant DI, Feingold M, Berkman MD (1971) Unusual facies, cleft palate, mental retardation, and limb abnormalities in siblings—a new syndrome, *J Pediat* **78**:686–9.

Pallister PD, Herrmann J, Spranger JW, Gorlin RJ, Langer LO Jr, Opitz JM (1974) The W syndrome, *Birth Defects Orig Art Ser* **X**(7):51–60.

Pena SDJ, Shokeir MHK (1974) Syndrome of camptodactyly, multiple ankyloses, facial anomalies and pulmonary hypoplasia: a lethal condition, *J Pediat* **85**:373–5.

Pena SDJ, Shokeir MHK (1976) Syndrome of camptodactyly, multiple ankylosis, facial anomalies and pulmonary hypoplasia: further delineation and evidence for autosomal recessive inheritance, *Birth Defects Orig Art Ser* **X(5)**:201–3.

Petajan JH, Momberger GL, Aase JM, Wright DG (1969) Arthrogryposis syndrome (Kuskokwim disease) in the Eskimo, *JAMA* **209**:1481–6.

Pierce ER (1974) Camptodactyly with associated malformations in the proband, *Birth Defects Orig Art Ser* **X**(5):201–3.

Pillay VK (1964) Ophthalmo-mandibulo-melic dysplasia, an hereditary syndrome, *J Bone Joint Surg* **46**:858–62.

Rabischong P (1962) L'innervation proprioceptive des muscles lombricaux de la main chez l' homme, *Rev Chir Orth* **48**:234–45.

Reardon W, Hall CM, Slaney S, Huson SM, Connell J, Al-Hilaly N, Fixsen J, Baraitser M, Winter RM (1993) Mesomelic limb shortness: a previously unreported autosomal recessive type, *Am J Med Genet* **47**:788–92.

Ritscher D, Schinzel A, Boltshauser E, Briner J, Arbenz U, Sigg P (1987) Dandy–Walker (like) malformation, atrio-ventricular septal defect and a similar pattern of minor anomalies in 2 sisters: a new syndrome?, *Am J Med Genet* **26**:481–91.

Rozin MM, Hertz M, Goodman RM (1984) A new syndrome with camptodactyly, joint contractures, facial anomalies, and skeletal defects: a case report and review of syndromes with camptodactyly, *Clin Genet* **26**:342–55.

Saffar P (1983) La teno-arthrolyse totale anterieure, *Ann Chir Main* **2**:345–50.

Salsbury CR (1936/37) The interosseous muscles of the hand, *J Anat* **71**:395–403.

Sanchez O, Yunis JJ (1974) Partial trisomy 8 (8q24) and the trisomy 8 syndrome, *Humangenetik* **23**:297–303.

Say B, Field E, Coldwell JG, Warnberg L, Atasu M (1976) Polydactyly with triphalangeal thumbs, brachydactyly camptodactyly, congenital dislocation of the patellas, short stature and borderline intelligence, *Birth Defects Orig Art Ser* **XII**(5):279–86.

Scharizer E (1979) Ein Beitrag zur Kamptodaktylie, *Handchirurgie* **11**:167–68.

Schmidt H-M (1990) Eine seltene Anomalie der oberflächlichen Beugesehnen am Kleinfinger, *Handchir Mikrochir Plast Chir* **22**:68–70.

Schmidt H-M, Lanz U (1992) *Chirurgische Anatomie der Hand* (Hippokrates: Stuttgart).

Schmidt R, Heinrichs H-J, Reissig D (1963) Die Mm. lumbricales an der Hand des Menschen, ihre Variationen in Ursprung und Ansatz, *Anat Anz* **113**:414–49.

Schmidt R, Kienast W, Sommer H, Dorn A (1965) Vergleich der Mm. lumbricales und ihrer Varietäten an der menschlichen Hand bei verschiedenen Völkern (Amerikanern, Deutschen, Franzosen und Russen), *Gegenbaurs Morph Jb* **107**:491–515.

Schubert WK, Partin JS, Partin JC (1976) Congenital cholestasis: clinical and ultrastructural study. In: Berenberg SR, ed.: *Liver Diseases in Infancy and Childhood*. Hauge: Martinus Nijhoff, 148–62.

Scott CI Jr (1971) Unusual facies, joint hypermobility, genital anomaly and short stature: a new dysmorphic syndrome, *Birth Defects Orig Art Ser* **VII**(6):240–6.

Senrui H (1998) Congenital contractures. In: Buck-Gramcko D, ed, *Congenital Malformations of the Hand and Forearm* (Churchill Livingstone: London).

Shrewsbury MM, Kuczynski K (1974) Flexor digitorum superficialis tendon in the fingers of the human hand, *Hand* **6**:121–33.

Shprintzen RJ, Goldberg RB (1979) Dysmorphic facies, omphalocele, laryngeal and pharyngeal hypoplasia, spinal anomalies, and learning disabilities in a new dominant malformation syndrome, *Birth Defects Orig Art Ser* **XV**(5B):347–53.

Siegert JJ, Cooney WP, Dobbyns JH (1990) Management of the simple camptodactyly, *J Hand Surg* **15B**: 181–89.

Silver HK (1964) Asymmetry, short stature, and varia-

tions in sexual development: a syndrome of congenital malformations, *Am J Dis Child* **107**:495–515.

Smith P, Breed C (1994) Central slip attenuation in Dupuytren's contracture: a cause of persistent flexion of the proximal interphalangeal joint, *J Hand Surg* **19A**: 840–43.

Smith PJ, Grobbelaar AO (1998) Camptodactyly: a unifying theory and approach to surgical treatment, *J Hand Surg* **23A**: 14–9.

Smith RJ, Kaplan EB (1968) Camptodactyly and similar atraumatic flexion deformities of the proximal interphalangeal joint of the finger, *J Bone Joint Surg* **50A**: 1187–1204.

Stedtfeld H-W, Brug E (1979) Beitrag zur Kamptodaktylie. *Handchirurgie* **11**: 161–65.

Stein A, Lemos M, Stein S (1990) Clinical evaluation of flexor tendon function in the small finger, *Ann Emerg Med* **19**:991–93.

Stewart JM, Bergstrom L (1971) Familial hand abnormality and sensori-neural deafness: a new syndrome, *J Pediat* **78**:102–10.

Stuve A, Wiedemann H-R (1971) Congenital bowing of the long bones in two sisters, *Lancet* **2**:495. (Letter).

Teebi AS, Shaltout AA (1989) Craniofacial anomalies, abnormal hair, camptodactyly, and caudal appendage, *Am J Med Genet* **33**:58–60.

Temtamy SA, McKusick VA (1978) *Genetics of Hand Malformations* (Alan Liss: New York).

Testut L (1884) *Les Anomalies musculaires chez l'homme expliquées par l'anatomie comparée et leur importance en anthropologie* (G Masson: Paris).

Tsipouras P, Del Mastro R, Safarazi M et al The international Marfan Syndrome Collaborative Study (1992) Genetic linkage of the Marfan syndrome, ectopia lentis, and congenital contractural arachnodactyly to the fibrillin genes on chromosome 15 and 5, *N Engl J Med* **326**:905–9.

Tubiana R, Thomine JM (1967) Le traitement chirurgical de la maladie de Dupuytren. In: *Maladie de Dupuytren* (GEM Monograph L'Expansion: Paris).

Urban MD, Rogers JG, Meyer WJ (1979) Familial syndrome of mental retardation, short stature, contractures of the hands, and genital anomalies, *J Pediat* **94**:52–5.

Van Maldergem L, Wetzburger C, Verloes A, Fourneau C, Gillerot Y (1992) Mental retardation with blepharo-naso-facial abnormalities and hand malformations: a new syndrome?, *Clin Genet* **41**:22–4.

Velores A, Lesenfants S (2000) Agenesis of the corpus callosum, camptodactyly and obesity, *Clin Dysmorph* **9**:107–9.

Weaver DD, Graham CB, Thomas IT, Smith DW (1974) A new overgrowth syndrome with accelerated skeletal maturation, unusual facies, and camptodactyly, *J Pediat* **84**:547–52.

Wilhelm A (1992) Zur Pathogenese und Behandlung der Kamptodaktylie. In: Buck-Gramcko D, Benatar N, Hoffmann R, Brüser P, eds, *Eine Festschrift zum 65 Geburtstag* (Druckhaus Mayer Verlag: Erlangen).

Wilhelm A (2000a) Operative treatment of campto-dactyly. In: *Congenital Differences of the Upper Limb*. Proceedings of the 5th International Symposium on Congenital Differences of the Upper Limb. Kyoto, Japan, 162–69.

Wilhelm A (2000b) Pathogenesis of camptodactyly. In: *Congenital Differences of the Upper Limb*. Proceedings of the 5th International Symposium on Congenital Differences of the Upper Limb. Kyoto, Japan, 156–61.

Wilhelm A, Kleinschmidt W (1968) Neue ätiologische und therapeutische Gesichtspunkte bei der Kamptodaktylie und Tendovaginitis stenosans, *Chir Plast Reconstr* **5**:62–7.

Wodniansky P (1957) Über die Formen der congeni-talen Poikilodermie, *Arch Klin Exp Derm* **205**:331–42.

Wood VE (1993) Camptodactyly. In: Green DV, ed, *Operative Hand Surgery*, third edition (Churchill Livingstone: London).

Zellweger H, Simpson J (1977) *Chromosomes of Man.* London: Simp.

11

Thumb hypoplasia: a spectrum of congenital disorders

Guy Foucher, Jose Medina, Giorgio Pajardi and Ricardo Navarro

The thumb develops from the radial aspect of the hand plate during the fifth to eighth week of gestation. Neglected during the first three months of life, the thumb is soon out of the palm, used as a nipple substitute and integrated for prehension as early as nine months of age. During growth, the average thumb reaches the distal half of the proximal phalanx of the index. Underdevelopment of the thumb is frequently seen but a short, a low-set or a slender thumb could have a near normal function and then only marginally interest the hand surgeon taking care of congenital conditions. For the pediatrician or the geneticist a short thumb could be a key entry to different syndromes (Table 1).

Hypoplasia is not simply a short thumb, but it is not easy to define thumb hypoplasia (TH) and even more difficult to classify the different types seen clinically. Even if not included *stricto sensu* in the definition we will partly include thumb aplasia in the discussion of pollicization. Some dysplasia accompanying TH also needs to be included. Reviewing our own series of 74 cases of TH and trying to classify them we soon realized that none of the existing classifications allowed a precise separation of a large spectrum of abnormalities. It seems more realistic at the time of surgical treatment to rely on a clinical assessment of each anatomical component of the thumb. Even intra-operative exploration is sometimes necessary to take a more precise decision.

General classification

In the IFSSH (International Federation of Societies for Surgery of the Hand) classification,

Table 1 Syndromes with short thumb

Edwards, 18q-, Aarkog-Scott, triploïdy, Apert, Carpenter, Pfeiffer, F-syndrome, Ashley, Christian brachydactyly, brachydactyly A1/C/D, cryptogenetic brachymetacarpalia, Cornelia Delange, diastrophic dysplasia, Duane, fibrodysplasia ossificans, hand-foot-uterus, Larsen, Tabaznik, Taybi-Linder, TAR, WL, WT, acro-pectoro-vertebral, Temtamy-Okihi, Temtamy-Meguid, BOD, Di George, Cooks, Richieri-Costas, Khalifa-Graham, Vilgoen-Kallis, Brunner-Winter, cheirolumbar dysostosis, Robinow

category 5 is hypoplasia but thumb is not mentioned. The majority of cases belong to category 1 or lack of formation either longitudinal or transversal (Table 2).

In *longitudinal radial deficiency*, the carpus and radius are frequently involved (Hall et al 1986) and thumb hypoplasia or aplasia is such a constant feature of the so-called radial club hand that a normal thumb evoked a special syndrome (thrombocytopenia with absent radii [TAR] syndrome).

In case of radial deficiency, a syndrome has always to be looked for, involving numerous organs and systems (haematopoietic, cardiac, gastro-intestinal, ophthalmic, otic, facial, skeletal, genito-urinary, spinal etc.; Table 3). Carroll and Louis (1974) in their review of 53 patients found that 77% had such an association, mainly in bilateral deficiency with 43% having gastro-intestinal localization, and 61% skeletal, but very few situated in the lower limb. This fact had already been stressed by Kato (1924), who found a single case of tibial aplasia in 253 reviewed cases. Such associations can occasionally be seen in syndromes like Roberts syndrome, VACTERL

Table 2 Classification of the IFSSH (modified from Swanson 1976, 1983) outlining only the categories with thumb hypoplasia

I   Failure of formation of parts (arrest of development)
    A   Transverse arrest
       7   Metacarpal (adactylia)
       8   Phalanx
    B   Longitudinal arrest
       I   Radial longitudinal
       II Ulnar ray deficiency
       6   absent / hypoplastic hypothenar muscles
       7   absent / hypoplastic extensor tendons
       8   absent / hypoplastic flexor tendons
II Failure of differentiation of parts
    A   Soft tissue involvement
       1   Disseminated
          a. Arthrogryposis
       4   Wrist and hand
          c. Thumb-in-palm
          d. Wind blow hand
    B   Skeletal involvement
       4   Wrist and hand
          a. Osseous syndactyly: mitten (Apert)
          b. Symphalangism: PIP, other
          c. Hypersegmentation: triphalangeal thumb, others
       5   Skeletal
          a. Osteochondromatosis (Bessel Hagen)
          c. Fibrous dysplasia
          d. Epiphyseal anomalies
          e. Other
III Duplication
       3   Radial segment
V   Undergrowth
       3   Hand alone: entire or partial
       3   Metacarpal
       4   Digit
          a. Brachysyndactyly
          b. Brachydactyly
VI Congenital constriction syndrome
VII Generalized skeletal abnormalities
    A   chromosomal

Table 3 TH part of a syndrome

Holt-Oram, VACTERL association, Blackfan-Diamond, thalidomide embryopathie, Nager, Goldenhar, Juberg Hayward, Levy-Hollister (LARD), Fanconi, Aase-Smith, Ives Houston, IVIC, Roberts, Rothmund Thomson, Say trisomy 18, Gerald, Cornelia Delange, acro-renal-ocular, Smith-Lemi-Opitz, Haas-Ofodile, Baller-Gerold, Sommer-Hines, Lewis, Keutel-Kindermann, radial malformation and Duane syndrome

and it is useful to mention that Manske and McCarroll (1995) have separated the group III in two sub-groups, A and B, according to the presence or absence of the first carpometacarpal joint (FCMCJ); Buck-Gramcko (1981) has even proposed to add a group IIIC when only the metacarpal head is present. In fact type IIIA corresponds to type II of Blauth (1967) and the latter did not separate intrinsic from extrinsic muscle involvement. Such successive modifications are explained by the difficulty of separation between the different types since many clinical cases show 'transitional' aspects. When the 'splitters' were unsuccessful, the 'groupers' had a go.

Table 4 Classification according to Muller (1937) and Blauth (1967)

TI	Slimness with thenar muscle hypoplasia
TII	Adducted thumb with thenar hypoplasia and occasionally MPJ laxity/joint dysplasia
TIII	Partial aplasia of the first metacarpal; thenar muscles nearly absent; severe abnormalities of muscles
TIV	First metacarpal absent with 'pouce flottant'
TV	Thumb aplasia

Table 5 Modified classification of Muller and Blauth by Buck-Gramcko and Manske

Type I	Minimal thumb hypoplasia
Type II	First web insufficiency, MPJ instability, thenar eminence muscle hypoplasia
Type IIIA	Same abnormalities as in type II, plus extrinsic muscles hypoplasia and slender first metacarpal bone
Type IIIB	In addition to IIIA abnomalies, absent first carpometacarpal joint
Type IV	Floating thumb
Type V	Absent thumb

association, and thalidomide embryopathy. Genetic study is mandatory in such cases and if isolated TH is mainly sporadic some syndromes have definite heredity (e.g. Holt-Oram, Fanconi). James et al (2001) have also demonstrated some proportionality between radius insufficiency and TH. Different types of TH have been described by Blauth (1967; Table 4) but many successive modifications have been proposed. The one described by Buck-Gramcko (1981) is the most frequently cited (Table 5).

Chapter 7 discusses some aspects concerning metacarpophalangeal joint (MPJ) instability (and the separation in type IIA and IIB [Smith 2000])

Thumb hypoplasia can also be seen associated with *longitudinal ulnar deficiency* and Cole and Manske (1997) put forward proposals to classify the hand aspects according to the first web. However, apart from first web involvement, the thumb can demonstrate a lack of opposition and/or pronation secondary to thenar muscle hypoplasia and in some cases a clear improvement after simple first web reconstruction led us to hypothesize that muscle hypoplasia could be secondary to lack of muscle development and that the insufficient pronation could also be due to the limited range of carpometacarpal joint (CMCJ) motion not allowing 'automatic' pronation which exists only in full opposition.

Thumb hypoplasia is also a frequent element of *transverse deficiency*. In such cases, the thumb could be reduced in length, presenting with only a proximal phalanx sometimes combined with hypoplasia of the thenar eminence. This aspect has to be distinguished from amniotic band syndrome where a true 'distal' amputation exists and the proximal anatomical structures do not show real hypoplasia. Recently IFSSH classification was modified by the International Committee to include symbrachydactyly, a spectrum of disorders that has long been recognized in German and Japanese literature (Manske 1993), after the descriptions by Müller (1937) and Blauth and Gekeler (1973). Many modifications were also provided (Ogino et al 1989) and we have put forward proposals (Foucher et al 2000a) for a further two separate groups in monodactyly type, calling them IIIB and IIIA, according to the absence or presence of first phalanx hypoplasia (brachymesophalangy) which is accompanied by instability of the thumb. But many other aspects of TH are present in symbrachydactyly: symphalangism, MPJ instability, clinodactyly, and thenar muscle hypoplasia.

Other categories of conditions can present with some forms of TH. *Radial polydactyly* (category 3) will not be discussed here but hypoplasia is a frequent or quite constant feature with reduced thumb size, nail hypoplasia, and thenar hypoplasia. Some dysplasia, like pollex abductus, that are frequently found in TH are also encountered in radial polydactyly (Lister 1991a).

The so-called *thumb-in-palm* or clench thumb can also present some hypoplasia of structures other than the extensor pollicis brevis. Weckesser (1955) proposed a classification, separating stiff from supple thumb-in-palm, and two other groups that were quite ill defined including Freeman Sheldon syndrome or orotalar syndrome and arthrogryposis. If in the first two groups hypoplasia or aplasia of the extensor pollicis longus were found more frequently, the two other groups would be entirely separate entities. When a child is seen early, a trial of orthosis worn constantly from the third month to the sixth and then only at night (to allow for normal development), has demonstrated that hypoplasia is more frequent than aplasia and that all the other components seen in late cases are secondary and can be avoided. Even in stiff cases, splinting has allowed us to avoid complex surgery, but we found that aplasia is more frequent in this group, leading to tendon transfer—perhaps such aplasia occurring early in foetal development could explain the difference in presentation.

Central deficiency can also show some aspects of TH, and not only be limited to first web insufficiency and some thumbs demonstrate a mixed appearance of *triphalangeal thumb* and TH. According to the classification by Buck-Gramcko (1998a), type IV and V could be considered in TH (Table 6), however many authors prefer to isolate type IV as a 'true' five fingered hand, and type V (as recognized by Tajima 1985), presents hypoplastic skeletal elements, joint instability, absent intrinsic muscles, rudimentary and inefficient extrinsics (with no active motion) and

Table 6 Classification of triphalangeal thumb according to Buck-Gramcko (1988a)

Type 1	Rudimentary phalanx, normal MP and CMC, normal thenar, normal length
Type 2	Short triangular; normal MP and CMC, normal thenar, ulnar more than radial deviation
Type 3	Larger transitional bone normal MP and CMC, no palmar abduction, supinated, tight first web, longer
Type 4	Long rectangular bone, restricted MP and CMC joints, very long, hypoplastic or absent thenar, deficient web, metacarpal hypoplastic, radial carpal hypoplastic
Type 5	Hypoplastic thumb, small phalanges, syndactyly with DII, association to radial dysplasia, normal joints, absent or hypoplastic thenar
Type 6	Associated to thumb duplication

Table 7 Classification of Tajima (1985)

TI	First ray aplasia
TII	Short first metacarpal or phalanx
TIII	Annular band with thumb amputation
TIV	Floating thumb
TV	TH adducted with hypoplasia/absence of thenar muscles
TVI	TH with five fingered hand
TVII	TH with cleft hand
TVIII	TH associated to radial polydactyly

frequently partial syndactyly and variable metacarpal epiphysis, sometimes with two plates (one proximal and one distal).

Finally, short or slender thumbs are frequently part of category 7 of complex syndromes (Tables 1 and 2) but in some cases, like diastrophic dwarfism, instability of the thumb due to hypoplastic ligaments needs some surgical reconstruction—no different than in other aspects of TH. Tajima (1985) did include in his classification some of the aspects already discussed (Table 7) but again it remains incomplete and we think that the best guide for surgical reconstruction is a careful clinical assessment of each anatomical structure of the thumb including: skin (skin envelope and first web), nail, joints (MPJ instability with hypoplastic ligaments, or interphalangeal joint (IPJ) symphalangism or CMCJ instability or hypoplasia), extrinsic tendons (extensor, flexor), intrinsic muscles (thenar muscles) and bone (distal defect, intercalated defect-brachymesophalangy-proximal metacarpal defect). Some of these elements have an aesthetic component (nail, thumb diameter) but the majority have a functional impact and frequently need surgical correction.

The true assessment is not always easy clinically and for example it is difficult to separate IP symphalangism from aplasia or dysplasia of the flexor pollicis longus (FPL) as some stiffness is not rare in flexor hypoplasia; indeed radiographic aspects in a young child do not always allow a clear distinction and clinical presentation is identical with absent dorsal and palmar creases. In such cases, we routinely perform a trial of dynamic splinting in flexion of the IPJ, but in cases of symphalangism we have found splinting useless. In FPL hypoplasia, active flexion could develop and in cases of dysplasia, passive flexion improves opening the possibility to

discuss surgical reconstruction with the patient and relatives. However, in most cases the full assessment is only obtained during surgery. We will discuss each surgical anatomical correction but the real issue is frequently to decide between amputation and pollicization or step-by-step reconstruction.

Joint hypoplasia

We have already discussed the differential diagnosis with instability due to brachymesophalangy. Here, we will discuss the IPJ, MPJ, and FCMCJ. We have not encountered instability at the IPJ but sometimes symphalangism. As already mentioned, absence of skin creases could also happen in cases of abnormal flexor pollicis longus (FPL). In cases of symphalangism, radiographical fusion is a late finding. To our knowledge, surgical correction has not been attempted at this level (contrary to the isolated long finger) mainly due to excellent compensation by the MPJ and FCMCJ. We have not found splinting in flexion successful and we use it more as a test to distinguish it from abnormal FPL.

At the MPJ level it is important to separate joint instability and instability due brachymesophalangy in symbrachydactyly. Radiographic distinction is relatively easy. We have encountered instability in longitudinal thumb hypoplasia and, less frequently, in symbrachydactyly. It could be unidirectional with insufficiency of the ulnar collateral ligament or multi-directional. When unidirectional, ligamentoplasty and capsulodesis could be sufficient. Ligamentoplasty could use the distal part of the opposition transfer. The most classical technique is the use of the flexor superficialis (FS) passed through holes. Su et al (1972) described a technique with two transverse tunnels in the distal part of the metacarpal and the proximal part of the first phalanx, to introduce the two slips of the FCS. Lister (1985) modified this technique by introducing the whole FS into the distal part of the first metacarpal and then either sutured it to the base of the first phalanx or, more securely, through a transverse canal taking care not to injure the epiphysis. Such a technique is contraindicated in cases of very slender metacarpal bone. Even when using the adductor digiti minimi (ADM) for opposition, proximal liberation of the muscle and more extensive distal harvesting allow for the tendon to be used to reinforce the ulnar collateral ligament. If the opposition is normal a free tendon graft or a capsulodesis is used. The capsular tissue on the ulnar side of the MPJ is variable; in some late cases the laxity is secondary to a tight first web but more frequently in our experience the tissue is hypoplastic but sufficient to be cut and sutured like a vest-over-pants.

When multi-directional, chondrodesis is an alternative but Manske said that it remains unpredictable. He described 'epiphyseal arthrodesis' (Kowalski and Manske 1988), carefully shaving the base of the first phalanx until the ossific nucleus is reached. The procedure was successful in 94% of the cases and is possible as soon as the x-rays show an ossification centre (2–4 years of age). In none of Manske's cases or in our experience has such a procedure interfered with growth. Finally classical arthrodesis is used when the patient is seen later, at the end of growth.

First carpometacarpal joint instability has not been frequently mentioned in the literature but we have seen it, not infrequently, as part of longitudinal hypoplasia. Two types deserve a special mention. The first is in so-called type II and IIIA, where the metacarpal is a bit slender but an FCMCJ is clearly seen in an adolescent. Laxity is perceived at palpation but also at simple inspection—a bump appearing in opposition. In two of our cases (patients aged 10–13 years) it was painful (Foucher et al 1999, 2000a–c). In one of these cases the pain was triggered by a flexor superficialis opposition transfer and the use of such a powerful muscle is contraindicated in cases of laxity since it creates a longitudinal force that could fail to compensate for any existing laxity. The second type is usually diagnosed much later and unveiled by an x-ray performed for FCMCJ pain in a young adult. On the anteroposterior view, a hypoplastic trapezium is seen with a tendency for metacarpal subluxation. It is important to recognize this clinical aspect since ligamentoplasty is usually insufficient and opening osteotomy at the trapezium level in these cases is a better option. We will discuss the replacement of this joint and base of the first metacarpal in the bone section.

One last point regarding a quite rare condition—the 'duck neck' deformity with hyperextension of the MPJ and secondary flexion of the IPJ. Contrary to Kobayashi et al (1976) who found a retracted extensor pollicis longus, we have operated on two children where we found a hypoplastic volar plate and managed to entirely reduce the deformity from the palmar aspect with a palmar capsulodesis.

Bone hypoplasia

Three types of bone hypoplasia can be discussed: longitudinal hypoplasia as seen in so-called type IIIB, transverse hypoplasia either distal (transverse deficiency), or intercalated deficiency as seen in brachymesophalangy (type IIIB of symbrachydactyly). Treatment options are quite different. In cases where the thumb is reduced to a first phalanx, function could be good enough when the FCMCJ and the opposition are normal. However, this condition is sometimes accompanied by the absence of a long finger and in some cases toe transfer is more useful for finger reconstruction. In our experience, due to limited flexion of the transferred toe, a longer thumb is sometimes necessary to obtain or maintain a good pinch during growth. It is rarely necessary to use a microsurgical toe transfer but three techniques are useful. The 'on-top plasty' consisting of the transfer in an island of an index stump, which allows thumb lengthening and first web deepening. Distraction lengthening (Kessler et al 1977, Foucher et al 2001a) performed either at the metacarpal (with secondary web deepening) or at the phalangeal level permits a limited additional length. It is out of the scope of this chapter to describe the technique but callostasis could be used, avoiding secondary bone graft. In cases of a thumb reduced to a segment of first phalanx with a skin pouch, transfer of a non-vascularized phalanx from a lesser toe, including the periosteum and the ligaments, could provide a sufficient length with some (but limited) growth potential (and mobility) if performed early. As a secondary measure, a distraction lengthening could be performed through the transferred phalanx (or the metacarpal) in case of insufficient growth.

In brachymesophalangy of the thumb, the instability of the first ray is a major functional issue. We have mainly encountered this problem in symbrachydactyly. The simplest technique is a non-vascularized transfer of a toe phalanx. However we found this technique unsatisfactory in some instances due to insufficient growth (Foucher 1997). This is also true in monodigital types (type IIIB) where a second toe is used for finger reconstruction. In two of our cases the patients lost the ability to pinch early on due to discrepancies in growth; the thumb becoming too short to join the tip of the toe. In such cases we favour the transfer of a vascularized epiphysis to keep the pace of growth (Foucher et al 2001c). In type IIB, with very hypoplastic fingers (without metacarpal support), a unique opportunity exists whereby one of the 'floating' fingers (usually the index) can be transferred whilst preserving the feeding artery. This quite demanding technique has the advantage of increasing the 'web', whilst at the same time providing thumb stability and some growth potential as demonstrated in our two clinical cases.

Finally a more controversial area is the reconstruction of longitudinal hypoplasia (Manske type IIIB). In such cases not only is the FCMCJ missing but also some carpal bones are hypoplastic or absent, namely the scaphoid and trapezium—the trapezoid is usually present. A distal implantation of the thumb is sometimes noticeable as well as some narrowing at the attachment level. There is little doubt that amputation followed by pollicization remains the best technique but there are two circumstances where an alternative should be considered. These alternatives can be a bone graft with no growth potential and no mobility, a non-vascularized metatarsophalangeal (MTPJ) transfer with limited growth (Tajima 1998) and some mobility, or a free-vascularized MTPJ compound transfer providing a skin flap, some tendons, and vascularized epiphysis. Yamauchi and colleagues (1979) seem to have published the first details of such a microsurgical technique. The MTPJ appears to be used the most, but Nishijima et al (1995) have used the proximal interphalangeal joint (PIPJ) of the toe. We have described our technique elsewhere (Foucher 1988, 1999, 2001c) so only a few technical points will be mentioned here.

The interposed metatarsophalangeal segment is difficult to position as well as the cutaneous flap. There is little risk of any distal Z deformity due to stiffness of the IPJ and the frequent

necessity for MPJ stabilization by chondrodesis, epiphyseal arthrodesis or classical arthrodesis. The position then has to be selected based on the sector of mobility in the MTPJ, which is demonstrated more in hyperextension than in flexion; in this position the lateral ligaments are relaxed allowing for some lateral motion mimicking the movement of circumduction. It seems logical to fix the joint at the recipient site, in such a position that flexion allows for pulp contact with the index finger and hyperextension allows abduction (and limited added pronation). It is not easy to interpose a sufficiently long segment without some collapse deformity of the intercalated joint, but it is possible to first increase the space using distraction lengthening. Our experience of five clinical cases with a long follow-up (up to 13 years) has been useful in decision-making (Foucher et al 1999, 2001b,c). In three of these cases the relatives had definitely refused pollicization despite 'doctor shopping' and we felt that there was no reason to punish the baby because of the parental decision. In these cases, we performed microsurgical reconstruction early as a first step, followed by operations to provide MPJ stability, sufficient first web, intrinsic, and extrinsic function.

The main conclusions are that first, the potential growth of the existing thumb is unpredictable and in one case the pinch was lost during growth and relatives had to be advised that a secondary distraction lengthening procedure would be necessary. Second, despite early operations (mean age 13 months), based on the modern conception of brain remodelling, integration in fine pinch was never obtained and if the thumb was used in grasping large objects, fine manipulation was maintained for the most part by the index and middle finger (with some rotation of these fingers). The other cases were performed at the request of patients (aged 13 and 11) who had some use of their unstable but quite well developed thumbs. Postoperatively, both showed improvement in their grasp function and continued to use the index and middle fingers for fine manipulation. Our conclusion is that early operations are not advisable, since they do not allow the patient to integrate the thumb in fine pinch and growth potential remains unpredictable. However there is a place for such reconstruction in the case of young patients asking for reconstruction when the thumb is sufficiently

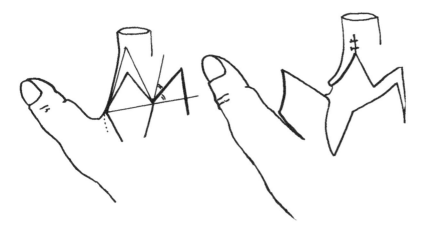

Figure 1

Illustration of the kite flap consisting in a pseudo-island, centred on the first dorsal metacarpal artery. The donor site is closed by an LLL Dufourmentel plasty.

developed and not cortically excluded. The patient has to be told that it is a multi-stage operation but two stages are usually enough for such a reconstruction. Our conclusions are then different than the ones proposed recently by Shibata et al (1998) but there is no doubt that culture has a definite bearing in such a decision and acceptance.

First web insufficiency

First web insufficiency is frequently present in congenital conditions. We do not consider its presence as a factor for inclusion in TH but it is frequently associated to longitudinal deficiency (radial, ulnar and central), symbrachydactyly, amniotic band syndrome, and thumb-in-palm, and in some cases, when seen late, it is a factor of secondary ulnar ligament laxity. Early correction is mandatory and frequently performed during the full correction of the disorder.

The surgical technique is composed of two steps; first web liberation and then covering by some sort of skin graft or flap. Liberation means cutting any abnormal bands (like the pseudo-intermetacarpal ligament [Lösch and Schrader 1978] or musculus lumbricalis pollicis [Lister 1991b]), aponeuroses of the adductor and first dorsal interosseous muscles and if necessary, partial de-insertion of these muscles. We prefer to free the adductor from its second (and if

necessary third) metacarpal and the first dorsal interosseous from the first metacarpal, so avoiding any transection of the muscles (Matev 1970). Skin grafting after such liberation is limited, but some full-thickness skin grafting could be combined with a flap. We do not believe that there is any specific 'favoured' flap to use (Foucher et al 2000b), or that one technique is the answer to an array of problems (Friedman and Wood 1997). We have compared the different techniques available (Table 6 and Fig. 1) and found that each flap has its own specific range of lengthening of the web fold and/or deepening of the web. Building an absent web (thumb-index syndactyly) is not the same as improving an existing one. Among the more useful flaps are include the four-flap Z-plasty described by Limberg (Lister and Gibson 1972) and popularized by Woolf and Broadbent (1972); this flap lengthens (164% with angles of 120°) more than deepens an existing and moderately deficient web. Ostrowski's flap (Ostrowski et al 1998) combines a rectangular flap on one side and two triangular flaps on the other and is mainly useful to deepen an existing web since it does not provide much lengthening of the fold. To create a web we found that two flaps are useful: the Tajima (1965) and Buck-Gramcko's flap (1998b) which is designed around a huge rotation flap from the dorsum of the hand. With suturing of the donor site limited deepening is obtained (Buck-Gramcko 1998b) but deepening could be provided by inserting full-thickness skin grafts on the ulnar aspect of the thumb and radial aspect of the index (Tajima 1965).

We have given up the use of a rotation flap from the dorsum of the hand (Flatt and Wood 1970) or index (Friedman and Wood 1997, Spinner 1969, Strauch 1975) and we think that a rotation flap from the dorsum of the thumb (Sandzen 1982) is contraindicated in cases of hypoplasia—both result in a conspicuous dorsal skin graft. We have described a technique called the 'pseudo-kite' flap (Fig. 1), which allows harvesting a losengic flap from the dorso-radial aspect of the index finger (Foucher et al 1992, 2001b). This axial-patterned flap contains the first dorsal metatarsal artery (Foucher and Braun 1979), which allows us to cut a narrow skin pedicle facilitating the rotation. The donor area is closed by a Dufourmentel 'LLL' flap (a modification of the Limberg design) (Dufourmentel 1962). Such a flap creates a web by covering the tetrahedral space opened through the first web liberation.

Other flaps could also be used mainly in case of failure of a previous flap with some scar tissue like the four and five flap Z-plasty (Hirshowitz et al 1975, Shaw et al 1973) or the Caroli's flap (Caroli and Zanasi 1989). We have never used tissue expansion or distant flaps in TH. Finally we often select a flap from an otherwise discarded part (radial duplication, central cleft) to provide a surgical approach for the different steps of the operation, without an additional scar. Translocation, and ray resection have also in some cases, improved the first web. The insertion of Kirschner wires (K-wires) to maintain the opening of the first web is optional and we prefer to avoid it, since removal is frightening for the babies. Dressing is frequently enough to maintain an open web space.

Extrinsic tendon hypoplasia (or dysplasia)

Extrinsic muscles and tendons are frequently hypoplastic, dysplastic or absent in TH. The condition is not unique to radial deficiency and could be isolated (in the absence of FPL or extensor pollicis brevis [Arminio 1979, DeHaan et al 1987, Koster 1984, Nakamura and Kubo 1993, Strauch and Spinner 1976, Tsuchida et al 1976]),

or associated to other conditions (ulnar deficiency and triphalangeal thumb). Some could argue about integrating isolated, absent or dysplastic FPL in TH but there is always Miura's (1981) case about a boy whose father presented a hypoplastic thumb with thenar hypoplasia.

Deficient FPL is frequently associated with other conditions such as absent thenar muscles, absent abductor pollicis longus (Neviaser 1979), MPJ instability, first web deficiency, and absent extensor pollicis), but it is also encountered as an isolated condition. Uchida et al (1985) put forward proposals to classify the disorder in two groups, separating those with and without thenar muscle hypoplasia. In the second group three sub-groups were identified: absent FPL, abnormal insertion to the transverse carpal ligament and abnormal connexion (pollex abductus [Fitch et al 1984, Lister 1991a, Tupper 1969]). In the group with muscle hypoplasia, the FPL could be absent or malpositioned (radial course, perforating the flexor retinacular ligament [Blair and Buckwalter 1983, Blair and Omer 1981]). Wood (personal communication 1996) has proposed a more extensive classification (Table 8). It is clinically difficult to separate the different types. Simple inspection demonstrates the absence of dorsal, as well as palmar creases. Some IPJ stiffness is frequently associated as relatives sometimes discover the condition at a later stage. Night splinting in flexion is useful as passive motion is frequently provided after a few months. In our series of 11 cases, three patients recovered a mean 35° of active mobility indicating that simple hypoplasia could occur and

Table 8 Classification of thumb dysplasia according to Wood (presented at the CHASG meeting)

Type 1	Absent FPL without hypoplasia of any other muscles
Type 2	Absent FPL with absent flexor pollicis brevis (Tsushida)
Type 3	Absent FPL with absent median innervated muscles (Dellon)
Type 4	Absent FPL with absent median innervated muscles and one absent neurovascular bundle
Type 5	Abnormal insertion of FPL
Type 6	Intact FPL with absent thenar muscles
Type 7	Intact FPL with absent thenar muscles and fixed adduction or abduction contracture
Type 8	Isolated unstable MPJ

spontaneously improve when strength to overcome joint stiffness (or underdevelopment) is decreased. Four patients did not wear the orthosis, two dropped out early in the programme and the remaining two achieved 30° of passive flexion but no active motion—relatives refused the offered surgical tendon reconstruction.

Some anecdotal cases of FPL reconstruction have been published with interesting results, such as section of abnormal insertion (Miura 1981), rerouting of the hypoplastic tendon (with an acceptable course [Blair and Buckwalter 1983]), and tendon transfers have been occasionally tried (Neal and Burke 2001) with variable but globally limited success. The last procedure encompasses a two-stage operation: the first step being the insertion of a silastic rod with pulley reconstruction and the second step being the insertion of the flexor superficialis of a long finger (usually the fourth). Ezaki (1996) prefers to insert a tendon graft and motorize it by sharing the flexor profundus of the index, but concluded that 'no treatment is indicated in the majority of these cases'. Traumatic FPL losses have extensively demonstrated that the loss is perfectly tolerated and partially compensated by MPJ flexion. We agree but we think that, mainly when hypoplasia of thenar muscles needs surgery, exploration of the FPL is worthwhile when IPJ has a passive range of motion exceeding 30°, and as in a few cases, liberation of abnormal insertion has provided some improvement. Even if the levels of abnormalities are multiple, traction through transverse incisions is helpful.

In radial insufficiency the problem is frequently associated to other conditions as in the so-called type IIIA where the MPJ is unstable, the first web insufficient, and the intrinsic and extensor are hypoplastic. Extensive dissection by Graham and Louis (1998) has proved that many adherences, abnormal insertions, and abnormal muscles could be found. In case of pollex abductus (Fitch et al 1984, Tupper 1969, Lister 1991a), a radial tilt of the thumb could sometimes be seen when attempting flexion and skin creases are absent. Surgery shows a band extending from the FPL to the extensor pollicis longus on the radial aspect of the thumb but resection is disappointing for flexion (and extension) recovery since the malformation is extensive with radial luxation of the FPL, absence or incompetent pulleys, abnor-

mal insertions more proximally, and abnormal or absent muscle. In our experience resection of the band as proposed by Tupper (1969) and Lister (1991a) was frequently insufficient to provide IPJ active mobility. We have not attempted any reconstruction of the FPL in such cases and it is not clear that even when combined with extensor pollicis longus (EPL) reconstruction that some flexion attitude could be prevented. We have not performed extensive dissection in our cases but in the nine cases with pollex abductus, six had no excursion when pulling proximally on the tendon. If there is some excursion, the tendon is best used as a transfer to reinforce opposition. In Tupper's series of four cases (Tupper 1969) and Lister's 11 cases (35.5% of type II TH, Lister 1991a) a mean range of 19.5° and 21° were obtained. In six cases Lister found an association with the musculus lumbricalis pollicis. The best results were reported by Fitch et al (1984) with three cases obtaining 45–50° of IPJ range of active motion. Again the result will be inversely proportional to the importance of the TH and when extensors are also hypoplastic such results could not be obtained as, even passively, the IPJ is quite stiff (Ezaki 1996).

Isolated hypoplasia or absence of extensor pollicis brevis (EPB) associated or not to EPL, is not a frequent congenital condition. It could be associated to some TH and McCarroll (1985) regularly found a gross laxity of the ulnar collateral ligament in fixed clasped thumb, which if not treated leads to the classical full-blown aspect of the thumb-in-palm condition with retraction of palmar thumb skin, first web retraction, and MPJ stiffness. However we have been impressed by the results of early splinting, proving that all the preceding signs are more often secondary and that hypoplasia of EPB is more frequent than aplasia. Indeed in a series of 11 patients seen in the first six months of life (thumb-in-palm is a physiologic position up until three months), splinting in extension was used either dynamically in cases of some MPJ stiffness or, more frequently, statically in cases of good passive extension. Ten cases including two patients with some stiffness on one side recovered full active extension after a mean delay of five months. The work of Crawford et al (1966) and later Miura's cases (2000) could explain the success rates of these findings; Muira (2000) stressed that in his series of 23 operated cases, none had an absent tendon. In our series of early splinting, only one case needed surgery on a supple thumb and absence of both extensors was proved at operation; an extensor indicis proprius (EIP) was transferred in this case but the surgeon (and the relatives) has to be prepared for the fact that this transfer may not be available and that another type of transfer may be necessary (Crawford et al 1966). In their anatomical study of the EPB, Dawson and Barton (1986) found frequent variations with only three of 16 dissections showing a classical aspect; the muscle was entirely absent in only one case. Few cases of absence of EPL have been published and such a condition could go unnoticed unless unveiled by a lesion of the EPB (Kobayashi et al 1976).

In four cases of radial longitudinal deficiency with a hypoplastic thumb maintained in flexed position that we ourselves have experienced, a transfer of the EIP resulted in more improvement in the position than in the range of motion due to poor FPL excursion. Reconstruction of extrinsic muscles in radial longitudinal deficiency remains for us, a surgical challenge with limited expectations for the patient.

Intrinsic muscle hypoplasia

Surprisingly in our series of 62 surgically explored cases of TH (excluding longitudinal deficiency Blauth type IV and V) we encountered only 12 cases where the adductor pollicis was absent. We have never attempted any reconstruction of this muscle and there is little in the literature about this special issue, whereas thenar eminence hypoplasia or aplasia is a well-covered subject with plenty of information on surgical correction. It must be noted however, with respect to clinical aspects of thenar hypoplasia, that even in cases of apparent muscle absence, good opposition can exist (through the superficial head of the flexor pollicis brevis) and usually only good pronation is missing. In such cases a pronation osteotomy is sufficient as strength is not necessary for opposition. Early articles have stressed that only median innervated muscles are absent in discrete TH (Su et al 1972). Another clinical problem is the apparent atrophy of the thenar eminence combined with a deficient first web, for example in a longitudinal ulnar deficiency. In some cases, surgical exploration has demonstrated the presence of the thenar muscle and we have found that first web improvement is the only operation needed—the muscles developing later on and the pronation improving by more ample motion at the FCMCJ.

Transfer of the adductor digiti quinti (ADQ) (Huber 1921) provides the best functional and aesthetic reconstruction for opposition. With careful dissection of this muscle, as elegantly explained by Littler and Cooley (1963), intrinsic muscles can be replaced 'by intrinsic muscle of similar excursion with adequate power transmitted directly, without intervening pulley or gliding tendon'. This muscle could be transferred to the dorsum of the first phalanx of the thumb to provide opposition (and pronation). Some technical points are worth noting however, such as the necessity to lift some of the distal extension (from the extensor aponeurosis), careful dissection of the proximal neurovascular pedicle, turning the muscle like a page to avoid twisting, and ensuring an ample subcutaneous tissue channel to accommodate the muscle bulk. Dissection could be more problematic when the ADQ has a common origin with the flexor digiti quinti. A simultaneous correction of the ulnar ligament insufficiency is necessary, but even after such a procedure careful patients follow-up is important since secondary deformities could occur (Wood and Skie 1997). Manske and McCarroll (1978) use both distal insertion transferring the aponeurosis expansion to the ulnar side to reinforce the ligament and Ogino et al (1986) have proposed a modification with proximal detachment of the muscle and fixation to the palmaris longus to improve appearance but at the risk of some traction on the pedicle. Reduction of digiti quinti abduction is minimal thanks to the compensation by extensors.

Many other types of opposition transfer could be performed and we have already mentioned the use of a flexor superficialis, which also allows for reconstruction of a strong ulnar MPJ ligament as already mentioned. Lister (1985) used the classical strip of flexor carpi ulnaris to reroute the tendon at the wrist level and Ezaki (1996) used a window in the transverse carpal ligament.

Pollicization

If everybody agrees on the benefit of pollicization in cases of thumb aplasia, its place in hypoplasia will remain controversial. The technical aspects of this operation (Littler 1952) are not discussed extensively here, but some data concerning its functional results are useful when making comparisons with reconstruction techniques.

Concerning the timing of such an operation—there are advantages and drawbacks for early versus late operation (Table 9). The pattern of pinch between the thumb and index develops at around 12 months but continues to improve in precision until about two years of age. Buck-Gramcko (1971) has championed an early operation stressing a better joint adaptation (of the new FCMCJ and the hypertrophy of the thenar muscle)—a policy that has been endorsed by the majority of surgeons in the field (Lister 1985, Ezaki 1996, Foucher et al 2000c) but Manske et al (1985, 1992) were not able to demonstrate any superiority in their results. The possibility of a syndrome (i.e. Fanconi anaemia, VACTERL, Holt Oram) or the associated radial club hand could delay pollicization. Some relatives could be reluctant to proceed with pollicization in presence of a TH at an early stage, but can be more easy to convince when the scissoring (due to index pronation) and the widening of the

Table 9 Advantages and drawbacks of early versus late correction of a congenital condition

Drawbacks
- Cardiopulmonary system development (1Y)
- Immune system (6 months)
- Embryogenic endosteal circulation involution (1Y)
- Surgical ease (size of structures, microsurgery, spasm and fat)
- Anaesthetic ease (easy drop in temperature, small body mass with higher anaesthetic concentration gas, lack of cardiac and pulmonary reserves, small size and irritability of the airway)
- Scar hypertrophy
- Cooperation (assessment, dressing, rehabilitation)

Advantages
- Brain integration (fine pinch 1Y)
- Growth remodelling (joint, muscles)
- Decreased parental distress

second space begin to be more obvious, secondary to the index-middle finger pinching habit.

Littler (1952) has covered the major steps. After skin incision we begin by carefully dissecting the palmar artery and nerves, allowing some time for the blood to fill the dorsal veins that were allowed to empty by partial exsanguination. A radial artery of the index finger, sometimes small in diameter, is present in the majority of cases and a Hartmann's boutonnière is often found in the 'second' space, one nerve forming a ring around the artery. Endoneurolysis avoids kinking of the vessel after the middle finger radial artery has been sacrificed. The intrinsic muscles are prepared, freeing the shaft of the second metacarpal. A proximal oblique bone section allows for the area to be prepared for fixing the new FCMCJ, while at the same time, preserving the insertions of the extensors and flexors of the wrist. The metacarpal is then cut through the distal epiphysis (with careful curettage of the growing plate) and discarded. Buck-Gramcko (1971) stressed the necessity of fixing the MPJ of the index in hyperextension to avoid a distal 'Z' deformity with flexion of the previous PIPJ. This has the added advantage of relaxing the lateral ligaments and so providing some lateral motion, mimicking circumduction. The head is fixed using a single absorbable stitch to the remaining second metacarpal proximal metaphysis. We have never encountered any proximal instability of the thumb. This technique allows us to precisely balance the thumb position using the tendon transfers alone and negates the need for a temporary K-wire, which artificially maintains it for a few weeks, and then needs removal. Ideally the thumb should be positioned in front of the middle finger, with full extension of the new MP and IPJ, and with full opening of the web with around 120° of pronation and 40° of abduction. The first palmar interosseous is used as an abductor pollicis brevis (sometimes reinforced by some remnants of thenar muscles) and the first dorsal as an adductor and fixation to a prepared band of the extensor hood at the new MPJ level is the best way to secure them with the appropriate tension. The extensor indicis proprius (not always present) is used as an abductor (and fixed dorso-ulnar to avoid supination of the thumb) and the extensor communis is simply freed from junctura and shortened. The majority of surgeons do not shorten the flexors (which adapt in some six months) but find opening of the A1 and part of the A2 pulleys to be useful. Due to excellent adaptation Manske et al (1992) do not always shorten the extensors and Zancolli (personal communication 1982) does not shorten the intrinsics either. To maintain the desired position at the end of the operation, we use a drop of strong glue to solidify the pulp of the new thumb to the one of the middle finger maintained in the intrinsic position with full abduction. We have tried quite a few of the incisions described in the literature but none result in a really physiologic web fold without visible dorsal incision. We prefer to have a huge dorsal flap to facilitate full opposition and decrease the amount of dorsal scar at the web level and for this purpose we have modified the Buck-Gramcko incisions. We agree with Lister (1985) that the web fold has to join the previous PIPJ.

This technique sometimes has to be adapted to the stiffness of the index and middle fingers as encountered in radial club hand. In such cases a longer thumb is less appealing but more functional in achieving a pinch between the two more radial fingers. Another situation where technique needs alteration is the pollicization of some transitional forms of triphalangeal thumbs, but it is important to inform the relatives that another operation may be necessary to improve appearance and function later on.

This is not the place to analyze the literature about pollicization. Many reports provided incomplete data (Buck-Gramcko 1981, Egloff and Verdan 1983, Kozin et al 1992, Sykes et al 1991). Manske et al (1992) gave useful and realistic data demonstrating that the range of motion is approximately 50% of normal, the pinch and grip strength 25% and integration in about 75% of the activities (ranging from 60% of activities requiring manipulation of small objects to 90% of those requiring the handling of large objects) takes the patients around 40% longer to perform. They recognized that results were not as good as in cases of index finger deficiencies such as that found in radial club hand. With this in mind, we isolated from our series of 35 patients having sustained 46 pollicizations, a group of 22 patients with 27 pollicizations performed in isolated hypoplasia or aplasia of the thumb but including one Rothmund syndrome associated to metacarpal M4M5 synostosis (Foucher et al 2000c). Eight hands needed some re-operation (30%)—a rate that is close to the 36% of Sykes et al (1991) and the 45% of Manske et al (1992)—these included adjustment of the first web (two cases), metacarpal shortening (three cases), opening osteotomy (one case) and opposition transfer (two cases). Mobility was assessed according to Kapandji's quotation (reduced to eight points due to absence of one long finger). The average score was five, with all patients reaching the auricular pulp. Eleven patients hit the maximum score. Mean active MPJ range of motion was 58° and IPJ 42°. Growth was satisfactory but excessive in three cases due to persistence growth of the metacarpal. Discrimination could only be assessed in 18 patients and reached 5 mm, but strength was more disappointing with 55% of grasp (on a Jamar dynamometer) and 42% for pinch compared to the standards according to age. In unilateral cases, grasp was 63% of contralateral and pinch 52%. In only five cases of unilateral involvement was the pollicized side dominant. Cosmetically the aspect of the hand was considered as excellent by 88% of relatives, explaining why allowing parents to meet another family where a child had a pollicization is probably the most significant factor to help them make an informed decision.

There are some contraindications but unfortunately it is in the more severe cases where the alternative is frequently simple abstention. A technical contraindication is evidently a hand with all fingers partially aplastic. In some radial club hands, the index could be missing and the majority of surgeons are reluctant to proceed with pollicization in a hand with only a few digits. However even in cases with quite stiff index fingers and absent thumbs or thumbs that cannot be reconstructed, the majority of surgeons will proceed with a pollicization, and in such cases a long thumb is usually more functional allowing the often stiff middle finger to come in contact with the thumb pulp. One difficult condition is a case where the fifth finger is used as a thumb. This is more frequent in radial club hand, again due to the presentation of the hand, but could be encountered in the absence of radial insufficiency. A thorough assessment is necessary but in teenagers, any improvements in pinch patterns seems logical and we have been pleased by the results of a modified Hentz and Littler operation (1977), performed on the little finger with shortening rotation osteotomy. We do not perform a true 'ulnar' pollicization but we combine metacarpal recession-rotation with a dorsal 'reverse' Buck-Gramcko flap to increase the web. Such an operation allows the hand to remain quite inconspicuous at rest but provides improvement of grasp for large objects.

Few surgeons will argue about the indication of pollicization in cases of very hypoplastic thumbs, but the limit between pollicization and reconstruction varies. Some surgeons have said that type IIIA is amenable to reconstruction and not type IIIB (Manske and McCarroll 1992, 1995), whereas others have limited reconstruction to type II (Lister 1985). We have difficulty in agreeing to this black-and-white view in light of a teratogenic sequence where classification as quoted by Buck-Gramcko (for the triphalangeal thumb) is just a snapshot 'of the most pronounced or frequent types of anomalies' (1998).

This is also not the place to discuss social and cultural factors but they bear great importance in countries where a hand with five digits is more important than a functioning four-fingered one. It is of importance to assess the 'potential' (Kleinman 1990) of the hypoplastic thumb as a whole since each hypoplastic component can be corrected with a quite simple procedure. However, the combined absence of extrinsic, intrinsic, and FCMCJ is, with the exception of cultural background or family refusal, an indication for pollicization. But is it a reason for refusing a child reconstructive surgery? Our answer is no. However, currently, we prefer to delay the reconstruction and reserve it for those young patients that actually ask for it, and have a sufficient development of the thumb. Indeed we have found that a too frequently forgotten aspect of TH is the potential growth, which is difficult to predict.

Hypoplasia or aplasia of one or several structures in a well developed and growing thumb is a good indication for reconstruction (or even abstention as in isolated hypoplasia of an FPL or an EPB). There are however difficult cases where the decision has to be tailored to the individual patient and when in doubt, we consider it less risky to proceed with an early pollicization if the family are in agreement, than to delay the treatment until the child is around 7–10 years old. We firmly believe that pollicization is a good compromise between function and appearance and that preservation of a very hypoplastic thumb requiring complex reconstruction can lead to limited function and a disappointing appearance.

Other techniques

Distraction lengthening could be combined to some of the techniques already described and could be used to prepare more space in longitudinal radial deficiency before interposing a joint transfer. We have also found that in some cases of type IIIB reconstruction, limited growth could lead to loss of distal pinch and in such cases distraction lengthening is useful.

We have already alluded to microsurgical partial toe transfer, providing epiphyseal transfer for TH in symbrachydactyly type IIIB and metatarsophalangeal toe transfer for TH with absent FCMCJ and there are only a few reported cases of great or second toe transfer in radial deficiencies (May et al 1981, Nyarady et al 1983). In trauma cases, reconstruction of a proximally amputated thumb without the thenar and FCMCJ remaining, is disappointing and gives, at best, some weak key pinch. In congenital cases, integration can also be a problem as seen in cases of reconstructed TH, and hypoplastic tendons and muscles explain the limited mobility of such transfers. One of the rare indications is a severe TH in symbrachydactyly and transverse deficiency. In symbrachydactyly type IIIA with intact thumb toe transfer onto the long fingers has provided impressive functional improvement. In more severe cases where generally a double transfer of the second toe from both feet is contemplated due to conjoined severe TH and absence of the long fingers, we have been disappointed by the inconstant distal contact of the two toes and in the case of such a contact the weakness of the pincer. We have given up such a transfer, favouring a modified Furnas-Vilkki operation (Furnas 1982, Vilkki 1995), which entails moving only one toe from the distal (distal to the epiphysis) and anterior (not radial) aspect of the radius. This so-called 'stub' operation (Foucher 1995) has the advantages of using only one toe, finding more tendon transfers to balance the toe, and compensating the limited mobility of the toe by the good one of the wrist.

On-top plasty using a hypoplastic finger could find exceptional indication in symbrachydactyly or transverse deficiencies. There are more indications of non-vascularized phalangeal transfers when excess of skin in the distal part is present. Growth in such cases has been a matter of debate. Carroll and Green (1975) found no growth whereas Goldberg and Watson (1982) found 90% normal growth; such a discrepancy depends on the preservation of the periosteum and joint ligaments as well as on the age at operation (less than a year).

Thumb hypoplasia has a large spectrum of congenital conditions. Some hypoplastic thumbs have good function and clinical diagnosis of a missing structure does not mean that a surgical replacement is necessary. Only a functional deficit needs to be compensated and in such cases, benefits need to be weighed against donor site morbidity and other consequences such as the loss of the flexor superficialis of one finger affecting not only the independence and strength of this finger but also that of the whole hand. In more advanced TH, the main issue is to decide between complex reconstruction versus pollicization of the index finger and only an individual approach can be taken in these instances.

Case studies

A simple case can be illustrated in a moderate form of TH that exhibits an absence of the thenar muscle and moderate first web insufficiency (without MPJ laxity) on the right side and a total absence of the thumb on the left. The first operation was performed on the right side at 14 months of age. It consisted of a four-flaps web plasty and an opposition transfer using the abductor digiti quinti. After preserving a long distal tendon taken from the extensor hood, the muscle was joined to the flexor brevis. The neurovascular pedicle was dissected and the insertion on the pisiform maintained on the radial aspect, giving sufficient length to attach the distal tendon to the dorsal capsule of the

thumb MPJ. We favour such an insertion in order to stabilize the MPJ in opposition and to provide some pronation in case of huge flexion range of this joint. Five months later a formal pollicization was performed on the opposite side. The final result was rewarding with good cortical integration and possibility of large and fine grip on both sides (Fig. 2).

A complicated case can be illustrated by a unilateral (right) thumb hypoplasia without intrinsic and extrinsic muscles and absence of the first carpometacarpal joint. The relatives had done some 'doctor shopping', refusing ablation of the hypoplastic thumb combined with a pollicization of the index finger. Such an operation was again advised, explaining that part of the amputated thumb would be used during the reconstruction. Both relatives definitely refused this operation, preferring a non-functional five-fingered hand. The complex multi-stages of reconstruction were explained in detail with reservation concerning the final function and potential growth. Attention was drawn to the type of pinch already used by the baby, between the index and middle finger, explaining rotation of the index. The sequelae at the donor site were also explained and the relatives finally elected to sacrifice the second ray to close the foot after discussions regarding the flail and short aspect of the second toe in case of preservation.

Five months later, at the age of 16 months the baby underwent the first stage of the operation—the free microsurgical metatarsophalangeal transfer. Dissection began at the donor site, isolating a 4 cm dorsal skin flap (2.5 cm wide), centred on the second metatarsophalangeal joint of the homolateral foot (with the pedicle on the ulnar side of the transfer to join either the radial artery, the superficial arch or even the ulnar artery). The dorsalis pedis artery was approached underneath the extensor hallucis brevis and dissected distally, so preserving the plantar origin, the dorsal artery of the first space and the origin of the plantar artery of the first space. As the ray was sacrificed, both extensors were maintained in the transfer and the second metatarsal was cut proximally to allow for dissection of the second plantar artery, which was found in its normal situation and of 1 mm diameter. The compound transfer was finally isolated on the great saphenous vein and two arteries (first dorsal and second plantar) taken in

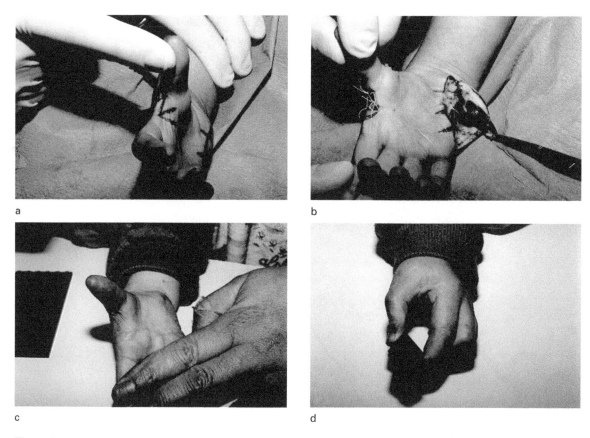

Figure 2

(a) Moderate deficit of the first web. (b) Huber-Littler opposition transfer. (c) Results at five months. (d) Result of pollicization on the opposite side with agenesia of the thumb.

continuity with the plantar arch and the dorsalis pedis. During foot revascularization, the hand was dissected and the absence of the intrinsic muscles with the exception of the adductor pollicis and absence of flexor pollicis longus and extensors was noted. A dorsal wrist vein was prepared through a separate transverse incision and a space was prepared for the joint transfer as well as the present radial artery (interrupted at the styloid radial process) and the brachioradialis, which was sutured to the extensor brevis as an abductor pollicis longus. The joint was maintained in flexion to provide range in hyperextension for abduction of the first ray. After completing the anastomoses, the skin flap

was inserted and both recipient and donor sites closed (with reconstruction of the intermetatarsal ligament at the foot level). The postoperative course was uneventful and three months later a 'pseudo-kite' flap was performed to provide a good first web. At the same stage, the extensor indicis proprius was transferred onto the base of the first phalanx (as an extensor brevis due to limited passive range of the IPJ), and the flexor superficialis of the fourth finger was used for opposition and MPJ stabilization; due to small diameter of the first metacarpal and proximal phalanx the classical technique was not used and one of the flexor bands was used for ligamentoplasty instead, taking care of the absence of

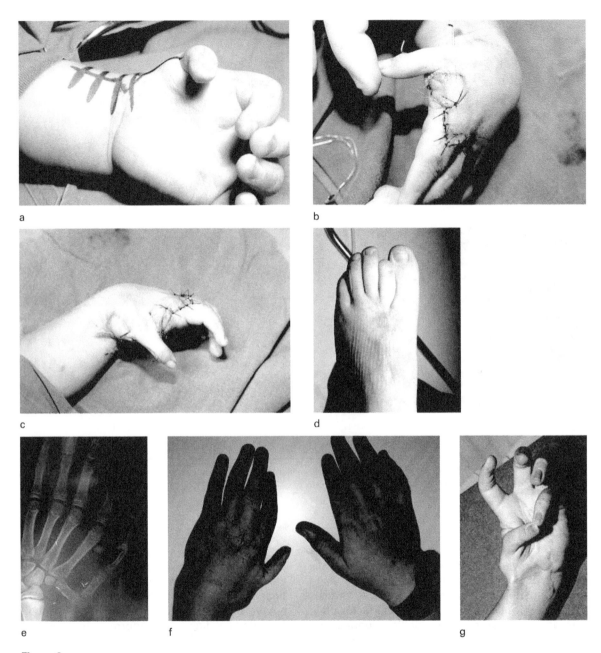

Figure 3

(a) Longitudinal thumb hypoplasia: Blauth-Manske type IIIB with absence of first carpometacarpal joint. (b and c) After transfer of the second metatarsophalangeal joint with microsurgical technique, a 'pseudo-kite' flap is used to reconstruct the first web and opposition is provided by the flexor superficialis of the fourth finger. (d) Aspect of the foot six months after the microsurgical joint and epiphysis transfer. (e) X-ray 10 years after the operation. (f and g) Clinical aspect at the 10–year follow-up stage showing the possibility of grasping large objects; the rotation of the index demonstrates the use of the pinch between the index and long finger for fine manipulation.

tension when pulling on the opposition transfer.

The patient was lost to follow-up after a year, due to their remote location, but was recontacted for assessment after five and 10 years post operation. At final assessment, growth was limited but the thumb tip reached the proximal third of the index finger; its diameter remained low compared to the opposite side. Rotation of the index finger was accentuated and the majority of pinch activity was between the index and middle finger. The large first web was used mainly for grasping large but light objects as the pinch strength could not be measured due to weakness. The child was able to grasp a cylinder of 8 cm (1 cm difference in the opposite side). The relatives were pleased with the final result but the child did express some concern regarding the cosmetic aspects (Fig. 3).

References

Arminio JA (1979) Congenital anomaly of the thumb: absent flexor pollicis longus tendon, *J Hand Surg* **4A**:487–8.

Blair WF, Buckwalter JA (1983) Congenital malposition of the flexor pollicis longus: an anatomy note, *J Hand Surg* **8A**:93–94.

Blair WF, Omer GE (1981) Anomalous insertion of the flexor pollicis longus, *J Hand Surg* **6A**:241–44.

Blauth W (1967) Der hypoplastische Daumen, *Arch Orthop Unfall Chir* **62**:225–46.

Blauth W, Gekeler J (1973) Symbrachydaktylien, *Handchirurgie* **5**:121–71.

Broadbent TR, Woolf RM (1964) Flexion-adduction deformity of the thumb-congenital clasped thumb, *Plast Reconstr Surg* **34**:612–16.

Buck-Gramcko D (1971) Pollicization of the index finger. Method and results in aplasia and hypoplasia of the thumb, *J Bone Joint Surg* **53A**:1605–16.

Buck-Gramcko D (1981) Hypoplasia and aplasia of the thumb. In: Nigst H, Buck-Gramcko D, Millesi H, eds, *Hand Surgery*, volume II, (Thieme: Stuttgart) 12–93.

Buck-Gramcko D (1998a) Triphalangeal thumb. In: Buck-Gramcko D, ed, *Congenital malformations of the hand and forearm*, (Churchill Livingstone: London), 403–24.

Buck-Gramcko D (1998b) Syndactyly between the thumb and index. In: Buck-Gramcko D, ed, *Congenital malformations of the hand and forearm*, (Churchill Livingstone: London), 141–47.

Caroli A, Zanasi S (1989) First web space reconstruction by Caroli's technique in congenital hand deformities with severe thumb ray adduction, *Br J Plast Surg* **42**:653–59.

Carroll RE, Louis DS (1974) Anomalies associated with radial dysplasia, *J Pediatr* **84**:409–14.

Carroll RE, Green DP (1975) Reconstruction of the hypoplastic digits using toe phalanges, *J Bone Joint Surg* **57**:727–32.

Cole RJ, Manske PR (1997) Classification of ulnar deficiency according to the thumb and first web, *J Hand Surg* **22A**:479–88.

Crawford HH, Horton CE, Adamson JE (1966) Congenital aplasia or hypoplasia of the thumb and finger extensor tendons, *J Bone Joint Surg* **48A**:82–91.

Dawson S, Barton N (1986) Anatomical variations of the extensor pollicis brevis, *J Hand Surg* **11B**:378–81.

DeHaan MR, Wong LLB, Petersen DP (1987) Congenital anomaly of the thumb: aplasia of the flexor pollicis longus, *J Hand Surg* **12A**:108–9.

Dufourmentel C (1962) La fermeture des pertes de substance cutanée limitées 'Le Lambeau de rotation en L pour Losange', *Annales de Chirurgie plastique* **7**:61–66.

Egloff DV, Verdan C (1983) Pollicization of the index finger for reconstruction of the congenitally hypoplastic or absent thumb, *J Hand Surg* **8A**:839–48.

Ezaki M (1996) Congenital anomalies: thumb dysplasia. In: Peimer CA, ed, *Surgery of the hand and upper extremity*, (McGraw-Hill: New York) 2145–64.

Fitch RD, Urbaniak JR, Ruderman RJ (1984) Conjoined flexor and extensor pollicis longus tendons in the hypoplastic thumb, *J Hand Surg* **9A**:417–19.

Flatt AE, Wood VE (1970) Multiple dorsal rotation flaps from the hand for thumb web contractures, *Plast Reconstr Surg* **45**:258–62.

Foucher G, Braun B (1979) A new island flap transfer from the dorsum of the index to the thumb, *Plast Reconstr Surg* **63**:28–31.

Foucher G (1988) Vascularized joint transfers. In: Green D, ed, *Operative hand surgery*, 2nd edn, (Churchill Livingstone:London) 1271–93.

Foucher G, Cornil C, Braga Da Silva J (1992) Le lambeau 'pseudo-cerf-volant' de l'index avec plastie LLL dans la reconstruction de la première commissure, *Ann Chir Plast Esthet* **37**:207–09.

Foucher G (1995) The 'stub' operation—modification of Furnas and Vilkki technique in traumatic and congenital and carpal hand reconstruction, *Ann Acad Med Singapore* **24**:73–76.

Foucher G (1997) Le transfert d'orteil dans les malformations congénitales, *Bull Acad Nationale Méd* **181**:1737–45.

Foucher G, Gazarian A, Pajardi G (1999) La chirurgie reconstructive dans les hypoplasies type III de Blauth, *Ann Chir Main* **1**:191–96.

Foucher G, Medina J, Pajardi G, Navarro R (2000a) La symbrachydactylie, classification et traitement. A propos d'une série de 117 cas, *Chir de la Main* **19**:161–68.

Foucher G, Medina J, Navarro R, Pajardi G (2000b) Apport d'une nouvelle plastie à la reconstruction de la première commissure dans les malformations congénitales. A propos d'une série de 54 patients, *Chir de la Main* **19**:152–60.

Foucher G, Navarro R, Medina J, Allieu Y (2000c) La pollicisation, vestige du passé ou opération d'actualité, *Bull Acad Nationale Méd* **184**:1241–53.

Foucher G, Pajardi G, Lamas C, Medina J, Navarro R (2001a) L'allongement par distraction progressive du squelette de la main dans les malformations congénitales. A propos de 41 observations, *Rev Chir Ortho* **87**:451–58.

Foucher G, Medina J, Navarro R, Khoury RK (2001b) Correction of first web space deficiency in congenital deformities of the hand with the pseudo-kite flap, *Plast Reconstr Surg* **107**:1458–63.

Foucher G, Medina J, Navarro R, Nagel D (2001c) Toe transfer in congenital hand malformations, *J Reconstr Micro* **17**:1–7.

Foucher G, Medina J, Navarro R (2001d) Microsurgical reconstruction of the hypoplastic thumb, type IIIB, *J Reconstr Micro* **17**:9–15.

Friedman R, Wood VE (1997) The dorsal transposition

flap for congenital contracture of the first web space: a 20–year experience, *J Hand Surg* **22A**:664–70.

Furnas DW (1982) Toe-to-radius transplant. Correspondence Newsletter of the ASSH 22.

Goldberg NH, Watson HK (1982) Composite toe (phalanx and epiphysis) transfers in the reconstruction of the aphalangic hand, *J Hand Surg* **7A**:454–59.

Graham TJ, Louis DS (1998) A comprehensive approach to surgical management of the type IIIA hypoplastic thumb, *J Hand Surg* **23A**:3–13.

Hall RF, Keuhn D, Prieto J (1986) Congenital hypoplasia of the thumb ray with absent navicular and hypertrophic styloid process of the radius: a case report, *J Hand Surg* **11A**:32–35.

Hentz VR, Littler JW (1977) Abduction-pronation and recession of second (index) metacarpal in thumb agenesis, *J Hand Surg* **2A**:113–16.

Hirshowitz B, Karev A, Rousso M (1975) Combined Z-plasty and V-Y advancement for thumb web contracture, *Hand* **7**:291–93.

Huber E (1921) Hilfsoperation bei medianuslahmung, *Dtsch Z Chir* **162**:271. *J Hand Surg* **4**:487–89.

James MA, Yinger K, McCarroll HR, Manske PR (2001) The association of radius deficiency with thumb deficiency. In: Ogino T, ed, *Congenital hand anomalies*.

Kato K (1924) Congenital absence of the radius, with review of the literature and report of three cases, *J Bone Joint Surg* **22**:589.

Kessler I, Baruch AD, Hecht OA (1977) Experience with distraction lengthening of digital rays in congenital anomalies, *J Hand Surg* **2A**:394–401.

Kleinman WB (1990) Management of thumb hypoplasia, *Hand Clin* **6**:617–41.

Kobayashi A, Ohmiya K, Iwakuma T, Mitsuyasu M (1976) Unusual congenital anomalies of the thumb extensors: report of two cases, *Hand* **8**:17–21.

Koster G (1984) Isolated aplasia of the flexor pollicis longus: a case report, *J Hand Surg* **9A**: 870–71.

Kowalski MF, Manske PR (1988) Arthrodesis of digital joints in children, *J Hand Surg* **13A**:874–79.

Kozin SH, Weiss AA, Webber JB, Betz RR, Clancy M,

Steel HH (1992) Index finger pollicization for congenital aplasia or hypoplasia of the thumb, *J Hand Surg* **17A**:880–84.

Lister G (1985) Reconstruction of the hypoplastic thumb, *Clin Orthop Rel Res* **195**:52–65.

Lister G, Gibson T (1972) Closure of rhomboid skin defects: the flaps of Limberg and Dufourmentel, *Br J Plast Surg* **25**:300–14.

Lister G (1991a) Musculus lumbricalis pollicis, *J Hand Surg* **16A**:622–25.

Lister GD (1991b) Pollex abductus in hypoplasia and duplication of the thumb, *J Hand Surg* **16A**: 626–33.

Littler JW (1952) The neurovascular pedicle method of digital transposition for reconstruction of the thumb, *Plast Reconstr Surg* **12**:303–19.

Littler JW, Cooley SGE (1963) Opposition of the thumb and its restoration by abductor digiti minimi transfer, *J Bone Joint Surg* **45A**:1389–96.

Lösch GM, Schrader M (1978) Connective tissue structures in the first intermetacarpal space in case of malformations of the hand with and without syndactyly, *Chir Plastica (Berl)* **4**:145–59.

McCarroll HR (1985) Congenital flexion deformities of the thumb, *Hand Clin* **1**:567–75.

Manske PR, McCarroll HR (1978) Abductor digiti minimi opponensplasty in congenital radial dysplasia, *J Hand Surg* **3A**:552–59.

Manske PR, McCarroll HR (1985) Index finger pollicization for a congenitally absent or non-functioning thumb, *J Hand Surg* **10A**:606–13

Manske PR, McCarroll HR (1992) Reconstruction of the congenitally deficient thumb, *Hand Clin* **8**:177–96.

Manske PR, Rotman MB, Dailey LA (1992) Long-term functional results after pollicization for the congenitally deficient thumb, *J Hand Surg* **17A**:1064–72.

Manske PR (1993) Symbrachydactyly instead of atypical cleft hand, *Plast Reconstr Surg* **91**:196.

Manske PR, Halikis MN (1995) Surgical classification of central deficiency according to the thumb web, *J Hand Surg* **20A**:687–97.

Manske PR, McCarroll HR (1995) Type IIIA hypoplastic thumb, *J Hand Surg* **20A**:246–53.

Matev IB (1970) Surgical treatment of flexion-adduction contracture of the thumb in cerebral palsy, *Acta Orthop Scand* **41**:439–45.

May JW, Smith RJ, Peimer CA (1981) Toe-to-hand free tissue transfer for thumb reconstruction with multiple digit aplasia, *Plast Reconstr Surg* **67**:205–13.

Miura T (1981) Congenital anomaly of the thumb-unusual bifurcation of the flexor pollicis longus and its unusual insertion, *J Hand Surg* **6A**:6613–15.

Miura T (2000) Flexion deformities of the thumb. In: Buck-Gramcko D, ed, *Congenital anomalies of the upper limb*, 425–29.

Müller W (1937) *Die angeborenen fehlbildungen der menschlichen hand*, (Thieme:Leipzig).

Nakamura R, Kubo E (1993) Bilateral anomalous insertion of flexor pollicis longus, *J Hand Surg* **18B**:312–15.

Neal NC, Burke FD (2001) Bilateral congenital absence of the flexor pollicis longus, *Hand Surg* **1**:191–94.

Neviaser RJ (1979) Congenital hypoplasia of the thumb with absence of the extrinsic extensors, abductor pollicis and thenar muscles, *J Hand Surg* **4**:301–03.

Nishijima N, Matsumoto T, Yamamuro T (1995) Two-stage reconstruction for the hypoplastic thumb, *J Hand Surg* **20A**:415–19.

Nyarady J, Szekeres P, Vilmos Z (1983) Toe to thumb transfer in congenital grade III thumb hypoplasia, *J Hand Surg* **8A**:898–901.

Ogino T, Minami A, Fukuda K (1986) Abductor digiti minimi opponensplasty in hypoplastic thumb, *J Hand Surg* **11B**:372–77.

Ogino T, Minami A, Kato H (1989) Clinical features and roentgenograms of symbrachydactyly., *J Hand Surg* **14B**:303–06.

Ostrowski DM, Feagin CA, Gould JS (1998) A three flap web plasty for release of short congenital syndactyly and dorsal adduction contracture, *J Hand Surg* **16A**:634–41.

Sandzen SC (1982) Dorsal pedicle flap for resurfacing a moderate thumb-index web contracture. *J Hand Surg* **7A**:21–24.

Shaw DJ, Li CS, Richey DG, Nahigian SH (1973) Interdigital butterfly flap in the hand, *J Bone Joint Surg* **55A**:1677–79.

Shibata M, Yoshizu T, Seki T, Goto M, Saito H, Tajima T (1998) Reconstruction of a congenital hypoplastic thumb with use of a free vascularized metatarsophalangeal joint, *J Bone Joint Surg* **80A**:1469–76.

Smith P, Hall R, Fleming A (2000) The Blauth II thumb hypoplasia. A re-evaluation of the classification and a new management algorithm. In: Ogino T, ed, *Congenital differences of the upper limb*. Proceedings of the fifth International Symposium on congenital differences of the upper limb, Department of Orthopedic Surgery, Yamagata University School of Medicine, 203–8.

Spinner M (1969) Fashioned transpositional flap for soft tissue adduction contracture of the thumb, *Plast Reconstr Surg* **4**:345–48.

Strauch B (1975) Dorsal thumb flap for release of adduction contracture of the first web space, *Bull Hosp Joint Dis* **36**:34–39.

Strauch B, Spinner M (1976) Congenital anomaly of the thumb: absent intrinsics and flexor pollicis longus, *J Bone Joint Surg* **58A**:115–18.

Su CT, Hoopes JE, Daniel R (1972) Congenital absence of the thenar muscles innervated by the median nerve, *J Bone Joint Surg* **54A**:1087–90.

Swanson AB (1976) A classification for congenital limb malformations, *J Hand Surg* **1A**:8–22.

Swanson AB, DeGroot Swanson G, Tada K (1983) A classification for congenital lin malformation, *J Hand Surg* **8A**:693–702.

Sykes PJ, Chandraprakasam T, Percival NJ (1991) Pollicization of the index finger in congenital anomalies. A retrospective analysis, *J Hand Surg* **16B**:144–47.

Tajima T (1965) Dorsal sliding skin flap for adduction contracture of the thumb. *Seikeigeka Orthop Surg* **16**:935–38.

Tajima T (1985) Classification of thumb hypoplasia, *Hand Clin* **1**:577–94.

Tajima T (1998) Reconstruction of the floating thumb. In: Buck-Gramcko D, ed, *Congenital malformations of the hand and forearm*, (Churchill Livingstone:London) 369–73.

Tsuchida Y, Kasai S, Kojima T (1976) Congenital absence of flexor pollicis longus and flexor pollicis brevis: a case report. *Hand* **8**:294–97.

Tupper JW (1969) Pollex abductus due to congenital malposition of the flexor pollicis longus, *J Bone Joint Surg* **51A**:1285–96.

Uchida M, Kojima T, Sakurai N (1985) Congenital absence of flexor pollicis longus without hypoplasia of thenar muscles, *Plast Reconstr Surg* **75**:413–16.

Vilkki SK (1995) Advances in microsurgical reconstruction of the congenitally adactylous hand, *Clin Orthop* **314**:45–58.

Weckesser EC (1955) Congenital flexion-adduction deformity of the thumb (congenital 'clasped thumb'), *J Bone Joint Surg* **37A**:977–80.

Wood VE, Skie M (1997) An unusual complication of the thumb abductor digiti minimi opponensplasty, *Hand Surg* **2**:183–89.

Woolf RM, Broadbent TR (1972) The four flap Z-plasty, *Plast Reconstr Surg* **49**:48–51.

Yamauchi Y, Fujimaki A, Yanagihara Y, Yoshizaki K (1979) Reconstruction of floating thumb, especially on the use of metatarsophalangeal joint grafting, *Seikeigeka Orthop Surg* **30**:1645–48.

12
Radial club hand

Paul J Smith and Gillian D Smith

Introduction

The first description of radial club hand was by Petit in 1733. He gave a detailed account of the autopsy findings of a newborn with bilateral absent radii. The term 'radial club hand' has been adopted to describe a spectrum of abnormalities of the preaxial border of the upper limb where the hand lies deviated radially, flexed and pronated at the distal end of the forearm. There is a combination of a lack of bony support on the radial side with carpal and musculotendinous abnormalities. This terminology is inaccurate and misleading. Many other descriptions applied to this deformity are equally so. A popular alternative 'radial dysplasia', with its emphasis on bony abnormality, fails to convey the spectrum of abnormality or the variety of tissues that may be involved. The best description is probably that of a longitudinal radial deficiency. This term encompasses underdevelopment, abnormal development, or absence of tissues of the radial aspect of the upper limb. There are frequently abnormalities in adjacent rays and the index finger may be hypoplastic. The radial digits may be stiff and the ulnar side digits progressively more mobile.

The spectrum of radial ray deficiency may range from a mildly hypoplastic thumb to complete absence of thumb, scaphoid, trapezium and, radius with a radially bowed ulna and short humerus. The milder deformities, types I and II, rarely need operative treatment whereas management of the more severe deficiencies, types III and IV, is difficult and controversial. The majority of work on radial club hand is related to types III and IV. The hand is displaced and lies on the radial side of the ulna. Preoperative measurements of motion are meaningless as the hand is floating without a wrist joint, and therefore, without any articulation of the ulna on the carpus. Ulnar growth may be limited to 60% of normal (Flatt 1994, Heikel 1959,). The long flexors of the fingers are at a mechanical disadvantage as the 'wrist' is flexed which limits grip strength. The combination of a stiff elbow, short forearm, radially deviated hand and hypoplastic or absent thumb limit hand function significantly. The functional disability is particularly problematic when the condition is bilateral. There is a frequent association with other anomalies or specific syndromes (D'Arcangelo et al 2000).

Epidemiology

The prevalence of this abnormality is estimated to be between 1 in 30,000 (Birch-Jensen 1949) and 1 in 100,000 (Flatt 1994) live births. The true incidence is unknown and will vary with the population studied. There is a slight preponderance of males (3:2) (Urban and Osterman 1990). Different authors disagree as to whether bilateral deformity is marginally more frequent (Bayne and Klug 1987, Heikel 1959, Lamb 1977, Pilz et al 1998) or less frequent (Flatt 1994) than unilateral. The right side is affected twice as often as the left (Flatt 1994).

Martini (1992) observed a seasonally higher incidence of longitudinal radial deficiency with a slight preponderance of female patients. Complete radial aplasia is more frequent than radial hypoplasia or partial radius aplasia (Bayne and Klug 1987, Lamb 1977, Urban and Osterman 1990). The severity of malformation of the humerus parallels the severity of the defect of the radius. Malformation of the carpal bones tends to decrease in a radial to ulnar direction.

Aetiology

The aetiology of radial club hand is still debated. In isolated cases, there is no evidence that the condition is genetically determined. Bilateral cases are more likely to have a syndromic association. There are a number of syndromes that include a radial ray deficiency, some of which may have a genetic basis (Fig. 2). These may be transmitted as an autosomal dominant or recessive condition but are usually the result of a sporadic mutation.

Multiple environmental factors have been implicated. There are theories suggesting in utero compression (Dareste theory), inflammatory processes (Virchow theory), nutritional deficiencies, radiation, and drugs all as aetiological factors (Flatt 1994). Thalidomide exposure in the first trimester (between days 38 and 45) is a known aetiological factor. Lamb (1977) found that 26 mothers of 68 cases he reviewed had ingested thalidomide. The anatomical findings and associated congenital abnormalities in cases with and without thalidomide exposure are similar but the incidence of other skeletal deficiencies is higher in the thalidomide group. Valproic acid is a known teratogen. There have been three reports of radial defects, supported by experimental evidence, after valproic acid exposure as part of the foetal valproic syndrome (Verloes et al 1990). Defects included the typical dysmorphism of the 'foetal valproic syndrome', bilateral radial ray aplasia, unilateral proximal phocomelia of the upper limb, kidney hypoplasia and brain atrophy. Phenobarbitone (Lindhout et al 1988) and ethanol (Pauli and Feldman 1986) are other drugs implicated in radial defects.

Matsuma (1994) demonstrated that in foetal white leghorn chickens, radial ray deficiencies could be produced by cauterization in the distal preaxial area, and ulnar ray deficiencies by cauterization in the distal postaxial area. The critical periods for both radial and ulnar ray deficiencies were the same—from immediately after the formation of the wing bud to before the formation of the digital plate. Kato et al (1990) demonstrated that busulfan, an anti-mitotic agent, given to pregnant rats induced defects similar to those seen in humans with radial club hand.

Tickle et al (1975) have proposed a model that suggests that the polarizing region, that deter-mines anteroposterior patterning in the limb, produces a morphogen that diffuses across the limb bud. The quantity of morphogen that a single cell was exposed to would determine the identity of the ray into which it developed. A deficiency would prevent ray development. Experimentally, similar defects have been created in chick wings and both retinoic acid (Tickle et al 1985) and expression of the sonic hedgehog gene (Riddle et al 1993) has been shown to reproduce signalling of the polarizing region.

Classification

The multitude of terms attached to radial club hand and its broad spectrum of abnormalities has not helped in its classification. In 1959, Heikel divided the condition into total radial aplasia, partial aplasia, and hypoplasia with carpal and thumb abnormalities. In 1976, the International Federation of Societies for Surgery of the Hand (IFSSH) classified radial deficiencies as 'Category 1: failure of formation of parts, longitudinal, radial complete or partial' (Swanson 1976). A sub classification expresses the severity and type of deformity (Table 1). In 1987 Bayne and Klug

Table 1 Classification of radial deficiency

Radial deficiency	Other features
Normal radius	Hypoplastic, functional thumb
	Hypoplastic, non-functional thumb
	Absent thumb
Hypoplastic thumb	Hypoplastic, functional thumb
	Hypoplastic, non-functional thumb
	Absent thumb
	Madelung's deformity
	Other deformities
Partial absence of distal radius	Hypoplastic, functional thumb
	Hypoplastic, non-functional thumb
	Absent thumb
Complete absence of radius	Hypoplastic, functional thumb
	Hypoplastic, non-functional thumb
	Absent thumb
Other	Absent or hypoplastic thenar muscles
	Absent or hypoplastic extensor muscles
	Absent or hypoplastic flexor muscles

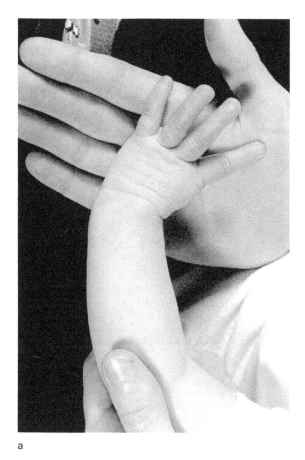

a

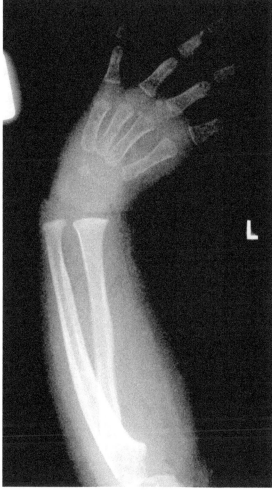

b

Figure 1

Photograph (a) and radiograph (b) of patient with radial club hand with a short radius (type I). Note associated thumb aplasia.

expanded on this classification, dividing radial deficiencies into four groups depending on the bony development of the radius as viewed on radiographs. Type I has a radius which is short distally but appears normal. The distal radial epiphysis is late to appear and associated thumb hypoplasia is common (Fig. 1). Type II has a short radius with defective epiphyses at both ends producing a hypoplastic radius (Fig. 2). Type III has partial radial dysplasia with the middle, distal (or rarely, the proximal) third absent and a short, thick radially bowed ulna (Fig. 3). In Type IV, the most common type

(67–90%; Manske et al 1981, Pilz et al 1998), the radius is completely absent (Fig. 4). This classification cannot apply to patients who have deficiencies of the carpus and thumb in the presence of a normal radius.

Other classification systems have attempted to incorporate the deficiency of the radius, carpal abnormalities, and hypoplastic thumbs. In the system suggested by James (1999), type N has a normal length radius and a normal carpus with thumb hypoplasia, type O has a normal length radius and radial side carpal abnormalities and type 1 has more than 2 mm shortening of the

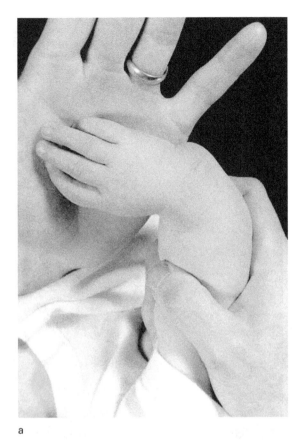

a

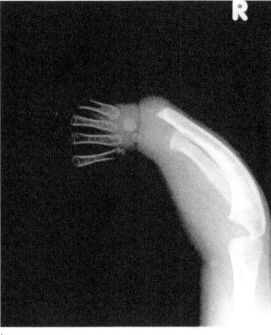

b

Figure 2

Photograph (a) and radiograph (b) of patient with radial club hand with short hypoplastic radius with defective epiphyses at both ends (type II).

radius compared to the ulna at the wrist. Type 2 has a hypoplastic radius with defective growth at the proximal or both ends, type 3 has a partial radius with absence of the distal physis, and type 4 has complete absence of the radius. In his series, all type 1 deficiencies had carpal abnormalities and 44% of type 1 and 11% of type O had proximal radio-ulnar synostosis or congenital dislocation of the radial head.

Patients with thrombocytopenia with absent radii (TAR) syndrome may not fit into any of these categories as they may have severe deficiencies of the radius with moderately hypoplastic thumbs. One suggestion has been to adopt a T (thumb), C (carpus), D (distal radius), P (proximal radius) system, (Allison 2000), similar to the tumour node metastasis (TNM) classification.

Anatomy

The classification of radial club hand is based on skeletal abnormalities but this oversimplifies the problem. The surgeon needs to be aware of the complex anatomical variations of this condition.

Bones and joints

Abnormalities are found along the whole length of the limb. Radial deficiencies appear to lie on a spectrum, which incorporates abnormalities of the radius, carpus, and thumb. Abnormalities of the thumb are normally associated with carpal abnormalities. Where the thumb and radius are

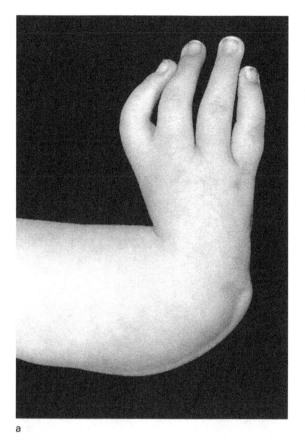

a

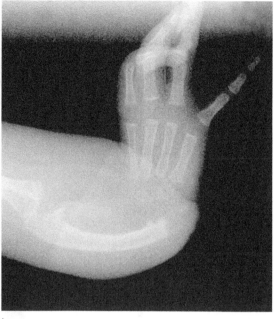

b

Figure 3

Photograph (a) and radiograph (b) of patient with radial club hand with partial aplasia of radius and marked bowing of ulna (type III).

involved, the carpus will invariably be abnormal. Only a small proportion of children with radial club hand have relatively normal thumbs, a significant proportion of whom have TAR syndrome.

Upper arm

In two-thirds the upper arm length is equal bilaterally. In the rest it is shorter on the side with more severe aplasia of the radius. The greater the severity of the radial defect, the more likely the distal humeral epiphysis will be involved. It is common for the olecranon fossa or trochlea to be small. Sometimes there is absence of the capitulum, the coronoid fossa, the medial condyle, the intertubercular sulcus or the whole distal end of the humerus.

Elbow movement

In type I radial club hand, elbow movement is normal. In the others it is limited. Flexion is affected more than extension and pronation-supination ranges from normal to zero. Lamb (1977) found 23% of elbows in radial club hand to have stiffness in extension. He was able to improve active elbow flexion to 90° in 20 of 27 cases by splinting the wrist straight. In light of this, the author has never failed to see patients regain a minimum of 90° of elbow flexion following wrist centralization, despite the presence of a stiff elbow preoperatively.

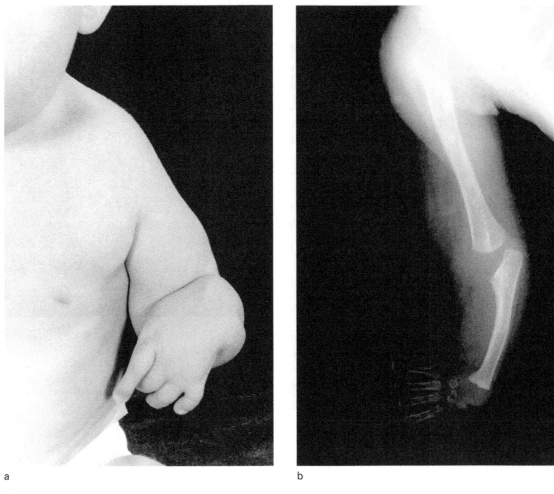

a   b

Figure 4

Photograph (a) and radiograph (b) of patient with radial club hand with complete absence of radius (type IV).

Forearm

This is always shorter on the affected side, the deficit worsening with increasing dysplasia. The ulna may be curved, short, and thickened. It may lack its styloid and coronoid processes. Except for the mildest cases, the ulna only grows to between 50% and 66% of the length of the normal ulna (Bora et al 1970, Heikel 1959, Lamb 1977). The distal radial epiphysis is delayed in appearance and closes early. Kelikan (1974) states that the distal epiphysis, responsible for

most of the length of the ulna, is reliant for development on functional stimulus. Usually, but not universally, there is curvature of the ulna, normally between 20–50° at varying sites along the bone. A few are curved at birth (3%; Lamb 1977) but bowing progresses with growth. There is usually moderate thickening of the bone after birth, which may represent a compensatory response to the stresses placed upon it.

The radius, if present, may have proximal abnormalities. Rarely, it is the proximal portion that is missing. The distal radius is often replaced by a fibrous condensation into which the dorsoradial muscles are both fused and inserted.

The range of supination-pronation is 24° actively and 83° passively. There is radial and volar displacement of the carpus in relation to the distal ulna. There is commonly no triangular fibrocartilage complex (Kelikian 1974), even in milder cases where there may be a fibrous connection between the ulna and carpus.

Carpal bones

The carpal bones are bound together by fibrous tissue and there is rarely any articular cartilage. O'Rahilly (1951) found an absent scaphoid in 65 of 80 cases of radial deficiency and an absent trapezium in 62 out of 73 cases. The capitate, hamate, and triquetrum are usually normal. In 1955, Riordan observed that in cases of radial deficiency, some of the carpal bones, most commonly the scaphoid, were often absent or fused to each other. Heikel (1959), examining 64 cases, noted the frequent absence of the scaphoid and trapezium and delayed ossification in the radial side of the carpus. Skerik and Flatt (1969) had similar findings with 21 cases. The scaphoid was absent in 17 and the trapezium in 14. Lamb (1977) examined 117 limbs in 68 patients. All had thumb hypoplasia and an absent trapezium and 98% had an absent scaphoid. He noticed an increasing number of carpal synostoses as the child matured. Deficiencies of the thumb and carpus in the presence of a normal radius may also be seen.

Digits

The first metacarpal and its phalanges are absent in 80% of cases (O'Rahilly 1951, Skerik and Flatt 1969). Where the thumb is hypoplastic, so is its metacarpal. The second to fifth metacarpals and their phalanges are usually present. The radial digits are more hypoplastic and stiffer than those on the ulnar side of the hand. Interestingly, the radial deviation of the wrist places the most functional fingers in an appropriate position for prehension. The index tends to pronate. In certain syndromes, such as Catel-Manzke syndrome, there is a delta phalanx present in the index finger or angulation at the proximal interphalangeal joints. These problems may require correction prior to pollicization.

The amount of movement in the joints varies. Typically metacarpophalangeal joints tend to flex poorly but do hyperextend (Heikel 1959). Proximal interphalangeal joints, particularly in the syndromic cases, tend to have fixed flexion deformities. All fingers tend to have a limited range of movement due to extensor tendon abnormalities (Heikel 1959), or joint and capsular abnormalities (Flatt 1994).

Muscles

Muscle variations in radial club hand are numerous, confusing and related to the severity of the skeletal deficiency (D'Arcangelo et al 2000). Postaxial muscles arising from the medial epicondyle are normal proximally, but may have aberrant insertions around the wrist. Preaxial muscles are more seriously affected. The muscles are often coalesced into a single functional muscle mass where the individual identity of the muscles is lost. With the exception of pectoralis major and coracobrachialis, muscles inserting on the humerus are usually normal. The abdominal origin of pectoralis major is often missing or its insertion may be aberrant. The deltoid may be abnormally inserted or fused with brachialis or triceps.

The long head of biceps is usually absent. If present, it has an abnormal origin and inserts into the lacertus fibrosus of the biceps. The short head is rarely normal, being fused either with the coracobrachialis or the forearm flexor musculature. It inserts into the joint capsule or the brachial fascia, sometimes dividing into two tendons distally to insert into the rudimentary radius, medial epicondyle or into the joint capsule. The median nerve directly innervates the biceps and anterior compartment muscles.

The brachialis can be normal or may fuse with the biceps with no specific insertion. The pronator teres is often fused with this muscle mass, with the palmaris longus or flexor carpi radialis. The supinator is usually absent. The brachioradialis is absent in type IV cases. If the radius is present, it inserts onto it; if not, it inserts either onto the carpus or with any muscle to which it is fused. The extensor carpi radialis longus may be absent or fused to adjacent extensor and the extensor carpi radialis brevis is infrequently present. Bora et al (1981) found neither of these muscles to be useful in any of their patients. The flexor carpi radialis, if present, is difficult to identify. The origin of flexor carpi ulnaris is normal but the insertion is aberrant. The extensor carpi ulnaris varies in its abnormality—it sometimes fuses with the extensor digitorum communis or with the flexor carpi ulnaris.

Extensor digitorum communis is frequently fused with the extensor carpi radialis longus or the extensor digiti minimi. The extensor indicis proprius is usually either absent, rudimentary or abnormal. It may insert into any bone of the index, middle, or ring finger or into the carpus.

The flexor digitorum superficialis is frequently abnormal with the radial head absent, the tendon to the index finger, and sometimes to the little finger, absent. The flexor digitorum profundus tendon to the index may be absent or have an anomalous insertion to the proximal or middle phalanges (Heikel 1959). Anconeus is rarely present. The palmaris longus, if present, is fused with the flexor digitorum superficialis and inserts more on the ulnar side than usual. The pronator quadratus is absent.

In the hand, the lumbricals may be part of the flexor digitorum profundus, be abnormally innervated or absent (usually the index lumbrical). The first dorsal interosseus may be absent. The other interossei and the hypothenar muscles are often hypoplastic or undifferentiated. The thenar muscles are rarely normal even in the presence of a thumb. The intrinsic muscles are particularly affected and may be abnormal in both their origin and insertion.

Accessory muscles are common but, with the muscle variability, it may be difficult to identify them. Flatt (1994) divides them according to their location. Accessory muscles arising on the humerus either arise distal to the deltoid insertion and insert into the lateral intermuscular septum or with brachioradialis, or arise from the lateral intermuscular septum and insert distal to the wrist. Accessory muscles arising on the ulna are extensors that lie deep in the wrist and finger extensors and insert into the carpus. Accessory muscles arising from soft tissue occur mainly from the long flexors, sometimes producing lumbrical muscles.

Nerves

Abnormal neural anatomy may be found from the brachial plexus distally, with fibres originating higher in the cervical cord than usual. The ulnar and axillary nerves are normal. The musculocutaneous nerve is frequently absent or abnormal, being joined with the median nerve. The radial nerve innervates triceps and then peters out. When the musculocutaneous nerve is absent, the median nerve supplies the anterior compartment of the arm. It divides into two (in 25–30% in the forearm), the radial branch providing sensation to the radial side of the hand and anastomosing with the ulnar nerve in lieu of the radial nerve. The median nerve is usually present, thicker than normal, but aberrant in its course. Stoffel and Strumpel (1909) have described eight variations in 16 cases.

Variations in nerve anatomy are most important distally at the 'wrist', where surgical intervention may place the aberrant median nerve at risk. It lies preaxially immediately below the deep fascia and forms a tight band which the unwary may divide during soft tissue release. Occasionally, it divides early into its distal branches but normally it is still large at the level of the wrist and may be mistaken for a fibrous anlage.

Vessels

The brachial artery is usually normal but it may divide high in the arm or fail to divide at the elbow. The degree of abnormality of the vessels distal to this corresponds to the severity of the deformity (Blauth and Schmidt 1969).

The ulnar artery is usually normal or enlarged. It may lie more radially and be the sole supply to the hand. The vessels lie radially at the distal end of the ulna (Heikel 1959). The interosseous arteries are well developed and may replace the radial or ulnar arteries. Arteriography showed an absent radial artery in 46%, hypoplastic radial artery in 38% and a persistent median artery in 77% of cases. The superficial palmar arch was absent in 15%, the deep palmar arch in 92% and the radial artery to the thumb in 38% (Inoue and Miura (1991). The palmar digital arteries are hypoplastic. Sometimes there is no radial digital artery to the index finger (8%). In pollicization then, the viability of the thumb is dependent on careful preservation of the single ulnar digital artery to the index finger.

Associated conditions

Radial deficiencies may be isolated, associated with congenital anomalies or with a specific syndrome. Bilateral cases are more likely to have other anomalies or be part of a syndrome. The incidence of associated anomalies varies in the literature from 25% (Lamb 1977) to 58% (Pilz et al 1998), with 40% in unilateral cases and 77% in bilateral cases (Kelikian 1974). Abnormalities of every organ system have been described in association with radial club hand (Table 2). A detailed physical examination by a paediatrician is mandatory and may need to be supplemented by further investigations.

Haematological abnormalities

Fanconi anaemia

With this autosomal recessive condition, the child develops a pancytopenia in childhood, usually between the ages of five and 10 years. They present small with skin pigmentation, cardiac, intestinal, or renal anomalies and mental retardation (20%). As the disease progresses the child develops bleeding, purpura and recurrent infections. It carries a dismal prognosis. Recently, sibling bone marrow transplant has provided a promising alternative to premature death. In the absence of a suitable bone marrow donor, any surgery indicated should not be postponed, as the haematological profile will deteriorate with time. The thumb is hypoplastic or absent and 15% have radial club hand (Goldberg and Bartoshesky 1985). Antenatal diagnosis is possible as there is an increase in spontaneous chromosome breaks in cultured cells (D'Arcangelo et al 2000).

Table 2 Syndromic associations with radial ray deficiencies

Haematological abnormalities	Fanconi anaemia TAR syndrome Aase-Smith syndrome
Congenital heart disease	Holt-Oram syndrome Lewis upper limb cardiovascular syndrome (ventriculoradial dysplasia)
Craniofacial abnormalities	Nager acrofacial dysostosis Hemifacial microsomia Goldenhar syndrome Juberg-Haywood syndrome (oro-cranio-digital syndrome) Baller-Gerold syndrome Rothmund-Thomson syndrome Duane-radial dysplasia syndrome Cleft lip and/or palate with radial dysplasia Goldblatt-Viljoen syndrome (radial ray-choanal atresia) Mobius syndrome (congenital facial diplegia) Hanhart syndrome (micrognathia and limb anomalies) Laryngeal atresia and laryngeal web with radial atresia Acro-renal-ocular syndrome Ophthalmo-mandibulo-melic dysplasia Roberts-SC phocomelia syndrome Levy-Hollister (LARD) syndrome
Skeletal abnormalities	VATER (or VACTERL) association Klippel-Feil syndrome Funston syndrome (cervical rib-radial ray defect) Keutel syndrome (costo-vertebral dysplasia/humero-radial synostosis)
Mental retardation	Seckel syndrome Cornelia de Lange syndrome
Renal abnormalities	Sofer syndrome (renal-radial ray aplasia)
Chromosome abnormalities	Trisomy 18 Trisomy 17 Trisomy 21 Trisomy 13 Chromosome 4 Deletion (4q- and 13q-) Ring chromosomes (B and D2)
Teratogenic syndromes	Aminopterin-induced syndrome Thalidomide embryopathy Varicella embryopathy
Miscellaneous	IVIC syndrome Smith-Lemli-Opitz syndrome with radial dysplasia

TAR syndrome

This autosomal recessive condition consists of bilateral type IV radial club hands with thumbs always present, but sometimes hypoplastic, and thrombocytopenia. Platelet count tends to improve with time, reaching normality around five years of age. Surgery should be deferred until platelet count exceeds 90,000. Platelet transfusion is needed perioperatively and may be required postoperatively. Up to 80% have lower limb defects needing orthopaedic attention (Christensen and Ferguson 2000) and 30% may have cardiac defects, especially Fallot's tetralogy (Goldberg and Bartoshesky 1985). Syndactyly, brachymesophalangia and clinodactyly may also feature.

Aase-Smith syndrome

This rare condition presents with a triphalangeal non-opposable thumb and mild radial hypoplasia. Hypoplastic anaemia and cardiac defects may occur.

Congenital heart disease

Holt-Oram syndrome

The cardiac septum, like the radius, forms in the fifth week of foetal life. Holt-Oram syndrome is an autosomal dominant condition with complete penetrance where both radial and cardiac defects occur. It manifests with increasing severity in successive generations consistent with anticipation. Skeletal defects affect the upper limbs exclusively and are always bilateral and usually asymmetrical. The radial ray is predominantly affected. In contrast to isolated radial club hand, this is more severe on the left than the right. The spectrum of associated abnormalities varies from clinodactyly, limited supination, and sloping shoulders to severe reduction deformities of the upper arm. Cardiac defects occur in 95% of familial cases and include both atrial septal defects (ASD, 34%) and ventricular septal defects (VSD, 25%); 39% have only ECG changes (Newbury-Econ et al 1996). Cardiac involvement ranges from asymptomatic conduction disturbances to multiple structural defects requiring surgery in infancy. Sudden death may be caused by heart block.

Lewis upper limb cardiovascular syndrome (ventriculoradial dysplasia)

This syndrome includes cardiac defects and multiple upper limb anomalies. It is debatable whether this is part of Holt-Oram syndrome or a separate entity.

Craniofacial abnormalities

Nager acrofacial dysostosis

This craniofacial dysostosis comprises maxillary and mandibular hypoplasia with ear deformities and cleft lip and/or palate. Some patients have radial ray defects, particularly hypoplasia and radio-ulnar synostosis.

Hemifacial microsomia

There is a maldevelopment of structures derived from the first branchial arch. Radial ray defects occur in a small minority.

Goldenhar syndrome

Oculo-auriculo-vertebral syndrome also has an association with cardiac, renal, and radial defects.

Juberg-Haywood syndrome (oro-cranio-digital syndrome)

This is an autosomal recessive condition where a hypoplastic thumb and short radius are associated with cleft lip and/or palate, microcephaly and syndactyly of the feet.

Baller-Gerold syndrome

This autosomal recessive condition combines craniosynostosis and imperforate anus with bilateral radial club hands and abnormal thumbs.

Rothmund-Thomson syndrome

This condition links acro-osteolysis, soft tissue calcification, and small hands with poikiloderma, congenital cataracts, and short stature. It is autosomal recessive.

Duane-radial dysplasia syndrome

This is an autosomal dominant condition where abnormal ocular movements are combined with deafness, vertebral and renal abnormalities, and radial club hand.

Roberts syndrome-secretory component (SC) phocomelia syndrome

Tetraphocomelia is associated with cleft lip and plate, other craniofacial abnormalities, genito-urinary, cardiac, and renal defects in this autosomal recessive condition.

Levy-Hollister (LARD) syndrome

Lacrimo-auriculo-radial-dental syndrome is of autosomal dominant inheritance. The patient has abnormal teeth and ears with no lacrimal appara-tus, radial ray defects, ulnar hypoplasia, syndactyly, and triphalangeal thumbs.

Skeletal abnormalities

VATER (or VACTERL) association

This is probably the most frequent syndromic association with radial club hand. It combines a minimum of three of the following: vertebral abnormalities, anorectal, cardiac, tracheo-oesophageal, renal, limb anomalies, and a single umbilical artery. The radial ray defects, being most evident, may be the initial presentation.

Klippel-Feil syndrome

The chief abnormalities in this sporadic condition are cervical fusions, cervical rib, kyphoscoliosis

and basilar artery insufficiency. Hands are only occasionally affected.

Mental retardation

Seckel syndrome

These patients have bird-headed dwarfism with radial deficiency, particularly affecting the thumbs, clinodactyly and dislocated radial head.

Chromosome abnormalities

Trisomy 18 (Edwards syndrome)

These patients have mental retardation, typical facies, cardiac and renal defects and foot abnor-malities. There are radial defects in 10% (D'Arcangelo et al 2000). Death is usually within a year of life.

Trisomy 21 (Down syndrome)

A single palmar crease is normal in this condi-tion but many other upper limb conditions have been described. Cardiac abnormalities are present in 40% or more.

Trisomy 13 (Patau syndrome)

These patients with cleft lip and palate, microph-thalmia, hypotelorism, cardiac defects and devel-opmental delay, mainly have a simian palmar crease and polydactyly. Radial ray defects also occur.

Miscellaneous

IVIC syndrome

This is named after Instituto Venzolano de Investigaciones Cientificas where it was first recognized. It is an autosomal dominant condi-tion with strabismus and deafness and radial ray deficiencies.

Management

Diagnosis

A new patient presenting with radial club hand must be investigated thoroughly to exclude other associated conditions. A full history must be obtained including a detailed family history, pregnancy history, and details of any consanguineous relationship. The child should undergo a detailed examination for other anomalies. Further investigations include a radiograph of the limb and a full blood count. Other tests depend on clinical findings but cardiac and renal investigations are frequently appropriate. Blood may be taken for chromosome analysis. Referral to a geneticist is helpful if there are other anomalies, both for establishing a diagnosis and counselling the parents regarding the risk of producing further affected siblings and the child's own risk of transmitting the condition.

Prenatal diagnosis

Routine prenatal ultrasonography may detect radial club hand. Certain groups such as those with an abnormal initial scan, with exposure to known teratogens in the first trimester, with obstetric problems or with a family history of congenital hand abnormalities undergo a more detailed scan during the second trimester. This should detect absence or hypoplasia of the radius or of the thumb or abnormal posture of the hand. If detected, this increases the index of suspicion for other anomalies. Amniocentesis, chorionic villus sampling, or cordocentesis allow chromosomal analysis, alpha-fetoprotein, and foetal blood sampling.

Treatment proposed

Untreated adults with unilateral deformities cope well with their disability. They use their normal hand for the majority of activities, with the affected one used for stabilization. In the bilateral case, the untreated adult may appear to function well but close questioning will reveal significant difficulties with activities of daily living. Buttoning clothes, attention to personal hygiene, turning keys, opening containers, riding bicycles, and driving may all be difficult. The apparently functioning individual is either avoiding these activities, has adapted to performing them in an alternative and inefficient manner, or needs the use of aids or an assistant to do so.

The aim of treatment, in the surgeon's eyes, is primarily to obtain functional improvement. Treatment attempts to correct the wrist deformity, maintain satisfactory wrist position and movement, preserve the maximum growth capacity of the forearm, and obtain an acceptable cosmetic result. Few authors would proscribe to the traditional view that these children should not be operated on or that surgery should always be confined to one limb. In the patients' view, the emphasis changes as they get older and cosmesis becomes their primary concern.

Wrist stabilization provides both functional and cosmetic improvement to the limb. It improves the mechanical advantage for the forearm musculature, hence improving finger motion and allowing increased grip strength. It effectively lengthens the arm by realignment and some suggest it stimulates distal epiphyseal growth (Kelikian 1974). By correcting the position of the hand on the forearm, the opportunity for pollicization to improve hand function is created. Pollicization in the presence of an unstable wrist will be ineffective.

Management options adopted will depend on the age of the patient, their functional disabilities, other associated anomalies and the severity of the deficiency.

Conservative treatment

Passive manipulation of the upper limbs by bending the elbow and distracting the tight radial tissues at the wrist should be initiated soon after birth. This needs to be repeated at every feed and should last approximately 10-min. It is important that it is explained to the parents that it will induce some discomfort in the child.

The elbow is frequently stiff but may improve with time. The accepted wisdom is that any surgery to correct the wrist position must be deferred until a reasonable range of flexion, ideally 90°, is obtained at the elbow. The concern is that failure to do so may result in a cosmetically acceptable, but functionally poor limb that is unable to reach the mouth to feed. We have never encountered this and found that wrist centralization leads to good elbow flexion within one month of surgery.

In type I and milder degrees of type II deficiencies, passive manipulation combined with splintage until skeletal maturity may be the only treatment required. In more severe deficiencies, this is an essential prelude to surgical intervention. This aims to progressively eliminate the contracture and improve the mobility and range of both the wrist and elbow.

Where the parents are reluctant to distract the wrists or the deviation is severe, serial casting may help to stretch the soft tissues or maintain the position. However, it is fraught with problems. It requires significant expertise, the shape of the child's arm does not accommodate casts well, pressure sores are a significant risk, and the cast needs frequent changes and cannot be used if the elbow is stiff in extension. The use of a brace with a ratchet holds similar problems. Correction does not address the entire deformity and tilts the carpus on the ulnar epiphysis rather than placing the hand in the correct relationship to the distal ulna. A combination of passive stretching to obtain the correct position and application of a brace to maintain that position gives better anatomical correction. Splintage should be continuous and be applied as soon as is feasible and this is only practical once the limb reaches a reasonable size.

Problems with serial casting and bracing are such that many surgeons prefer to emphasize manipulation and have abandoned these techniques in the baby. The use of neoprene braces (Kennedy 1996) may obviate some of these problems but, in some centres, new techniques of soft tissue distraction have superseded these.

Lamb (1997) has demonstrated that the wrist, if in a good position, encourages the development of elbow flexion in a proportion of those patients with stiff extended elbows. Once the deformity is easily correctable or fails to improve further, wrist stabilization or centralization should be performed. There is some confusion in the literature as to when to discontinue splintage, with some authors recommending continuation until growth is complete, even after surgery.

Contraindications to surgical treatment

There are instances where surgical treatment may not be appropriate. These have been detailed by Dobyns et al (1993):

- Children who have adequate function and other anomalies that shorten their life expectancy or have severe mental retardation.
- Patients less than six months old where major anomalies or blood dyscrasias may not have become apparent.
- Adults who have adapted to their deformity, establishing entrenched functional patterns using an ulnar prehensile pattern.
- Patients with severe contractures and neurovascular deficiencies that make correction impossible.
- Patients with type I or mild type II deficiencies who may be adequately treated conservatively.

In addition, patients with poor elbow flexion bilaterally are generally stated to be unsuitable candidates as surgery may restrict their functionality still further. This is not our experience at Great Ormond Street Hospital where we have seen an improvement in elbow flexion following wrist centralization or stabilization procedures.

Operative treatment

In type I or mild type II deficiencies, if the wrist remains unstable, surgery may be recommended to lengthen the radius. More severe type II, type III and IV deficiencies require operative realignment of the hand on the forearm. This entails realignment of the carpus on the ulna with or without preoperative soft tissue distraction and/or release, rebalancing of deforming forces by tendon transfers and correction of the ulna curvature with actual lengthening when necessary.

Those who believe that wrist stabilization should not be attempted without an adequate range of elbow flexion suggest posterior elbow capsulotomy or tendon transfers to assist weak elbow flexors (Menelaus 1976). We do not believe this at Great Ormond Street Hospital. We have seen a rapid improvement in range of elbow movement following soft tissue distraction and wrist stabilization and have never performed surgery on the elbow in these cases and see no requirement for it.

Surgery for an absent or hypoplastic thumb should be considered but the results are dependent on the severity of the deformity affecting the surrounding digits and are inferior to those with an isolated thumb hypoplasia (Buck-Gramcko 1998, Sykes et al 1991).

Soft tissue release

Flatt (1994) advocates early soft tissue release when a fibrous anlage is present at birth, the ulna is markedly curved, or soft tissue contracture is not passively correctable. A radially sited Z-plasty incision provides access for release of the deep fascia and sometimes a fibrous anlage found deeper. Care must be taken as the median nerve lies immediately beneath the deep fascia in an aberrant position. It is usually the tightest structure remaining and may need to be mobilized from the fascia to obtain full correction.

Sometimes correction may require release of the dorsoradial muscle mass. Ideally they should be reattached in a dorsoulnar position, which will produce a dynamic internal tendon transfer that reinforces the stability achieved by other procedures such as wrist stabilization.

Carpal realignment

Procedures to realign the carpus can be broadly divided into two groups: procedures that add a strut to replace the missing radius and those that attempt to realign the carpus on the remaining ulna. The myriad of procedures described, with further modifications of each, confirms that no single procedure is established as the definitive answer to this problem. Within the literature, there is ambiguity concerning the terminology of procedures to realign the carpus on the ulna in type III and IV deformities. These may be divided into:

- Carpal resecting procedures.
  - Centralization—where a carpal slot is created for the ulna head opposite the third metacarpal.
- Carpal preserving procedures.
  - Radialization—where the whole carpus is preserved and the ulna is placed opposite the second metacarpal and maintained there by rebalancing with tendon transfers.
  - Stabilization—where, following soft tissue distraction, the intact carpus is aligned with the distal end of the ulna opposite the third metacarpal together with tendon transfers.

Bone struts

Historically, attempts were made to replace the missing radius with bone struts. This did not address the other components of this deformity. The non-vascularized graft failed to grow leading to a late recurrence of the deformity associated with a short ulna. Bone struts using tibial, ulna or fibular grafts have been used to provide a bony support for the carpus in lieu of the radius. Albee (1928) inserted bone graft into the radius; Antonelli (1904) split the ulna longitudinally and fitted the carpus in the resultant notch; Ryerson (cited by Kato 1924) used an ulna graft complete with the distal epiphysis and Define (1970) used the periosteum of the ulna with the distal epiphysis attached. Starr (1945) transferred the fibular head as a non-vascularized epiphyseal transfer, but in 1963 Riordan reported his experience with poor growth in the fibular head and abandoned the procedure. Tsuge and Watari (1985) described their use of the first metacarpal as a radial support when they combined realignment of the carpus and pollicization in one procedure but have not published long-term results.

Centralization

Centralization was first described by Sayre in 1893 who placed a sharpened distal ulna in a notch in the carpus created by excision of the lunate and capitate. It became popular after Lidge (1969) described a modification that preserved the distal ulnar epiphysis. The purpose is to stabilize the carpus on the distal ulna whilst maintaining a functional range of wrist movement within the midcarpal joint. For the normal individual wrist flexion of 10°, extension of 30°, 10° of radial and 14° of ulnar deviation is sufficient for most activities. Most authors report results similar to these after centralization.

At Great Ormond Street Hospital, following centralization, we have had a maximum of 20° of flexion-extension that occurs at the midcarpal joint but never had radial and ulnar deviation unless the centralization had failed completely. We believe that high ranges of motion in the literature may represent failure of centralization.

Areas of advancement with centralization have been in preoperative stretching of the soft tissues to limit the surgical release required, the technique of centralization and in the maintenance of a satisfactory position with continued growth. Traditionally, stretching of the tissues has been by manual stretching exercises combined with serial casts and splints. More recently soft tissue distraction using external fixators has emerged. For long-term maintenance of a satisfactory position, rebalancing of the deforming forces on the wrist must be performed by the use of tendon transfers at the time of centralization.

Operative details differ amongst different authors, particularly in the incisions used for exposure (Pilz et al 1998). Access is required to the radial side of the wrist for soft tissue release and to the ulnar side for excision of fibro-fatty tissue and tendon transfers. When exposing the ulna, a distally based capsular flap is raised, preserving the epiphyseal blood supply. Care is taken to avoid damaging the ulnar nerve, its dorsal branch, or the ulnar artery. The radial artery is commonly absent. The extensor retinaculum and the insertion of the extrinsic radial flexors and extensors, which are usually joined, are released. When approaching the radial side of the wrist, the median nerve lies radially just beneath the deep fascia. Sometimes a deeply lying radial fibrous anlage needs release.

After the palmar capsule is released, the carpus can usually be realigned over the distal ulna. The cartilaginous joint surfaces are gently refashioned with a scalpel. Care is taken not to damage the distal ulna epiphyseal growth plate. A notch is created in the carpus that is as deep as the width of the ulna head. This has been shown to be a stable construct (Lamb 1977), but may require dissection of fibrous tissue from the distal ulna and resection of both the proximal and distal carpal bones, especially in cases of long-standing deformity. In the severely curved ulna, an osteotomy may be required simultaneously for the bone to accommodate a Kirschner wire (K-wire). It is possible to be more conservative in carpal resection and obviate the need for an ulnar osteotomy if preoperative soft tissue distraction has been utilized.

The K-wire is passed retrogradely through the shaft of the third metacarpal to emerge through the metacarpal head. It is then driven antegradely through the ulna epiphysis and into the ulnar shaft. The ulna dorsal capsule must be firmly reattached in a vest-over-pants fashion. Tendon transfers may be performed. It has been suggested that, in the bilateral case, ideally one forearm should be placed in 45° of pronation and the other in 45° of supination (Urban and Osterman 1990). This is not our normal practice.

When the K-wire is removed, the arm is put in a thermoplastic splint continuously. Individual regimes for removal of the K-wire vary from six weeks to two years postoperatively. Periods of splintage vary; most suggest splintage until age six and others suggest continuing until skeletal maturity. Complications include the inability to proceed due to vascular compromise, pin tract infections, skin necrosis and pin migration, or fracture. Lamb (1977) in his five year follow-up of 117 cases in 68 patients post-centralization found radial deviation decreased from 78° to 22° with minimal change in finger range of motion and without a detrimental effect on ulnar growth. Bora et al (1970) treated 31 wrists by centralization of the carpus on the ulna with 72% having satisfactory improvement of the deformity. Recurrence of the deformity occurred in three cases, which they attributed to muscle imbalance. No significant impairment of ulnar growth occurred and straightening of the wrist did not affect function adversely (Watson et al 1984).

Stabilization

Watson et al (1984) described a modified centralization procedure, preserving carpal bones but emphasizing excision of the fibrotic radial anlage from the centre of the wrist and forearm to allow the hand to move into the new position. We would term this procedure stabilization to differentiate it from classical centralization. Watson and colleagues described 12 procedures using this technique with good 10–year results. Remodelling of the ulna occurred after 2–6 years, which broadened distally, resembling a radius and giving greater support to the carpus.

Bayne and Klug (1987) followed up 64 patients with 101 radial deficiencies for a mean of 8.6 years, with a range of 1–27 years. Results of stabilization were good in 21, satisfactory in 20, and unsatisfactory in 10. They attributed their poor results to failure to adhere to outlined principles of soft tissue release and adequate centralization. None of their patients had a decrease in finger function or increase in flexion contracture after stabilization. Ulnar growth continued, the ulnar length remaining two-thirds of that of the normal ulna after stabilization unless severe epiphyseal damage had occurred. They advocated early surgery as 54% of those treated under the age of three had good results whilst those treated later had only a 24% success rate.

Damore et al (2000) examined 19 cases of radial club hand in 14 patients who had stabilization or centralization of the carpus at a mean age of 3.2 years (range, 0.7–8.1 years). Those undergoing centralization were the more severe where stabilization was not felt to be possible. They were followed up for a mean of 6.5 years (range 1.5–22.2 years). These procedures corrected the angulation initially by an average of 58° (range 15–95°) but there was a later relapse of 38° (range 5–105°). They found significant correlations between the preoperative angle and the amount of correction, the amount of correction obtained at surgery and the recurrence of the deformity, and the age at time of initial surgery and the amount of recurrence.

Current surgical options favour stabilization without resection of carpal bones, stabilized by tendon transfers. We favour firstly preoperative soft tissue distraction. Following this, 50% of our patients require centralization, due to insufficient muscle mass, which we always supplement with tendon transfers if possible. The other 50%, where there is more substantial muscle bulk, we treat with a combination of stabilization and tendon transfer.

Tendon transfers

Long-term maintenance of the corrected position is related to balancing the deforming forces acting on the wrist. Increasingly with carpal preserving stabilization, tendon transfers are considered vital to prevent recurrence of the deformity. Balance is achieved by providing more pull in the dorsoulnar direction. Centralization alone is frequently followed by a recurrence of the deformity (Bora et al 1981).

The common insertion of the radial flexors and extensors is reattached to the ulnar carpus dorsally or to the extensor carpi ulnaris tendon in centralization, as in radialization. The extensor carpi ulnaris is shortened or advanced distally to the shaft of the fifth metacarpal. The flexor carpi ulnaris may also be moved and sutured to the extensor carpi ulnaris to improve wrist dorsiflexion.

Some authors reattach the origin of the hypothenar muscles, dissecting them from the pisiform and attaching them proximally to the ulna. Manske and McCarroll (1978, 1998) have not found this useful and express concerns regarding interfering with the abductor digiti minimi which may be required for a later opponensplasty.

Bora (1970) also uses the flexor digitorum superficialis tendons to the middle and ring fingers, which he passes around the ulnar border of the forearm and the shafts of the second and third metacarpal to attach back on themselves. This may be carried out primarily or as a secondary procedure. Unfortunately, these tendons may not be present in those severe cases that would benefit most from this transfer.

Radialization

Buck-Gramcko (1985) introduced the technique of radialization and suggested its use at between six and 12 months of age. This procedure repositioned the hand and radial carpal bones over the distal end of the ulna with excision of all fibrotic tissues. No carpal bones were excised. The hand was fixed with a K-wire in an overcorrected position of moderate ulnar deviation. The conjoined radial wrist extensor and flexor were transposed to the extensor carpi ulnaris tendon to improve muscle balance. His results in 30 hands (23 patients) were similar to those of Watson et al (1984) using stabilization.

Radialization, theoretically, allows greater protection for the distal ulnar epiphysis thereby maintaining maximal length, and allows optimal wrist motion. Placing the ulna radially decreases the moment arm of the radial soft tissues. Release and transposition of the radial muscle mass, which acts as a deforming force may be the most important part. More recently, Buck-Gramcko has suggested that those with more severe deformities do not do so well with this procedure.

Arthrodesis

Wrist arthrodesis corrects the position of the hand and stabilizes the wrist but limits the range of motion, and potential function, of an already compromised limb (Heikel 1959). It is not recommended in the bilateral case (Lamb 1977). To avoid further reduction in growth potential, it should be deferred in the unilateral case until the distal ulnar epiphysis has completed its growth around the age of 12 years. By then, the child has well-established patterns of prehension using the deformed hand. Most surgeons reserve arthrodesis for salvage cases in the adolescent or adult patient, although this may often be the inadvertent result of attempted centralization.

History of distraction lengthening

Distraction lengthening is a confusing term in the literature as it is applied to three different procedures, all of which use external fixation to distract tissues. In distraction osteogenesis, popularised by Ilizarov (1990), a corticotomy and distraction stimulate new bone formation, which consolidates in time. In rapid distraction and bone grafting, popularised by Matev (1979), an osteoid bed is formed which usually requires bone grafting to fill the gap. Soft tissue distraction allows stretching of all the soft tissues only limited by neurovascular compromise.

Soft tissue distraction

Kessler (1989) applied the techniques of distraction using external fixators to the soft tissues in the radial club hand. He used a device, previously used for distraction osteogenesis, to distract the soft tissues pre- or perioperatively for centralization. The main objective is to reduce radial angulation but it also avoids the need for a Z-plasty to the skin and bone resection. An advantage of this technique over traditional techniques of serial casting or bracing is its ability to simultaneously distract and correct radial deviation of the wrist.

Nanchahal and Tonkin (1996) confirmed the efficacy of this technique. They found that preoperative distraction of soft tissues allowed radialization without excision of a part of the carpus in five out of six patients whilst centralization with carpal excision was necessary in five out of six patients not treated by preoperative distraction. Average improvements in radial angulation and radial translation were 19° and 16 mm in the non-distraction group and 38° and 17 mm in the distraction group. It is still uncertain what rate of neural lengthening and increase in length is permitted without causing intraneural damage.

Bone lengthening

Radial lengthening

In type I or mild type II deficiencies, the wrist may be stable but with a radially deviated hand. Kessler (1989) and Manske and McCarroll (1998) have treated some of their patients by distraction osteogenesis of the radius. The osteotomy is performed at the midshaft of the radius and the proximal pins inserted so as to transfix the ulna to avoid proximal radial distraction. Manske and McCarroll (1998) gained 18–20 mm of increased length but were circumspect about the degree of relapse that might be expected with growth.

Ulnar lengthening

The short forearm, typical of radial club hand, is both a functional and a cosmetic problem. Carrying things and heavy work is awkward with limbs of disparate length. Driving a manual gearbox car may be impossible if the forearm is too short to reach the gear stick. The space in which the affected arm can function is limited by its length, and the movement of the shoulder. Once the forearm is lengthened, the elbow movement becomes more important in placing the hand in space. With a good shoulder and elbow and reasonable forearm length, wrist movement is less important and primary arthrodesis may be suitable for those with very deficient musculature. Traditional techniques used in osteotomies and bone grafting often had donor site morbidity and were only able to provide small improvements in length.

In 1977 Dick et al reported on two cases that had had bilateral lengthened forearms by distraction lengthening using an Abbott-Anderson device. This required two lengthening cycles to gain 5.4 and 6.4 cm and they experienced significant problems with non-union. They succeeded in lengthening the ulna by 50%.

The Ilizarov technique, developed in the Soviet Union, gradually gained acceptance in lower limb trauma. Slowly reports in the literature of its use in the upper limb began to emerge (Smith and Greene (1995), initially, for a variety of pathologies. Villa et al (1990) reported lengthening of 13 cm (130%). Tetsworth et al (1991), despite functional and cosmetic improvement in 92% of their patients, reported a complication rate of 86%.

With distraction in radial club hand, there are the specific problems of angulation of the proximal fragment under the stress of lengthening and angulation of the wrist, necessitating separate fixation of the hand. Seitz and Froimen (1991) considered that the full circular frame was not essential, a half-frame lengthening device being adequate. Even the most successful centralization, radialization or stabilization will, at best, result in a relatively stiff wrist with interference with growth distally. Ulnar lengthening, using the Ilizarov technique, may be suitable after wrist centralization in neglected cases or those with recurrent deformity or growth disturbances. It is used when there is residual shortening and bowing of the ulna with recurrent radial deviation of the hand causing functional and cosmetic problems. Two full rings are applied to the ulna and a subperiosteal ulnar osteotomy is performed. Distraction is commenced on the concave side at seven days and continued at 0.5 mm per day. Once the angular correction is made, bone lengthening is continued until the ulna length matches that of the contralateral side. Weekly radiographs monitor callus formation and the distraction rate is altered to avoid premature consolidation or poor callus formation. Bayne and Klug (1987) do not suggest osteotomy if the angular deformity is less than 30°.

It has been suggested that ulnar bowing and ulnar length remain stable postoperatively and patients retain cosmetic and functional improvement (Damore et al 2000). Others suggest that only 57% of the angular correction is maintained at a mean of 3.6 years postoperatively (Bora et al 1981). This discrepancy may be related to uncorrected muscle imbalance. Kawabata et al (1998) achieved mean lengthening of 51% although at follow-up length had deteriorated to 83%. Whether this is due to the ulnar physis having intrinsically poor growth or distraction osteogenesis itself restricting growth by applying a compressive force on the ulnar physis is uncertain. Paley and Herzenberg (1998) reviewed the technique and found that it was possible to lengthen 5–8 cm in 6–8 year olds and 10–13 cm in 12–16 year olds.

Catagni et al (1993) used the Ilizarov technique for ulnar lengthening in five adults with radial hemimelia and previous wrist centralization. Although successful with a gain in ulna length from 4–13 cm all procedures were prolonged (7–25 months) and all patients had complications. Four of the five patients had stiff digits afterwards but their hand function was improved. Villa et al (1990) performed 13 forearm-lengthening operations in 12 patients for a variety of problems, gaining between 2 cm and 13 cm (10–143%) in 3–19 months. Eleven of the 12 patients were functionally and cosmetically improved. In nine patients, the cosmetic improvement made a significant psychological difference. Complication rates were high and included three temporary deep radial nerve palsies, one sympathetic dystrophy, one malunion, one delayed malunion, two refractures, and three mild losses of motion.

Ulnar lengthening should not be performed until stability has been obtained at the wrist. The timing of this varies between individuals and the age at which the child will tolerate this treatment varies considerably. Different series describe distraction from a mean of six years onwards until adulthood. The argument for delaying this treatment comes from the uncertainty of the effect distraction has on epiphyseal growth. Late distraction will remain stable whereas early distraction may lose some gain, as the contralateral limb growth is greater. However, it frequently produces stiffness and younger children may recover function quicker.

Ulna curvature

Curving and hypoplasia of the ulna is an integral part of the more severe radial deficiencies, especially when untreated. If curved at birth, some authors suggest this is due to an anlage of the radius and suggest early release. There is controversy as to whether ulna curvature is static or progressive but several authors (Damore et al 2000) have shown no evidence of progression following centralization with tendon transfers, when the deforming forces have been removed. Closing wedge osteotomies may be performed, proximal to the intramedullary pin stabilizing the wrist, at the time of centralization or radialization. This is easier to do when the radius is rudimentary or absent but shortens the ulna further.

Glossop and Flatt (1995) used a computer-simulated model looking at opening or closing wedge osteotomies to straighten the curved ulna in radial club hands. They applied this to 68 lateral x-ray films of curved ulnae in 39 children. Closing wedge osteotomies yielded only millimetres gain in length, many decreased it. Opening wedge osteotomies of reasonable angle lengthened the ulna by 5 mm or more. They suggested that no more than two wedges should be used. We have found that, by using soft tissue distraction for three months preoperatively, the ulnar bowing corrects spontaneously, avoiding the requirement for osteotomies. This is due to bone remodelling in response to the longitudinal forces exerted on the bone.

Microsurgical reconstruction

Microsurgical techniques have rekindled an interest in the provision of a bony strut to stabilize the hand against the ulna. Modifications of Starr's fibula transfer technique to incorporate microvascular transfer have been made with descriptions of microvascular transfer of distal fibula epiphyseal grafts. Tsai et al (1986) used vascularized epiphyseal transfer in eight patients, two of whom had radial club hand. Of these two, one underwent premature epiphyseal closure whereas the other grew only slightly less than expected. Pho et al (1988) used free vascularized epiphyseal transfer of the proximal fibula in three patients that showed signs of longitudinal growth and epiphyseal adaptation.

Vilkki (1998) has described a technique for Bayne type IV radial club hands using preoperative soft tissue distraction to achieve proper alignment of the hand on the ulna followed by microvascular epiphysis transfer of the second metatarsophalangeal joint with the whole of the metatarsal. He suggests performing this in the second year of life as it is technically demanding procedure and to limit damage to the epiphysis, ischaemic time should not exceed 3–4 hours. His six-year results are promising but the long-term results will be dependent on continued growth so follow-up until skeletal maturity is necessary.

Results of surgery

Radial deformity

Objective measurements of improvement in radial club hand are difficult. Measuring angles is problematic (Heikel 1959) as are obtaining standardized radiographs in a child with limited motion in the limb. With growth the surgical correction of the hand position on the forearm is not always maintained.

Lamb (1977) reported an improvement from 78° radial deviation preoperatively to 22° following centralization. Bora et al (1981), looking at the maintenance of correction over 10 years following centralization with tendon transfer, found that there was a measurable, but functionally insignificant, increase in the hand-forearm angle and a decrease in ulnar bowing. There were no significant changes in ulnar length, wrist position of wrist or elbow motion.

Manske et al (1981) described specific measurements to assess his results. The hand-forearm angle lies between the longitudinal axis of the third metacarpal and that of the distal ulna. The hand-forearm position is the length of the perpendicular from the proximal pole of the fifth metacarpal to the longitudinal axis of the distal ulna. The latter was considered a more valid assessment of surgical improvement than hand-forearm angle. Manske and colleagues (1981) reported a change in hand-forearm position from an average of 10 mm radial to the longitudinal axis of the distal ulna to an average of 12 mm ulnar to it. He used a single ulnar approach and did not release radial structures.

Geck et al (1999) showed a statistically significant correction of hand-forearm angle and hand-forearm position with radialization similar to modified centralization in 29 limbs in 23 patients with a mean follow-up of 50 months. Final wrist position was not affected by age, severity of deformity, or the performance of an ulnar osteotomy. The survivorship rate at five years was 67%. Significant risk factors for revision included radial or positive hand-forearm angle and early surgery. There was a suggestion that small postoperative hand-forearm position, or radial translation, increased the risk of revision.

Ulnar Length

Heikel (1959) showed that in patients with radial club hand the growth of the distal ulnar epiphysis is slowed and that surgery may further adversely affect distal ulnar growth. Bora et al (1981) noted that the retardation in length with radial club hand was not significantly worsened by surgery unless the physeal plate was damaged. Hippe and Blauth (1979) found that 17% of their patients had growth disturbance postoperatively. Lamb (1977) failed to show growth disturbance if centralization was performed prior to eight years of age and Frankel et al (1971) found poor growth if centralization was performed after the age of five years.
Heikel (1959) and Manske et al (1981) both demonstrated that surgery does not alter the curvature of the ulna and nor does it spontaneously correct. Bayne and Klug (1987) state that in patients with elbow webbing it is difficult to obtain sufficient soft tissue release and they are more likely to sustain epiphyseal damage. Likewise older children > 12 years are more diffi-

cult to centralize and so epiphyseal damage is more likely. They consider the ideal timing for centralization to be between six months and one year old. In their series over 50% of the good results were treated at less than three years old and their good results also had adequate preoperative soft tissue stretching, surgical goals attained, proper postoperative bracing and less severe soft tissue contractures and hand defects. They believed that inadequate soft tissue release creates a pressure effect that produces unequal ulnar epiphyseal growth leading to distal ulnar bowing (more distal than that seen at birth which is mid-diaphyseal). In their series of 101 radial deficiencies in 64 patients, 15 of the 26 ulnar osteotomies performed were necessary because of unequal growth and angulation.

Function

Demonstrating functional improvement in the unilateral case may prove difficult since the children are functionally well adjusted preoperatively. Lamb (1997) noted functional benefits in bilateral cases. Following radialization, active wrist flexion ranges between 40–90°, extension is to neutral, active ulnar deviation to neutral, and radial deviation from 30–55° (Buck-Gramcko 1985). The expected improvement in range of motion of the digits has not been found (Heikel 1959, Lamb 1977) but Bora et al (1981) found that operated patients had 54% of the normal digital range of motion compared to non-operated patients who had only 27%. Heikel (1959) could find no difference in grip strength between untreated and treated extremities.

Thumb hypoplasia

The incidence of thumb hypoplasia or aplasia in radial club hand varies from 17–100% (Allison 2000) in different series. Management depends on the severity of thumb involvement, the severity of the proximal defect and whether it is unilateral or bilateral. Thumb hypoplasia may require a flexor digitorum superficialis (FDS) opponensplasty for Blauth type IIA (Lister 1985) or a chondrodesis and an abductor digiti minimi

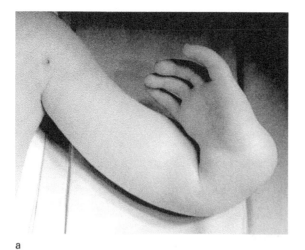

a

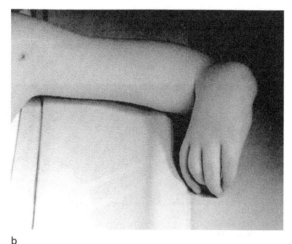

b

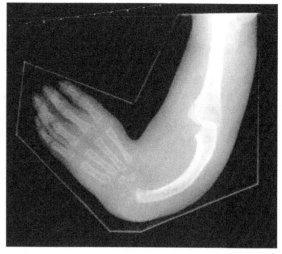

c

Figure 5

Preoperative photograph (a) and radiograph (b) of patient with type IV radial club hand when limb is of sufficient size to apply fixator (has associated thumb aplasia).

transfer for Blauth type IIB (Manske and McCarroll 1978). Thumb hypoplasia of Blauth type IIIB, IV, or V requires pollicization on a minimum of one side if the condition is bilateral. Many authors believe that pollicization is not worthwhile in the unilateral case and should only be carried out on the dominant side in the bilateral case. We would agree with Lamb (1977) that pollicization should be carried out if the overall condition of the limb and hand suggest that worthwhile functional benefit may be achieved.

Pollicization for isolated thumb hypoplasia usually gives excellent functional results. Pollicization in an isolated radial club hand with thumb hypoplasia also gives results that are

good although it is essential to stabilize the wrist first and assess the index finger which may be hypoplastic and may be missing its flexor and extensor tendons (Manske et al 1972).

Patients with syndromic radial club hand behave differently and do not do so well (Buck-Gramcko 1998, Manske and McCarroll 1992, Sykes et al 1991). They frequently have stiff adjacent digits, which limit the functional improvement they can obtain from a pollicization. In addition, they demonstrate specific problems such as a flexion contracture of the proximal interphalangeal joint of the index finger and radial deviation of the finger that need to be addressed prior to pollicization. Deciding which patients will do sufficiently well to justify pollicization in these cases can be difficult. Pollicization narrows the palm but this may not alter their function significantly. In this group of patients, poor grip strength is normal and they are unlikely to adopt heavy manual occupations. There have been reports of pollicization of the most ulnar digit (Harrison 1970, Wood 1988) rather than the index finger but this is not standard practice.

Our approach to radial club hand

Initially the patient is assessed by a paediatrician to check for other birth defects, particularly those which need to take precedence over the operative management of the limb problems. During this time the parents are encouraged to perform stretching exercises, both to the wrist and to the digits, prior to each feed. This allows maintenance of joint mobility and gradual distraction of the wrist by stretching to maintain length of radial tissues.

As soon as is practicable splints are fitted which are used at night. These need adjusting every 2–4 weeks, until the patient is operated on. When the forearm is large enough, we apply a Pennig fixator across the wrist to perform soft tissue distraction (Fig. 5). This is normally at a minimum of 10 months old. If the child is learning to walk, it is deferred until they are stable on their feet.

Generally, it is possible to stretch the wrist sufficiently at the time of surgery to apply the fixator. Rarely, the wrist is very tight and the flexion of the hand on the forearm is greater than the maximum flexion of the distractor. In these cases, open release of the deep fascia overlying the radial structures is required to apply the fixator. Sometimes the brachioradialis, radial extensors, and the flexor carpi radialis are divided distally. Two pins are placed transversely, distally through a minimum of two metacarpals (four cortices) and two are placed transversely, proximally through the ulna. The longest fixator that will fit is applied. Care is taken to ensure that it is not interfering with elbow flexion (Fig. 6). A radiograph confirms satisfactory pin placement (Fig. 7). We have

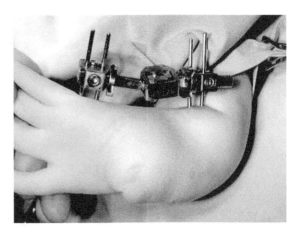

Figure 6

Application of longest Pennig fixator possible to the radial side of the forearm and hand of the patient in Figure 5. Care is taken to avoid interfering with elbow flexion but the fixator bar must extend proximally to achieve maximum distraction length with each fixator.

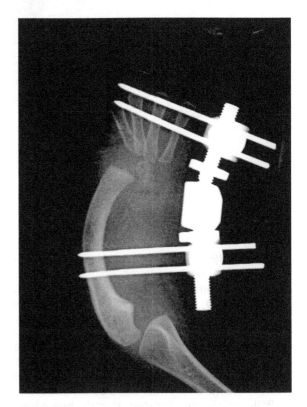

Figure 7

Radiological confirmation of satisfactory pin placement in the patient in Figures 5 and 6.

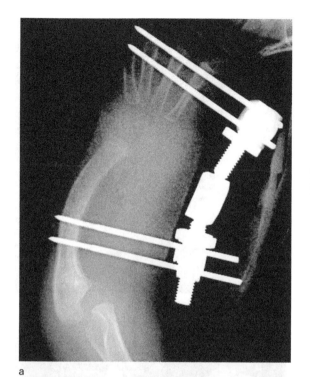

a

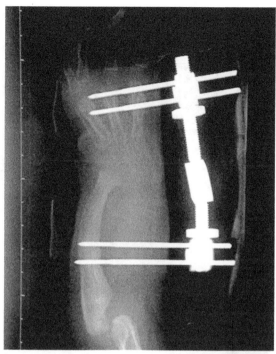

b

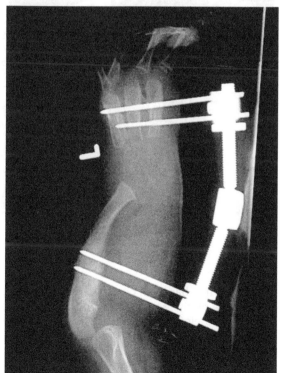

c

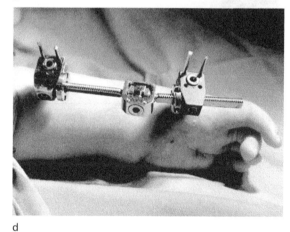

d

Figure 8

Radiological series of forearm during soft tissue distraction in the patient shown in Figures 5–7. (a) Radiograph taken after three weeks of distraction. (b) Radiograph taken after two months of distraction. (c) Radiograph taken four months after application of Pennig fixator, following completion of distraction and short period of remodelling. Note periosteal reaction on concave side of ulna with early remodelling. (d) Clinical photograph taken four months after application of Pennig fixator, after completion of distraction.

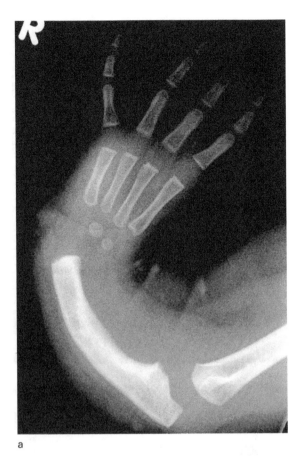

a

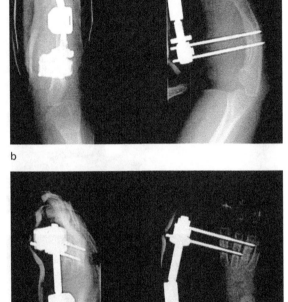

b

c

Figure 9

Radiological changes and ulnar remodelling occurring with soft tissue distraction. (a) Preoperative radiograph of type IV radial club hand with marked ulnar bowing. (b) Radiograph of same patient six weeks post application of Pennig fixator showing marked periosteal reaction on the concave side of the ulna as reaction to stress loading. (c) Radiograph of same patient, following completion of distraction, five months after application of fixator. Note the ulna straightening following remodelling resulting in an ulna less likely to require osteotomy.

found that in children with stiff elbows, their range of motion at the elbow improves after the wrist has been straightened.

After 48 hours, the dressing is changed and the children and parents are taught how to clean the pin sites. Distraction is delayed for a week postoperatively and then begun at 1 mm/day. When the bone has been distracted the whole length of the bar, the bar is exchanged for a longer one on the ward. Distraction usually takes about six to eight weeks. Figure 8 demonstrates the distraction process to the full length of the longest fixator. The fixator is left on longer if the ulna is bowed as we have observed that, with distraction, periosteal reaction occurs on the concave surface and the bone appears to

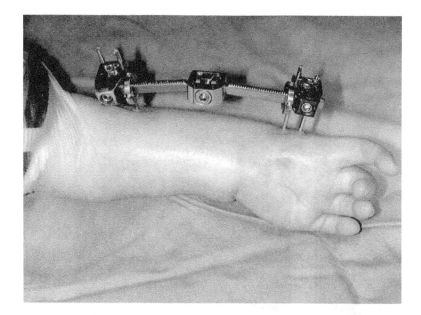

Figure 10

Photograph of patient shown in Figures 5–8, post distraction, ready for wrist stabilization or centralization.

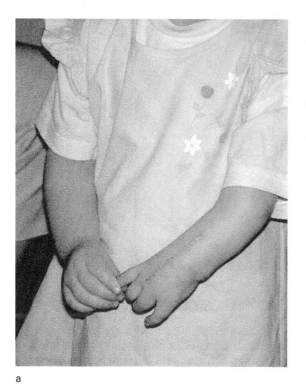

a

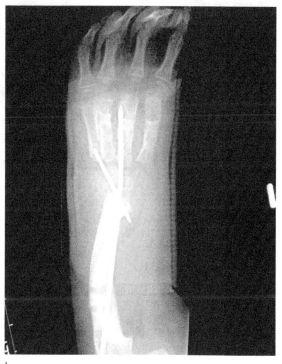

b

Figure 11

Early postoperative result following wrist centralization of patient shown in Figures 5–8 and 10. (a) Photograph demonstrating dorsal incision and corrected position of hand on forearm. (b) Radiograph of same patient immediately post wrist centralization.

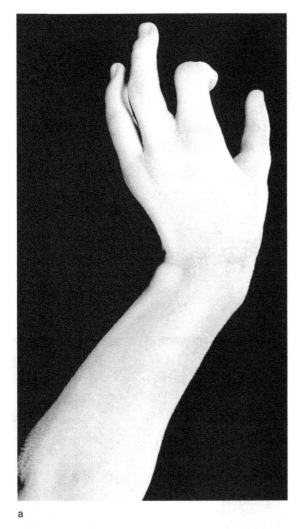

a

Figure 12

(a) Clinical photograph and (b) radiograph showing y-shaped distal ulna that can arise with distraction.

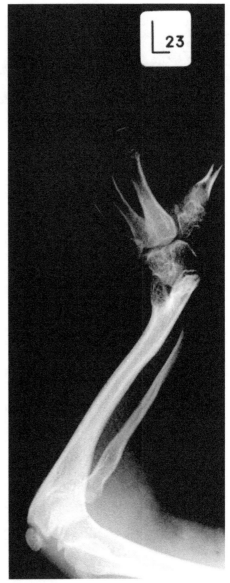

b

remodel straighter. This may take several months. Figure 9 demonstrates the bony changes and remodelling that occur radiologically with the distraction process.

When we are satisfied with the position of the hand and the ulna remodelling, the patient is admitted for wrist centralization or stabilization and tendon transfer (Fig.10). At operation, if the patient is found to have good muscle mass,

stabilization is performed with carpal preservation and transfer of the radial muscle mass to extensor carpi ulnaris. A single axial K-wire is passed across the wrist through the third metacarpal shaft. This is removed one year later. If the muscle mass is found to be poor, the ulna is placed into a carpal slot and the wrist is fixed with an axial K-wire and an oblique one (Fig. 11). Tendon transfer is performed if possible. The oblique wire is removed when it loosens whilst the axial one is left indefinitely.

Since we have started using preoperative soft tissue distraction, we have rarely needed to perform ulnar osteotomies. Seven of our patients have developed a y-shaped distal ulna with distraction (Fig. 12) although this has not caused any functional impairment. We usually pollicize the index finger on the best side in bilateral cases and repeat the procedure on the other side if the patient requests it or has done reasonably well from the first procedure.

The single most important development within the management of radial club hand, which has changed our practice at Great Ormond Street Hospital, is the use of preoperative soft tissue distraction. We consider it provides several distinct advantages:

- It negates the problem of excessive soft tissue on the ulnar side of the wrist at stabilization. This avoids the problem of designing incisions and raising flaps to redistribute the skin and reduces the visible scarring. We use a dorsal straight-line incision (Fig.13).
- It permits lengthening of the radial soft tissues.
- It maintains normal ulnar length because it protects the distal epiphysis. We have found that the ulna growth obtained in those who have undergone soft tissue distraction exceeds that in those who have not.
- If the distractor is maintained in position for three months, angulatory correction of the ulna occurs (Fig. 9). This is due to bone remodelling because of the longitudinal forces applied to the bone. It avoids the need for ulna osteotomies.
- We have found that elbow flexion improves shortly after distraction has commenced.
- In total, 50% of our patients undergo wrist stabilization and tendon transfer, maintaining some wrist motion. The rest require centralization with the creation of a carpal slot. Either procedure is made easier when the child has undergone distraction.

Conclusion

Radial club hand is an aesthetically distressing condition initially for the parents and later the

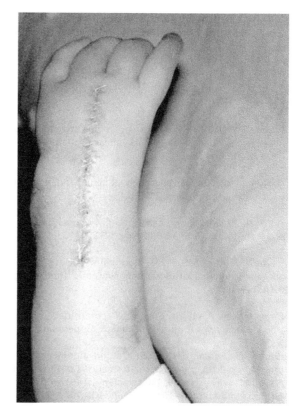

Figure 13

Dorsal straight-line approach to the wrist is possible where preoperative soft tissue distraction has been employed.

child. Functionally there is good adaptation to the deformity, despite the forearm shortening, deviated wrist and stiff digits. With hypoplastic or absent thumbs often a dorsal prehensile pattern is established which may be quite precise, although inefficient and relatively weak. Frequently the child has other abnormalities that may also affect the physical and mental development and therefore, hand function.

There is no universal agreement on the management of those children with the more severe deformities but most authors would suggest addressing the wrist initially, either with radialization or centralization. We have found that soft tissue distraction has a number of advantages in these patients and may improve their long-term functional outcome. We would advocate the use of this prior to open procedures on the wrist and would suggest combining the latter with tendon transposition wherever possible.

References

Albee FH (1928) Formation of radius congenitally absent: condition seven years after implantation of bone graft, *Ann Surg* **87**:105.

Allison M (2000) The spectrum of radial longitudinal deficiency, *J Hand Surg* **25A**:984.

Antonelli I (1904) Su un caso macanza congenita bilaterale del radio, *Gazz Med Italiana* **55**:501–13.

Bayne LG, Klug MS (1987) Long-term review of the surgical treatment of radial deficiencies, *J Hand Surg* **12A**:169–79.

Birch-Jensen A (1949) *Congenital deformities of the upper extremities* (Ejnar Munksgaard: Copenhagen).

Blauth W, Schmidt H (1969) On the significance of arteriographic diagnosis in malformations of the radial marginal ray (radial dysplasia). *Zeitschrift für Orthopaedie und Ihre Grenzgebiete* **106**:102–10.

Bora FW, Nicholson JT, Cheema HM (1970) Radial meromelia. The deformity and its treatment, *J Bone Joint Surg* **52A**:966–79.

Bora FW Jr, Osterman AL, Kaneda RR, Esterhai J (1981) Radial club-hand deformity: long-term follow-up, *J Bone Joint Surg* **63A**:741–45.

Buck-Gramcko D (1985) Radialization as a new treatment for radial club hand, *J Hand Surg* **10A**:964–68.

Buck-Gramcko D (1998) Pollicization. In: Buck-Gramcko D, ed, *Congenital malformations of the hand and forearm* (Churchill Livingston: London) 379–402.

Catagni MA, Szabo RM, Cattaneo R (1993) Preliminary experience with Ilizarov method in late reconstruction of radial hemimelia, *J Hand Surg* **18A**:316–21.

Christensen CP, Ferguson RL (2000) Lower extremity deformities associated with thrombocytopenia and absent radius syndrome, *Clin Orthop Rel Res* **375**:202–6.

D'Arcangelo M, Gupta A, Scheker L (2000) Radial club hand. In: Gupta A, Kay S, Scheker L, eds, *The growing hand*, (Mosby: London) 147–70.

Damore E, Kozin SH, Thoder JJ, Porter S (2000) The recurrence of deformity after surgical centralization for radial club hand, *J Hand Surg* **25A**:745–51.

Define D (1970) Treatment of congenital radial club hand. *Clin Orthop* **73**:153.

Dick HM, Petzoldt RL, Bowers WR, Rennie WRJ (1977) Lengthening of the ulna in radial agenesis: a preliminary report, *J Hand Surg* **2A**:175–78.

Dobyns JH, Wood VE, Bayne LG (1993) Congenital hand deformities. In: Green DP, ed, *Operative hand surgery*, Volume 1, 3rd edn, (Churchill Livingstone: New York) 288–303.

Flatt AE (1994) Radial club hand. In: Flatt AE, ed, *The care of congenital hand anomalies*, 2nd edn, (Quality Medical Publishing: St. Louis) 366–410.

Frankel ME, Goldner JL, Stelling FH (1971) Radial club hand: is centralization necessary? A rational surgical approach. In: Proceedings of the American Academy of Orthopaedic Surgeons. *J Bone Joint Surg* **53A**: 1026.

Geck MJ, Dorey F, Lawrence JF, Johnson MK (1999) Congenital radius deficiency: radiographic outcome and survivorship analysis, *J Hand Surg* **24A**: 1132–44.

Glossop ND, Flatt AE (1995) Opening versus closing wedge osteotomy of the curved ulna in radial club hand, *J Hand Surg* **20A**:133–43.

Goldberg MJ, Bartoshesky LE (1985) Congenital hand anomaly: aetiology and associated malformations, *Hand Clin* **1**:405–15.

Harrison SH (1970) Pollicization in cases of radial club hand, *Br J Plast Surg* **23**:192–200.

Heikel HVA (1959) Aplasia and hypoplasia of the radius: studies on 64 cases and on epiphyseal transplantation in rabbits with the imitated defect, *Acta Orthop Scand* **39**:1–154.

Hippe P, Blauth W (1979) Experience in club hand surgery. *Zeitschrift fur Orthopadie und Ihre Grenzgebiete* **117**:863–72.

Ilizarov GA (1990) Clinical applications of the tension-stress effect for limb lengthening, *Clin Orthop* **250**:8–26.

Inoue G, Miura T (1991) Arteriographic findings in radial and ulnar deficiencies, *J Hand Surg* **16B**: 409–12.

James MA, McCarroll HR Jr, Manske PR (1999) The spectrum of radial longitudinal deficiency: a modified classification, *J Hand Surg* **24A**:1145–55.

Kato H, Ogino T, Minami A, Ohshio I (1990) Experimental study of radial ray deficiency, *J Hand Surg* **15B**:470–76.

Kato K (1924) Congenital absence of the radius: review of literature and report of three cases, *J Bone Joint Surg* **6A**:589–626.

Kawabata H, Shibata T, Masatomi T, Yasui N (1998) Residual deformity in congenital radial club hands after previous centralization of the wrist. Ulnar lengthening and correction by the Ilizarov method, *J Bone Joint Surg* **80B**:762–65.

Kelikian H (1974) *Congenital deformities of the hand and forearm* (WB Saunders: Philadelphia) 780–824.

Kennedy SM (1996) Neoprene wrist brace for correction of radial club hand in children, *J Hand Ther* **9**:387–90.

Kessler I (1989) Centralization of the radial club hand by gradual distraction, *J Hand Surg* **14B**:37–42.

Lamb DW (1977) Radial club hand. A continuing study of 68 patients with 117 club hands, *J Bone Joint Surg* **59A**:1–13.

Lidge RT (1969) Congenital radial deficient radial club hand, *J Bone Joint Surg* **51A**:1041–42.

Lindhout D, Stewart PA, Reuss A et al (1988) Prenatal ultrasound in anti-epileptic drug exposure [abstract], *Teratology* **37**:473–74.

Lister G (1985) Reconstruction of the hypoplastic thumb, *Clin Orthop Rel Res* **195**:52–65.

Manske PR, McCarroll HR (1978) Abductor digiti minimi opponensplasty in congenital radial dysplasia, *J Hand Surg* **3A**:552–59.

Manske PR, McCarroll HR, Swanson K (1981) Centralization of the radial club hand: an ulnar surgical approach, *J Hand Surg* **6A**:423–33.

Manske PR, McCarroll HR (1992) Reconstruction of the congenitally deficient thumb, *Hand Clin* **8**:177–96.

Manske PR, Rotman MB, Dailey LA (1992) Long-term functional results after pollicization for a congenitally deficient thumb, *J Hand Surg* **17A**:1064–72.

Manske PR, McCarroll HR (1998) Radial club hand. In: Buck-Gramcko D, ed, *Congenital malformations of the hand and forearm* (Churchill Livingston: London).

Martini AK (1992) Morphology and systematic aspects of the longitudinal radial defect. *Handchirurgie, Mikrochirurgie, Plastische Chirurgie* **24**:16–22.

Matev IB (1979) Thumb reconstruction in children through metacarpal lengthening, *Plas Reconstr Surg* **64**:665–69.

Matsumura T (1994) Congenital hand malformation-local disturbance in the limb bud and longitudinal deficiency: an experimental study on the pathogenesis. *Seikeigeka Gakkai Zasshi* [*J Jap Ortho Ass*] **68**:234–49.

Menelaus MB (1976) Radial club hand with absence of the biceps muscle treated by centralization of the ulna and triceps transfer. Report of two cases, *J Bone Joint Surg* **58B**:488–91.

Nanchahal J, Tonkin MA (1996) Preoperative distraction lengthening for radial longitudinal deficiency, *J Hand Surg* **21B**:103–7.

Newbury-Ecob RA, Leanage R, Raeburn JA, Young ID (1996) Holt-Oram syndrome: a clinical genetic study, *J Med Gen* **33**:300–7.

O'Rahilly R (1951) Morphological patterns in limb deficiencies and duplications, *Am J Anat* **89**:135–93.

Paley D, Herzenberg JE (1998) Distraction treatment of the forearm. In: Buck-Gramcko D, ed, *Congenital malformations of the hand and forearm* (Churchill Livingston: London) 73–117.

Pauli RM, Feldman PF (1986) Major limb malformations following intrauterine exposure to ethanol: two additional cases and literature review, *Teratology* **33**:273–80.

Petit JL (1733) Remarques sur un enfant nouveau-ne', dint les bras e-taient difforme's. *Mem d l'Acad Roy d Sci* (Paris) 17.

Pho RW, Patterson MH, Kour AK, Kumar VP (1988) Free vascularized epiphyseal transplantation in upper extremity reconstruction, *J Hand Surg* **13B**:440–47.

Pilz SM, Muradin MS, Van der Meulen JJ, Hovius SE (1998) Evaluation of five different incisions for correction of radial dysplasia, *J Hand Surg* **23B**:183–85.

Riddle RD, Johnson RL, Laufer E, Tabin C (1993) Sonic hedgehog mediates the polarizing activity of ZPA, *Cell* **75**:1401–16.

Riordan DC (1955) Congenital absence of the radius, *J Bone Joint Surg* **37A**:1129–40.

Riordan DC (1963) Congenital absence of the radius: a 15–year follow-up. In: Proceedings of the AOA, *J Bone Joint Surg* **45A**:1783.

Sayre RH (1893) A contribution to the study of the club hand, *Trans Am Ortho Ass* **6**:208.

Seitz WH, Froimen AI (1991) Callotasis lengthening in the upper extremity: indications, techniques and pitfalls, *J Hand Surg* **16A**:932–39.

Skerik SK, Flatt AE (1969) The anatomy of congenital radial dysplasia: its surgical and functional implications, *Clin Orthop Rel Res* **66**:125–43.

Smith AA, Greene TL (1995) Preliminary soft tissue distraction in congenital forearm deficiency, *J Hand Surg* **20A**:420–24.

Starr DE (1945) Congenital absence of the radius: a method of surgical correction, *J Bone Joint Surg* **27A**:572.

Stoffel A, Strumpel E (1909) Anatomische Studien uber die Klumphand, *Zeitschrift Orthopedic Chirurgie* **23**:1–15.

Swanson AB (1976) A classification for congenital limb malformations, *J Hand Surg* **1A**:8–22.

Sykes PJ, Chandraprakasam T, Percival N (1991) Pollicization of the index finger in congenital anomalies: a retrospective analysis, *J Hand Surg* **16B**:144–47.

Tetsworth K, Krome J, Paley D (1991) Lengthening and deformity correction of the upper extremity by the Ilizarov technique, *Orthop Clin North Am* **22**:689–713.

Tickle C, Summerbell D, Wolpert L (1975) Positional signalling and specification of defects in chick limb morphogenesis, *Nature* **254**:199–202.

Tickle C, Lee J, Eichele G (1985) A quantitative analysis of the effect of all trans-retinoic acid on the pattern of chick wing development, *Dev Biol* **109**:82–95.

Tsai T-M, Ludwig L, Tonkin M (1986) Vascularized fibular epiphyseal transfer: a clinical study, *Clin Orthop* **210**:228.

Tsuge K, Watari S (1985) New surgical procedure for correction of radial club hand, *J Hand Surg* **10B**:90–94.

Urban MA, Osterman AL (1990) Management of radial dysplasia, *Hand Clin* **6**:589–605.

Verloes A, Frikiche A, Gremillet C, Paquay T, Decortis T, Rigo J, et al (1990) Proximal phocomelia and radial ray aplasia in fetal valproic syndrome, *Eur J Paediatr* **49**:266–67.

Vilkki SK (1998) Distraction and microvascular epiphysis transfer for radial club hand, *J Hand Surg* **23B**:445–52.

Villa A, Paley D, Catagni MA, Bell D, Cattaneo R (1990) Lengthening of the forearm by the Ilizarov technique, *Clin Orthop Rel Res* **250**:125–37.

Watson HK, Beebe RD, Cruz NI (1984) A centralization procedure for radial club hand, *J Hand Surg* **4A**:541–47.

Wood VE (1988) Small finger pollicization in the radial club hand, *J Hand Surg* **13A**:96–99.

13
Cerebral palsy

Caroline Leclercq, Giorgio Pajardi, Jole Colombelli, Paolo Zerbinati and Maurizio Calcagni

Cerebral palsy is a general term that includes all the sequelae of infantile encephalopathies occurring during the perinatal period or during infancy. This chapter will discuss infantile cerebral hemiplegia, which is the only type of cerebral palsy possibly amenable to surgical functional improvement in the upper limb. It is characterized by unilateral cortical and subcortical involvement, particularly in the pyramidal tract, which causes a motor deficit and various degrees of spasticity in the contralateral limbs. It can be associated with epilepsy and mental retardation. It manifests progressively during growth, but once established, follows a non-progressive course, which makes it amenable to surgical treatment.

Clinical examination
Caroline Leclercq

Clinical examination is of the utmost importance. It will allow the physician to:

- Evaluate the motor and sensory deficit in the upper limb.
- Evaluate spasticity.
- Evaluate the existing function and functional needs of the upper limb.
- Perform a complete general examination in order to seek associated neurologic disorders, and seek for contraindications to surgery.

This examination is lengthy, and requires detailed knowledge of neurology and physiatry. It is best performed with all the specialists involved in the child's care (physiatrist, physical therapist, occupational therapist, pediatrician, and surgeon).

It must be performed in a warm, quiet, and friendly environment. Trust must be established by the examiner at the beginning of the evaluation; this is essential since the child's cooperation is vital for the sensory-motor evaluation, and because spasticity may increase considerably if the child is frightened or recalcitrant. If painful procedures (i.e. injections) are necessary, they must be left for last. Symptoms may vary with the child's emotional state and fatigue level; even the weather can modify the clinical picture. Therefore it is not wise to decide on surgery after a single examination. Some children cannot cooperate throughout the entire examination, and a second session may be necessary to complete it. Video recording of this examination is most helpful, both in the decision-making and in the evaluation of surgical outcome.

Resting posture of the upper limb

Inspecting the limb at rest prior to examination provides information on the amount of spasticity. If predominant, spasticity usually leads to a resting posture in shoulder adduction and internal rotation, elbow flexion, forearm pronation and severe wrist flexion (Fig. 1). The fingers may assume varied positions, either in a clenched fist, or sometimes in a swan-neck type of deformity. This can be a result of either excessive traction on the extensor tendons due to excessive wrist flexion (extrinsic swan-neck) (Fig. 2) or to spasticity of the interossei muscles (intrinsic swan-neck). The fingers may also assume a claw type deformity, with the metaphalangeal (MP) joints hyper-extended and the proximal interphalangeal (PIP) joints flexed, due to a combination

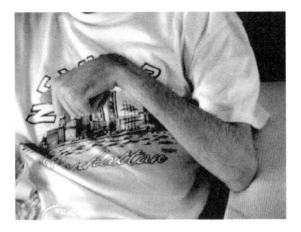

Figure 1

Typical spontaneous posture in shoulder internal rotation, elbow flexion, forearm pronation, and wrist hyperflexion.

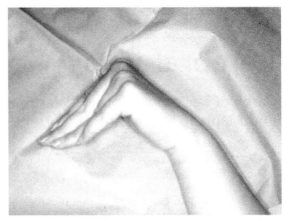

Figure 2

Swan neck deformity of the intrinsic type.

of excessive traction on the extensor tendons and paralysis of the intrinsics. A boutonnière type of deformity is less common. The thumb can assume either an adducted posture or an adducted and flexed posture. The adducted thumb is often in a slight retro-position, with the MP and interphalangeal (IP) joint extended. The 'flexus-adductus' thumb, often referred to as thumb-in-palm, is embedded in the palm with full opposition and full flexion of MP and IP joints (Fig. 3). Often the clenched fist is curled around the thumb. Any factor that aggravates spasticity will increase these deformities.

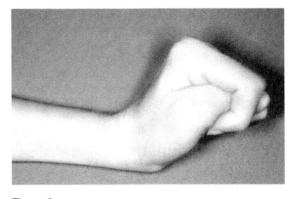

Figure 3

Flexus-adductus thumb.

Evaluation of spasticity

Spasticity is a muscle hypertony, defined by five classic characteristics. (1) It is selective, predominant on flexor and adductor muscles, responsible for the characteristic 'flexion-pronation' deformity of the upper limb described above. (2) It is elastic. Attempts at reducing the deformity meet with a resistance, which increases with the strength applied. Unlike 'plastic' contractures, the limb returns to its initial position as soon as the imposed movement is stopped. However if the opposing force is maintained long enough, the limb usually yields, sometimes abruptly. (3) It is present at rest, and exaggerated with voluntary movement, emotion, fatigue, and pain. (4) The osteotendinous reflexes are exaggerated, brisk, diffuse, and polykinetic. Clonus is infrequent in the upper limb. (5) Synkineses may be associated. Synkineses is 'the phenomenon whereby paralyzed muscles incapable of a certain voluntary movement, execute this movement in a voluntary fashion by accompanying intact muscles' (Lhermitte sign). For example, Souques synkinesis is the extension and abduction of the fingers with voluntary shoulder abduction.

Motor assessment

Motor examination of the upper limb is not easy in children, especially before five years of age. The child should be provided with toys of different forms and colours, and be observed at play (Goldner 1974). Each muscle or muscle group is evaluated for (1) voluntary control (2) fibrous contracture, and (3) joint motion.

Voluntary motor control

The palsy (or 'pseudo palsy') usually predominates in the extensor and supinator muscles, and in the distal part of the upper limb. Motor examination of the extensors and supinators may be made difficult when the antagonist flexors and pronators are severely spastic (Fig. 4). More than a true paralysis, there is a deficit in voluntary control linked with the pyramidal tract involvement. This deficit predominates in the distal muscles spared from spasticity (wrist and finger extensors, abductor and extensor pollicis longus, and supinators). The proximal muscles (shoulder external rotators and elbow flexors) are involved to a lesser degree. The lack of control varies with limb position. For instance, voluntary movement of the thenar muscles is facilitated by elbow extension. In some cases these muscles may be present, but made ineffective by the spastic antagonist or by elongation caused by a severe deformity. The flexor, adductor, and pronator muscles, mostly spastic, usually retain some voluntary control. Their examination is made difficult when synkineses or co-contractures are present. In difficult cases, motor blocks and electromyogram (EMG) studies are helpful (see below).

Fibrous contracture

Fibrous contracture may involve spastic muscles. Unlike spasticity, fibrous contracture is permanent and cannot be overcome (Fig. 5). Shortening the articular segment involved can alleviate it. For example posturing the wrist in flexion relieves contracture of the finger flexors. Clinical distinction between contracture and spasticity may be difficult to establish. In such cases nerve blocks with lidocaine can be helpful

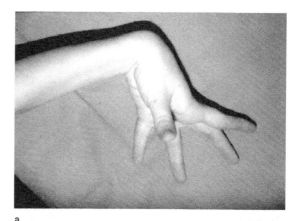

a

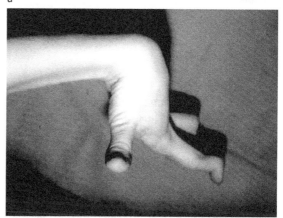

b

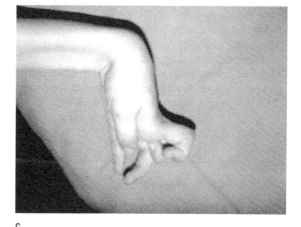

c

Figure 4

Three successive attempts at active finger extension, leading to different finger positions (a) (b) and (c) due to spasticity of the antagonists and lack of muscle coordination.

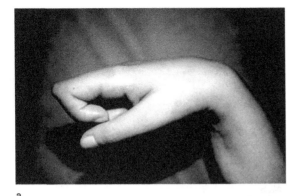

a

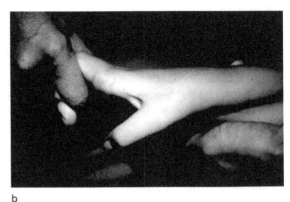

b

Figure 5

(a) Spontaneous resting posture. (b) Maximal passive extension, demonstrating a fibrous contracture of the flexor muscles.

(Roper 1975). The anaesthetic may be injected either in the nerve trunk or in the motor point of the muscle(s) involved. Spasticity yields completely whereas contracture persists (Braun et al 1970). These blocks also allow the antagonist muscles (i.e. extensors and supinators) to be evaluated in cases where spasticity is severe. Over the past few years, botulin toxin has gradually replaced nerve blocks. Botox is now approved for children, and is much easier to use, as it is injected directly into the muscle body. It is helpful both as a diagnostic tool to distinguish between spasticity and contractures, and as a therapeutic tool (see later: Surgical treatment). The only drawback is the duration of its effectiveness, which lasts from the second week until 3 to 4 months after the injection, which is too long for a diagnostic purpose alone, and too short for a therapeutic purpose.

Joint range of motion

Passive range of motion of the involved joints may be difficult to assess, not so much because of spasticity but because of muscle fibrous contractures. It is tested with the involved muscles fully relaxed. Motor blocks are of no help here, as they do not alleviate muscle contracture. Sometimes it is so difficult that it is not until preoperative examination under anaes-

thesia that the actual range of motion can be evaluated (Fig. 6). Some joints of the fingers and thumb may have an increase in passive motion, resulting in joint instability. This occurs mainly at the thumb MP joint, and at the fingers MP and PIP joint (hyperextension).

General motor assessment

Finally a general motor assessment is performed, in order to evaluate the global motor control of the upper limb, such as the head-to-knee test where the patient is asked to place his hand on his head and then to move it to the contralateral knee. The speed and precision of the movement are recorded. These non-specific tests involve many of the elements susceptible to perturbation (hypertonia and muscle contracture, ataxia, apraxia, and extrapyramidal lesions).

Primitive reflexes are also sought. They are due to an abnormal sensory motor development, and impair greatly the functional capacity of the limb. The best known of these primitive reflexes is the asymmetric neck reflex; when the head is turned actively or passively to one side, it produces abduction of the shoulder, and extension of the elbow, wrist and fingers of the ipsilateral upper limb while the contralateral limb flexes in all joints.

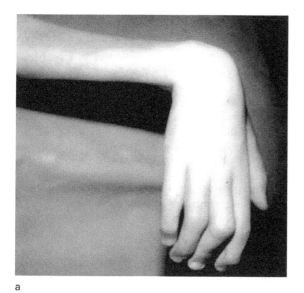

a

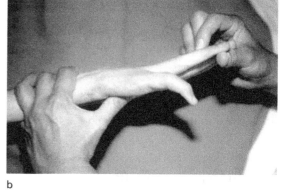

b

Figure 6

(a) Severe wrist spasticity. (b) Testing under general anesthesia brings the wrist to neutral only, demonstrating fibrous contracture of the wrist extensors, but no contracture of the finger flexors.

Once the motor examination has been completed, an attempt at classification can be made, using, for instance, Zancolli's classification (Zancolli 1979) where:

- Type I includes the spastic 'intrinsic-plus' hands, in which spaticity of the interossei and lumbrical muscles causes flexion of the MP joints and extension of the IP joints, sometimes associated with a swan-neck deformity. In this type a wrist flexion deformity is rare.
- Type II includes the spastic 'flexion-pronation' hands with (hyper) flexion of the wrist and pronation of the forearm. Three groups are individualized depending on the degree of active finger extension. In the first group, with the wrist in neutral or near neutral, there is full active extension of the fingers. In the second group there is nearly complete active extension of the fingers, but with some degree of wrist flexion. This group is further subdivided based on the presence (subgroup A) or absence (subgroup B) of an active wrist extension. In the third group there is no active finger extension, even with maximum wrist flexion.

We did not find any of the available classifications particularly helpful, since the clinical picture varies greatly from one child to the other depending on the amount and extent of both spasticity and paralysis, and often did not fit into any specific classification.

Sensory examination

Sensory examination is practically impossible in the small child; it becomes feasible at age four to five (and two-point discrimination at age six to seven). It requires, besides the child's cooperation, a certain level of intellectual capacities and language ability (Tardieu 1984). The basic sensory functions (light touch, pain, temperature) are essentially intact in cerebral palsy, while complex sensations (epicritic sensibility, proprioception, gnosis) are more readily affected.

Light touch is explored with a smooth point or a finger, pain with a needle, and temperature with tubes of hot (40°C) and cold (melting ice) water. Epicritic sensibility is explored with discriminatory tests such as two-point discrimination. Proprioception is tested by vibration (tuning fork) and by the sense of position of the limb: the patient is blindfolded, the unaffected limb is placed in one position, and he is asked to reproduce it with the affected limb. Proprioception is usually more disturbed in the distal part of the limb. Gnoses are the most affected. Placing an object in the child's hand and asking him to identify it tests stereognosis. Graphesthesia is tested by drawing figures or forms in the patient's palm. Sensation is considered satisfactory when the child identifies at least three out of five objects, can recognize large figures drawn in the palm, and has a two-point discrimination test no greater than 5–10 mn (according to the child's age) (Hoffer 1979a).

Functional examination

This part of the examination tests the actual use of the upper limb. It should be video-recorded. Handing objects of different sizes and volumes to the child tests prehension. The pollicidigital pinch is often limited to a lateral 'key-grip' type of pinch because of the lack of fine voluntary control and of the adducted thumb. Grasp is generally preserved, although not always functional because of the finger flexor contractures and extensor weaknesses.

Bimanual activities (such as carrying a container with two handles or holding one object into which another one should be placed) give the most information on the child's actual functional ability. The child and family are also asked to describe precisely how the hand is used in activities of daily living such as dressing and eating. In a number of cases the upper extremity is neglected by the child in spite of a true functional capacity. In these cases, the child may persist in ignoring the limb whether functional ability can be improved through surgery or not. Several charts have been designed to assess the functional value of the upper limb (Goldner 1974, Tardieu 1984). We have chosen to use that described by Hoffer (1979a), which tests dressing, personal hygiene, feeding, bimanual activities, grasp and release, and the lateral pinch.

General preoperative examination

The aim of this general examination is to evaluate the real benefice the child will get from surgery, taking into account other neurological impairments, the patient's age, intelligence, motivation and environment.

Other neurological impairments

As these children are hemiplegic, the lower limb deficit must also be assessed, and it is especially important to know about the child's walking ability, and the possible need for a walking aid (wheelchair, crutch). If operations are necessary for improvement of the lower limb, they are usually planned before any upper extremity surgery.

Associated extrapyramidal signs should also be detected. These include the following:

- Athetosis, which is made of unexpected, non-voluntary movements causing a slow oscillation of the limbs. It is reduced at rest, abolished at sleep, increased by noise, fatigue, and emotions.
- Chorea is made of brisk rapid and anarchic non-voluntary movements, of variable amplitude, which can involve all territories. In the upper limb, these contortions of the forearm, hand, and fingers make activities of daily living impossible.
- Parkinson syndrome is characterized by the classic triad: resting tremor, plastic hypertonia (predominant in the proximal muscles) with the cogwheel sign, and akinesia.

If these extrapyramidal signs are predominant, they preclude surgical treatment, since the child is unable to use his hand because of these non-voluntary movements. But when they are mild, they do not contraindicate surgery.

The capacity of the child to communicate must be evaluated, seeking for visual, hearing and language problems. Behavioural problems such as irritability, inability to concentrate, and emotional instability may also constitute contraindications to surgical treatment when they are predominant. Intelligence is evaluated through the intelligence quotient (IQ). It is usually stated that rehabilitation surgery is not indicated when IQ is lower than 70, but this is not absolute, and in any event surgical procedures aimed at improving comfort, cosmesis and personal hygiene are still indicated.

Age

Because the neurological deficit in cerebral palsy is not evolutive, early surgery can be planned.

Sometimes it is necessary to operate very early because of an increasing deformity. But in most cases one can wait until the child is old enough that motor and sensory capacities can be evaluated accurately and he or she can cooperate through surgery and postoperative rehabilitation. Sequelae of cerebral palsy in adults should be evaluated very cautiously before surgical planning, because usually the patients have already adapted functionally and socially to the handicap, and surgery may be more disturbing than beneficial.

Motivation and environment

Evaluation of motivation should take into account the patient's ability to understand the modalities and benefice of the proposed treatment, and to participate actively in the postoperative regimen. Understanding and motivation on the parents' part are also mandatory. Environmental factors during the surgical period are also important, such as a rehabilitation centre with an integrated school system and physiotherapists specializing in such treatments.

Electromyography

EMG studies are often very helpful. Both static and dynamic studies are necessary, which requires cooperation on the child's part (Hoffer 1979b). This may be difficult to achieve in children younger than five. In spastic muscles, EMG studies give information on the voluntary control, the possibility of relaxation, and possible co-contractures of the antagonist muscles. In other muscles, such studies are able to identify voluntary control that is not clinically detectable (spastic and/or retracted antagonists, joint deformity and/or stiffness). When needed, EMG studies can help in determining the most appropriate muscles for transfer.

Radiography

X-rays are part of the preoperative evaluation. They are aimed at assessing any growth distur-

bance and joint deformity linked to the spasticity, however satisfactory views may not be easy to achieve when there is a severe deformity such as wrist hyperflexion. Contralateral views in the same position may then be helpful.

Surgical treatment options

Giorgio Pajardi, Jole Colombelli, Paolo Zerbinati and Maurizio Calcagni

Making surgical decisions for patients with cerebral palsy is challenging for many different reasons. The condition is heterogeneous in degree, as well as type of involvement, and a multitude of factors affect motor function, including spasticity, dysphasic muscle activity, poor motor planning, balance problems, impaired spatial perception and poor proprioception. General factors, such as environment, motivation, obesity, intelligence, and age also affect treatment outcome.

Accurate assessment of the outcome of treatment has been limited by the lack of objective measurement tools, as well as by the long period of time required to assess the ultimate outcome. Some limitations in the outcome assessment in cerebral palsy have been partially overcome in the past decade through the availability of computer-based gait analysis, which is an excellent, objective, and functional assessment tool. Computer-based decision-making constitutes just one of the three types of examination that are necessary to accurately assess a patient with cerebral palsy. The other two are the standard clinical examination and the examination under anaesthesia that takes places just before the start of corrective surgery. In addition computer-based decision-making fulfils a useful role after surgery, in that it accurately and objectively documents the outcome, which in turn, allows meaningful comparison between the pre- and postoperative status of the patient.

The decision for treatment rests on some conditions. First, what is the mean objective of intervening into the natural course of cerebral palsy? The child with cerebral palsy wants to be pain-free and able to sit well, even if it is necessary to use a special chair. It is important to be able to move around, but it is not absolutely necessary to walk. Therefore any additional steps taken to obtain walking capacity are open to debate.

The principles for decision-making in spastic patients are essentially the same as for other problems in pediatric orthopaedics. Spasticity adds a special difficulty because it aggravates an existing disharmony between the agonist and antagonist muscles. Even after a successful operation there will still be a motor function disability, which is pejorative to the final result. Indications for surgery in cerebral palsy are never limited to a single muscle or body region. All parts are related to the whole and it is their individual and cumulative effects that make surgical decision-making extraordinarily challenging.

The majority of children with cerebral palsy are included in physical and/or occupational therapy programmes. These include passive motion exercises, active use training and static or dynamic splinting. In many cases botulin toxin A muscle blocks are used for diagnostic and therapeutic purposes. After botox injection muscle spasticity subsides and it is possible to assess better antagonistic function and joint stiffness. Moreover during the time span of reduced muscle hypertonicity, physical therapy can be more effective in overcoming joint contracture or in obtain muscle lengthening (Koman et al 1994).

The aim of upper limb surgery in cerebral palsy patients is to improve, if possible function, or at least hygiene and cosmesis. It is not the purpose of this chapter to draw guidelines for treatment indications, but we would like to underline the importance of clarifying with the patient and his/her parents the results that are achievable through surgery—when cognition, hand placement and sensibility (or eye control) are poor, surgery can only achieve hygienic and cosmetic results. There are a number of surgical procedures that can correct muscle imbalance.

Nerve procedures

Muscle tone can be ameliorated by reduction or elimination of nerve supply. Exact recognition and dissection of single muscle branches with peroperative electric stimulation allow for selective and precise hyponeurotization (Brunelli and

Brunelli 1983). Neurotomy is a definitive procedure to be reserved for more severe cases.

Muscle-tendon procedures

Procedures addressing the muscle-tendon unit can be roughly divided into the following:

- Proximal origin sliding.
- Intra-muscular lengthening (or fractional lengthening).
- Distal tendon lengthening.
- Tenotomy.
- Tendon transfer.

The effects of these procedures are threefold: muscle contracture release, reduction of deforming forces on bone and reduction of centripetal proprioceptive signals. Moreover tendon transfer permits reduction of original spastic contracture altogether with antagonistic reinforcement.

Bone and joint procedures

Some cases of established and extremely severe deformities have to be corrected with osteotomies when soft tissue release procedures fall short of the surgical goal (cosmetic or functional). Arthrodesis and/or bone resection (e.g. proximal row carpectomy) are definitive procedures necessary in many severe cases in order to achieve a durable result especially in patients with only cosmetic expectations. They are rarely indicated in children under 15.

Capsulodesis is often necessary in order to correct joint deformities secondary to muscle imbalance and to improve the result after tendon transfer.

Specific procedures

Like in other surgical fields there is no single answer for the spastic upper limb, but an armamentarium of procedures. We will try here to outline those used most frequently with topographic criteria.

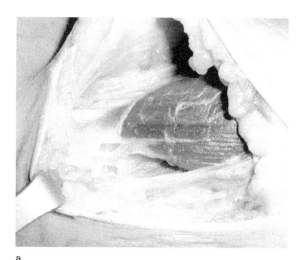
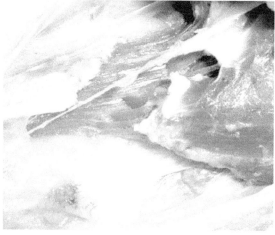

a   b

Figure 7

(a) Intra-muscular lengthening of biceps-preoperative. (b) Intra-muscular lengthening of biceps-peroperative.

Shoulder

Typical shoulder deformity is in adduction and internal rotation. When the passive range of motion (PROM) is less than 45° of abduction and 15° of external rotation there is an indication for surgery. Also chronic pain, not central or secondary to an orthopaedic pathology, can be successfully treated.

In the past the commonly proposed procedures were humeral osteotomy and subscapularis lengthening, nowadays preferred methods are subscapularis tenotomy and pectoralis major tenotomy or intra-muscular lengthening. Surgical approach is through the delto-pectoralis groove, isolation of the cephalic vein, dissection of the subscapularis tendon near the circumflex humeral vessels; after careful protection of shoulder capsule in order to preserve joint stability, the tendon is released at the level of the musculo-tendinous junction. The pectoralis major can be transected near its humeral insertion or lengthened at the musculo-tendinous junction. In rare cases the shoulder is abducted during run attempt and spasticity of the deltoid muscle brings the arm at almost 90° of abduction with the elbow flexed. The deltoid muscle

can be lengthened through a small linear incision after protection of the axillary and radial nerves (Tachdjian 1972).

Elbow

Spastic elbow flexion deformity is present in almost all cases of cerebral palsy and is due to spasticity of the biceps, brachialis and brachioradialis muscles (Keenan et al 1990). When limited it has no functional importance, but in more severe cases (i.e. 90° flexion contracture) it impairs object reaching and two-handed activities.

The Scaglietti medial epicondyle muscle release, the first proposed in literature, is now obsolete especially as a single procedure. All flexor muscles are carefully detached from their bony insertion up to the pronator quadratus and allowed to slide distally. The modern surgical option includes resection of the lacertus fibrosus, fractional lengthening of the biceps (Fig. 7) and brachialis and release of the brachioradialis origin, giving an average improvement of 40° (Mital and Sakellarides 1981). With severe contracture, tenotomy of the biceps or Z-plasty lengthening is necessary.

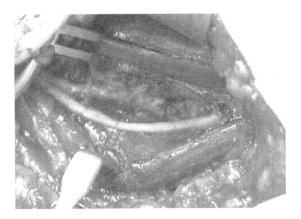

Figure 8

Hyponeurotization of the musculocutaneous nerve.

When the flexion contracture is less severe and the botulin blocks have demonstrated that there is no fibrous muscle contracture, hyponeurotization of the musculocutaneous nerve is an alternative procedure (Fig. 8). Through a linear incision on the medial aspect of the upper arm the nerve is exposed and the motor component isolated and almost 80% is transected.

Forearm pronation deformity

This deformity is a major impairment in bimanual activity and the patient is often obliged to use the dorsum of the hand or even the forearm. Surgical procedures that sometimes have to be combined (e.g. pronator quadratus release and flexor aponeurotic release) are:

- Pronator quadratus release: through a palmar approach the pronator quadratus is detached from its radial insertion and elevated from the interosseous membrane.
- Flexor aponeurotic release: through a transverse incision distal to the epicondyle 2 cm of forearm fascia is excised and all fascial septa of the flexor and pronator muscles are divided down to the ulna and interosseous membrane (Zancolli 1979).
- Pronator teres (PT) release or transfer: the PT tendon is incised in a Z fashion and then

sutured after rerouting from the radial to the ulnar side. This procedure enables the PT to become an active forearm supinator (Bleck 1987).

- Flexor carpi ulnaris (FCU) transfer: the FCU tendon is transferred subcutaneously to the wrist extensors around the ulna. While deforming forces in wrist flexion and ulnar deviation are eliminated and antagonistic muscles reinforced (Colton et al 1976), the new direction of FCU tends to supinate the forearm.

Wrist

Wrist arthrodesis is usually associated with a proximal row carpectomy in order to gain additional length for the flexor tendons. Fixation can be obtained with a carefully contoured plate or with Kirschner wires and a long arm cast (Pinzur 1996). Wrist arthrodesis is always associated with soft tissue procedures in order to achieve a good resolution of flexor contracture (Rayan and Young 1999).

Many different tendon transfers can be performed either through the interosseous membrane or through a subcutaneous tunnel. The most commonly performed are the flexor carpi ulnaris (FCU) to the extensor digitorum communis (EDC) (Fig. 9) and the flexor carpi radialis (FCR) to the extensor carpi radialis brevis (ECRB)(Zancolli and Zancolli 1981). Wrist flexors can be lengthened at the musculo-tendinous junction when the patient has residual active control or transected in case of cosmetic procedures.

Fingers

Intra-muscular lengthening of all finger flexors (Fig. 10) in functional cases gives adequate length to the musculo-tendinous unit retaining function (Waters and Van Heest 1998). Superficialis to profundus (STP) transfer gives maximum tendon lengthening (5–8 cm), but it is not functional and therefore should be reserved for cosmetic purposes (Keenan et al 1987a). Hyponeurotization of the motor branch of ulnar nerve at Guyon's tunnel (Fig. 11) alleviates intrinsic muscle contracture (Keenan et al 1987b). Arthrodesis of PIP joint is a definitive procedure

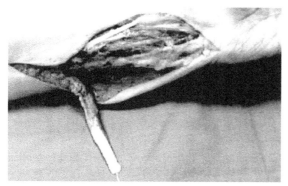

a

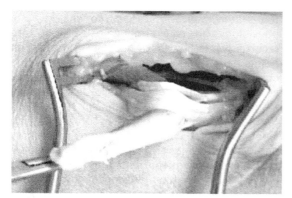

b

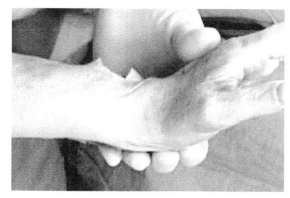

c

Figure 9

(a–c) Transfer of the FCU to the EDC.

that is very stable and without risk of recurrence, but is mostly indicated for cosmetic purposes. It can be also useful in order to prevent swan-neck deformity secondary to STP transfer.

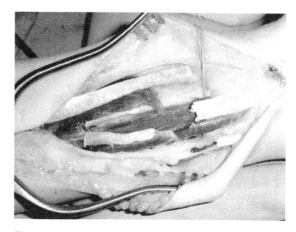

Figure 10

Intra-muscular lengthening of the finger flexors.

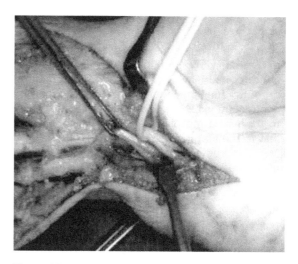

Figure 11

Hyponeurotization of the motor branch of ulnar nerve.

Thumb

Thumb-in-palm is one of the most common deformities in cerebral palsy patients (House et al 1981). One surgical option is adductor and first dorsal interosseous muscle release from the first metacarpal. In rare cases of extreme deformity with TM joint stiffness, an opening osteotomy of the metacarpal may be necessary. The release

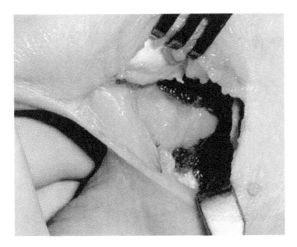

Figure 12

Surgical release of the adductor pollicis muscle.

starts with a cutaneous Z-plasty; then a myotomy of the transverse portion of the adductor muscle is performed leaving the oblique fibres intact in order to retain pinch function (Fig. 12). When the contracture is extreme the myotomy is extended to the whole muscle belly at the bone insertion and to the first interosseous muscle. In this case MP arthrodesis or capsulodesis is also performed in order to prevent MP hyperextension.

Intra-muscular lengthening of thumb long flexor (FPL) is performed through the same palmar incision used for finger tendons release. In cosmetic cases a simple tenotomy is also possible.

Tendon transfers have been proposed such as the brachioradialis (BR) to the thumb long extensor (EPL) and the palmaris longus (PL) to the abductor pollicis longus (APL). A limited, but very useful procedure is the transfer of the radial part of FPL to the EPL. Rerouting of the EPL in a more radial and palmar position reduces its adductive effect, reducing IP extension. The tendon is withdrawn from the third compartment and sutured after a passage under the APL and extensor pollicis brevis (EPB) tendons, which act as a pulley (Rayan and Saccone 1996). In case of hyperflexion of the IP joint, the FPL can be transferred subcutaneously to APL insertion. Simple spasticity without fibrous muscle contracture can

be overcome with neurotomy of the distal motor branch of the median nerve (Keenan et al 1987b).

Arthrodesis of the MP joint is 10° of flexion and pronation, and of IP joint is 5° of flexion and is rarely indicated in children.

Indications

Distinction of the aforementioned techniques in cosmetic and functional, or else more invasive and irreversible (but also more stable and with lower risk of recurrence of the deformity, and more functional with respect to anatomy and physiology, but with a higher risk of long term recurrence), is nowadays obsolete. Two relevant points have to be considered; first of all it is the combination of different procedures that define a cosmetic or a functional protocol (e.g. fractional lengthening of a finger flexor can be, alone, a functional procedure, but it becomes cosmetic when associated with a proximal row carpectomy and wrist arthrodesis). The second consideration is the evolution of the pathology together with child growth. The combination of these aspects exposes affected children to a high risk of deformity recurrence and it is relevant for surgical planning. Our point of view on surgical decision-making is based on the following considerations:

- Extensive use of botulin toxin, which gives better results in children than in adults, as it can be an efficient, and often definitive, alternative to surgery.
- Always evaluate the possibility of staging surgery in order to allow for spontaneous improvement, helped by limited surgery (e.g. fractional lengthening of finger flexors and delay of transfer for extensors).
- Use of selective denervation as a first choice method as often as possible (importance of careful assessment).
- Limit bone procedures to the wrist, and only in case of fully stabilized deformity.
- Always give preference to less invasive procedures with shorter recovery times, less pain and shorter immobilization in order to reduce the risk of downgrading overall function of the upper limb as a whole.
- Regarding thumb-in-palm correction, preference should be given to dynamic procedures

because they allow for a spontaneous evolution towards a useful pinch (EPL rerouting, FPL transfer to APL, for example).

In conclusion we think that it is very important to carefully combine different surgical procedures in each clinical case in order to obtain a very predictable result. We have also to keep in mind that modern surgery for spastic patients aims, through early procedures, towards functional rehabilitation and not towards stabilization of a highly compromised situation.

References

Bleck EE (1987) *Orthopedic Management in Cerebral Palsy* (JB Lippincott: Philadelphia).

Braun RM, Mooney V, Nickel VL (1970) Flexor-origin release for pronation-flexion deformity of the forearm and hand in the stroke patient, *J Bone Joint Surg* **52A**:907.

Brunelli G, Brunelli F (1983) Partial selective denervation in spastic palsies (hyponeurotization), *Microsurgery* **4**:221–24.

Colton CL, Ransford AO, Lloyd-Roberts GC (1976) Transposition of the tendon of the pronator teres in cerebral palsy, *J Bone Joint Surg* **58B**:220.

Goldner JL (1974) The upper extremity in cerebral palsy, *Orthop Clin North Am* **5**:389.

Hoffer MM (1979a) The upper extremity in cerebral palsy, AAOS Instruct Course Lecture, 133.

Hoffer MM (1979b) Dynamic electromyography and decision-making for surgery in the upper extremity of patients with cerebral palsy, *J Hand Surg* **4A**:424.

House JH, Swathmey FW, Fidler MO (1981) A dynamic approach to the thumb-in-palm deformity in cerebral palsy, *J Bone Joint Surg* **63A**:216.

Keenan MA, Korchek JI, Botte MJ et al (1987) Results of transfer of the flexor digitorum superficialis tendons to the flexor digitorum profundus tendons in adults with acquired spasticity of the hand, *J Bone Joint Surg* **69A**:1127–32.

Keenan MA, Todderud EP, Henderson R et al (1987) Management of intrinsic spasticity in the hand with phenol injection or neurotomy of the motor branch of the ulnar nerve, *J Hand Surg* **12A**:734–39.

Keenan MAE, Haider TT, Stone LR (1990) Dynamic electromyography to assess elbow spasticity, *J Hand Surg* **15A**:607.

Koman LA, Mooney JF, Smith BP et al (1994) Management of spasticity in cerebral palsy with botulinum A toxin; report of a preliminary randomized double blind trial, *J Pediatr Orthop* **14**:299.

Mital MA, Sakellarides HT (1981) Surgery of the upper extremity in the retarded individual with spastic cerebral palsy, *Orthop Clin North Am* **12**:127.

Pinzur MS (1996) Carpectomy and fusion in adult-acquired hand spasticity, *Orthopedics* **19**:675–77.

Rayan GM, Saccone PG (1996) Treatment of spastic thumb-in-palm deformity: a modified extensor pollicis longus tendon rerouting, *J Hand Surg* **21A**:834–39.

Rayan GM, Young BT (1999) Arthrodesis of the spastic wrist, *J Hand Surg* **24A**:944–52.

Roper B (1975) Evaluation of spasticity, *Hand* **7**:11.

Tachdjian MO (1972) *Pediatric Orthopedics* (WB Saunders: Philadelphia).

Tardieu G (1984) *Le dossier clinique de l'IMC. Méthodes d'évaluation et applications thérapeutiques.* 3rd edn. Paris.

Waters PM, Van Heest A (1998) Spastic hemiplegia of the upper extremity in children, *Hand Clin* **14**:119–34.

Zancolli E (1979) Surgery of the hand in infantile spastic hemiplegia. In: Zancolli EA, ed, *Structural and Dynamic Bases of Hand Surgery*, 2nd edn (JB Lippincott: Philadelphia) 263.

Zancolli EA, Zancolli ER Jr (1981) Surgical management of the hemiplegic spastic hand in cerebral palsy, *Surg Clin North Am* **61**:395–406.

14
Volkmann's ischaemic contracture

Piero L Raimondi, Roberto M Cavallazzi and Steven ER Hovius

Introduction

The ischaemic contracture described by Volkmann in 1881 is the final consequence of a compartment syndrome in the upper arm, due to different aetiological causes. The pathophysiology of a compartment syndrome consists of a rapid increase of the interstitial tissue pressure (ITP), (Seiler et al 2000) in an unyielding muscular compartment that leads to a progressive reduced capillary perfusion, which can provoke if the compressive cause is not rapidly removed, a severe irreversible damage of the flexor muscles and nerves in the forearm. The deep flexor compartment in the forearm is the most frequently affected site due to its position next to the bone and for its especially tight surrounding fascia (Inoue et al 1996). This situation can develop classically in supracondylar fractures in children where a tight bandage or plaster has been applied. This had been the principal cause in the past but it decreased dramatically in the last 20 years in most developed countries thanks to the prevention of compartment syndrome in traumas, especially in children (Mubarak et al 1979, Holden, 1979).

The prevention of tight bandages or plasters, the close clinical observation of an increased ITP (eventually applying compartment pressure measurements) and the early wide fasciotomy where indicated, helped to decrease the morbidity of compartment syndromes (Pirone et al 1988). Nevertheless in the last few years new causes of compartment syndromes have been observed: direct injection of toxic agents in the forearm, prolonged compression of the forearm in drug addicted or in coma patients, and severe forearm trauma that is not adequately treated in total brachial plexus lesions where the patients' lack of sensibility and pain can hide the clinical signs for a correct early diagnosis.

Compartment syndrome: prevention and treatment

As already mentioned humeral supracondylar fractures, forearm and diaphyseal humeral fractures or elbow luxations can provoke a compartment syndrome; the mechanism is ITP augmentation caused either by haematoma or direct compression of the brachial artery and/or by external compression due to a tight bandage or plaster (Mubarak et al 1979). It is a sort of combined reduction of the continent space and an increase in volume of the contained structures. This progressive and rapid unbalance produces a reduction of the tissue perfusion with a more or less severe ischaemic muscular damage (Eaton et al 1975). Other possible causes are a prolonged compression of the forearm in coma patients (mostly in drug addicted patients) or a direct injection of a toxic agent in the forearm muscles in the proximity of the humeral artery (Seyfer 1994). Despite the differences in aetiology the mechanism of the compartment syndrome development is the same.

The pressure necessary to produce permanent damage to muscles and nerves has been disputed by many authors and supported by many different experimental methods. It seems that the critical pressure beyond which a circulatory obstruction starts to develop is 13 mmHg (Matsen et al 1976). Other experimental studies in dogs (Sheridan et al 1976) prove that muscular and nerve lesions start to develop beyond 30 mmHg and that at 70 mmHg the cell necrosis is complete. Nerves are particularly sensitive to ischaemia. Experimental studies (Hargens et al 1998) show that at 30 mmHg disturbances of nerve conduction start to develop, while beyond 50 mmHg the nerve conduction stops completely. Mubarak et al (1978) states that 30 mmHg is the limit beyond which a compartment syndrome can develop.

The duration of compression is obviously an important factor in provoking the gravity of lesions. Whitesides et al (1975), in a experimental study in dogs, demonstrated that with a period of four hours of ischaemia only 5% of muscle cells were damaged, while after an eight hour period of ischaemia nearly 100% of muscle cells were damaged. Therefore the rate of ITP pressure alone must not be taken as an absolute factor in determining the diagnosis of a compartment syndrome, but it must be integrated with all the other clinical data (Bleton 1996).

In clinical practice the most characteristic sign in an impending compartment syndrome is pain. The pain is progressively increasing, often out of proportion in relation to the injury. The pain is aggravated with passive movements of the affected muscular group and is not relieved with analgesic drugs or by elevating the arm. This apparently paradoxical sign is due to the reduced inflow in the antigravity position of the arm by the diminished arteriolar pressure with a consequent reduction of muscular perfusion and therefore an aggravation of the symptoms (Bleton 1996, Lanz et al 2000). Sensory disturbances are also present with a progressive marked tension of the forearm, which is highly painful at palpation. The active finger mobility is also reduced. The radial pulse may be absent or markedly reduced.

In such clinical situations the first step is to remove all bandages or plasters which can be responsible for an external compression as soon as possible. This can improve a possible arterial spasm and produce a progressive return to normal perfusion, and if, after 45 minutes (maximum one hour) no changes in symptoms occur, there is an indication to perform a wide and complete fasciotomy.

The operation is performed under general anaesthesia or axillary block anaesthesia in adults and with a tourniquet. The use of a tourniquet allows a better evaluation of the reperfusion of the affected muscles and nerves after the release. A long sinuous incision is made at the volar aspect of the forearm as the anterior compartment is most frequently affected (Tsuge 1975, 1982). This allows a complete decompression of the flexor compartments and one must be sure to completely open the deep flexor compartments, which comprise the main affected muscles. Special care must be taken to spare all veins even in the superficial plane.

If the radial pulse has disappeared, the anterior elbow region is systematically opened in order to expose the humeral artery and vein and to decompress them. Sometimes the blood flow recovers immediately; in other circumstances a trombectomy is necessary and in some severe cases a repair with a vein graft must be performed. It is surprising that only a few papers recommend this vascular step of emergency treatment of compartment syndrome (Copley et al 1996, Gulgonen 2001, Petrolati et al 1978, Raimondi et al 1987).

When the compression time has been prolonged, the muscles after fasciotomy may show a lack of normal oxygenation, with a brown colour and a scarce or absent bleeding. Some authors (Bleton 1996), despite this aspect of the muscles, do not recommend debridement in this early phase since there is a possibility of muscular regeneration and moreover at this time it is very difficult to recognize the real limit of healthy from dead tissue. It would seem more prudent to make debridements on a step-by-step basis until a possible granulating tissue formation develops. Other authors (Gulgonen 2001) recommend an early debridement of all the apparently non-viable muscular tissues after fasciotomy.

Once the fasciotomy has been performed the oedematous muscles herniate through the incision and the wide distance between the skin margins demonstrates the amount of muscle compression in the area. The skin incisions are kept opened and after a few days, when the acute compartment syndrome has been solved, the skin margins can be closed again by suturing or the granulating muscles can be covered by split thickness skin grafts. In severe crush syndromes a hyperbaric oxygen treatment seems to be effective in helping the revitalization of the borderline vascularized muscles after fasciotomy (Gulgonen 2001).

The ischaemic Volkmann's contracture

Different clinical classifications on the established Volkmann contracture have been suggested by Seddon (1956), Tsuge (1975), Zancolli (1979) and Benkeddache et al (1985). Between them we use the Tsuge classification, which consists of three types: mild, moderate and severe. In the mild type the deep flexor muscle degeneration is localized more frequently in the long and ring fingers; even the little and index fingers can be affected to some extent. Sensory disturbances are absent and the main characteristic aspect is the tenodesis effect of the affected fingers. In the moderate type also called 'classical type', all the finger flexors including the flexor pollicis longus are affected; even the superficial flexors and the wrist flexors are affected with a more severe flexion contracture of fingers and wrist. In this type nerve deficits are present to a different extent, more frequently in the median nerve but often in both the median and ulnar nerves. The severe type presents with extensive degeneration of all flexor muscles with a concomitant involvement of the extensor muscles, with a quite complete lack of active muscle contraction and median and ulnar nerve paralysis.

This classification has the advantage of being simple but if we want to be more specific as regards the nerve deficit in the hand we can use Zancolli's classification. There are four types in Zancolli's classification depending on the intrinsic muscle function: normal intrinsic muscles (type I), paralytic intrinsic muscles (type II), retracted intrinsic muscles (type III) and combined type (type IV). None of the classifications take into account the vascular situation, i.e. the presence of the radial pulse. We suggest that the vascular conditions of the arm are always tested in order to plan an eventual secondary vascular reconstruction.

Clinical examination has to start with the assessment of the active and passive range of motion of all the joints of the fingers and the wrist. Electromyography can be useful to determine the state of muscle function and nerve conduction velocity. Angiography is always performed when the radial pulse is absent or weak. Some authors have suggested a CT scan or MRI to predict the condition of muscle tissue and the amount of fibrous degenerated tissue (Hovius et al 2000, Landi et al 1989).

Treatment

Rehabilitation and the use of dynamic splints are systematically carried out from the beginning irrespective of the severity of the contracture. In mild cases a correct and early rehabilitation treatment with dynamic splinting may solve a limited flexor retraction without the need for surgery. In all cases better conditions are created for surgical treatment. Surgery is indicated three to four months after injury. This time seems necessary in order to reach a stabilization of the lesions and allow an eventual muscular regeneration to occur; also nerve lesions are more manageable at this point (Gulgonen 2001).

Surgical treatment varies depending on the severity of the contracture and the amount of muscle tissue still functioning. The operations can be briefly divided into two groups depending on the presence of functioning muscles; in the first group we can put the muscle slide operation or tendon lengthening operation, which can be applied to cases in which flexor muscles still exist even if partially functioning. From this operation we can expect a useful result due to active function of the flexor muscles. In the second group are the most severe cases in which, due to the fibrous substitution of the muscular mass, only tendon transfers from the dorsal not involved compartment and the free muscle transfers can give some active function to the hand.

Tendon lengthening

In moderate types there is an indication to lengthen eventually after having removed the infarcted tissue and retracted tendons (Seddon 1956). The lengthening that can be obtained by an intramuscular tenotomy is generally around 2–2.5 cm. The disadvantage of this type of operation is that it increases the weakening in the muscles with a substantial impairment in function. When the deep flexor tendons are fibrotic but the superficial flexor tendons are spared there is an indication for a special lengthening obtained by sectioning the profundi tendons very proximally (at the musculotendinous junction) and the superficial ones more distally. This allows the flexion retraction to be eliminated and the transfer of the active force of the superficial flexor tendons to the distal tendons of the deep flexor tendons. To recover a useful active flexion of the fingers one of the most difficult challenges of this operation is to correctly evaluate the tension of the tendon sutures. If necessary a lengthening of the wrist flexor tendons and of the long flexor to the thumb may be added. The rate of recurrence of flexion contraction from a pure tendon lengthening type of operation is very high (Hovius et al 2000) and therefore not advocated.

Epitrochlear muscle slide operation (Page-Scaglietti operation)

Page described the epitrochlear muscle slide operation in 1923 and in 1957 Scaglietti added the neurolysis as a systematic step to the operation. The ideal indication for this operation is in a moderate or classic type of Volkmann's contracture in cases in which it can be expected that an important part of the muscle mass is still functioning. The distal sliding of the epitrochlear muscles will allow the muscles to actively contract, so eliminating the flexion contracture of the fingers and wrist (Gulgonen 2001, Petrolati et al 1978, Raimondi et al 1987, Tsuge 1975).

The operation is performed either under general anaesthesia in children or with an axillary nerve block or general anaesthesia in adult patients. The skin incision goes from the inner side of the elbow to the distal epiphysis of the ulna following a wide flap on the anterior elbow region in order to allow the exposure of the humeral artery and veins and the median nerve. The ulnar nerve is isolated and anteriorly transposed. Furthermore the epitrochlear muscles are detached at their bony insertion from the medial epicondyle, from the ulna, from the interosseous membrane and from the radius until the distal tendons are reached. Subsequently, a forced extension of wrist and fingers is performed in order to break all the possible adhesions which may still exist and in so doing obtain a complete extension of wrist and fingers. The detached muscles will slide distally where the muscles reinsert spontaneously. During the operation an extirpation of an infarcted zone is performed. External neurolysis is carried out on both nerves and, if an evident stenosis of the nerve is present, an interfascicular neurolysis is performed. In severe cases the damaged tract of the median nerve will have to be resected followed by repair with a nerve graft. If the brachial artery is compressed by fibrous tissue an adventitiectomy is performed; this can produce an improved distal vascular supply. If the artery is occluded we suggest a resection of the thrombotic tract and to substitute it with a saphenous vein graft. Due to the extension of the surgical exposure two drains are recommended and the arm is immobilized with a plaster for four weeks.

The experience of Petrolati et al (1978) and Raimondi et al (1987) with the vascular secondary repair together with the Page-Scaglietti operation demonstrates that the quality of results are considerably better in terms of recovery of motor and sensory function; moreover the trophism of the limb seems better. The main improvement however, has been the reduction of recurrence of contracture, which is the typical complication in the long-term treatment of Volkmann's ischaemic contracture.

Tendon transfers

These operations are generally indicated when no active, or only a poor muscular function is present (Zancolli 1965, 1979). The extensor muscles must have been spared by the ischaemia and must have sufficient strength to be transposed to flexors. Generally good motors to be transposed are the brachioradialis muscle and the extensor carpi radialis longus, which are transposed to the flexor pollicis longus and flexor profundus of the fingers, respectively. The hand may need transfers to treat the claw deformity due to the ulnar palsy. The extensor indicis proprius, the extensor digiti quinti or the extensor carpi ulnaris can be used in these cases. Prior to the tendon transfer the resection of all fibrotic retracted tissue has to be performed in order to put the hand and wrist in the ideal condition for the transfers. Due to the presence of scar tissue a frequent complication in this type of surgery may be the adhesions of the transfers, which may require a secondary tenolysis. Naturally, the rehabilitation is of paramount importance in the achievement of the final functional result.

Free vascularized innervated muscle transfer

Since the publication of the first results of free muscle transfer (Ikuta et al 1976, Manktelow et al

1978, 1984) this operation has now become quite routine (Ercetin et al 1994). Its ideal indication is in the severe type in which no functioning muscle has been spared. It is obvious that the only functional chance in these cases is to revascularize and reinnervate a new muscle. The most frequently used muscles are the gracilis muscle and the latissimus dorsi. These muscles can offer only a limited part of the contracting force of the finger flexors and actually the gracilis seems to be the weakest when compared for instance to the latissimus dorsi or to the rectus femoris muscle. On the other hand the reduced morbidity of the donor site, the reliability of the vessels and the good distal tendon of the gracilis muscle makes it the first choice for transfer in severe Volkmann's ischaemic contracture.

From the technical point of view the muscle insertion is done proximally, directly on the medial epicondyle and distal to the deep flexor tendons. Tension is of paramount importance to obtain a good balance in the hand; at the end of the operation all the finger joints (metacarpophalangeal, MP; proximal interphalangeal, PIP; distal interphalangeal, DIP) must be flexed with the wrist in neutral position. With respect to the vascular anastomosis, it is very important to know in advance, the vascular condition of the elbow and forearm region and to this end, it is suggested that an angiography be performed (Hovius et al 2000). Generally the anastomosis takes place in the forearm but in case of doubt we have to move more proximally, at the brachial artery level, with an interpositional vein graft. The appropriate nerve for the reinnervation of the transfer is the anterior interosseous nerve, which is normally spared in Volkmann's ischaemic contracture. The functional results we obtained by this reconstruction are not excellent. The average strength of finger flexion obtainable by a free muscular flap is approximately 40% of normal.

Conclusions

The prevention of compartment syndrome is the best way to reduce the development of Volkmann's ischaemic contracture. In recent years, in most developed countries, the incidence of ischaemic contracture has decreased following the classical supracondylar fracture in children. Conversely, other types of causes have increased the number of Volkmann's ischaemic contracture. The surgical treatment depends on the clinical situation regarding type and severity of the contracture. In this field there is not a single specific operation that can be done to solve the problem for every different clinical situation. All the treatment options should be considered in order to select the best option, however in the last 10 years, there is little doubt that microsurgery has provided new opportunities to assure some function, even in the worst cases for whom in the past there was little or no possibility for functional improvement.

Volkmann's ischemic contracture: case studies and discussion
Steven ER Hovius

Case 1

A 3-year-old girl was seen nearly two months following a supracondylar fracture, repositioning, and Kirschner wire (K-wire) fixation. She presented with a claw hand on the right side but our investigations were made more difficult by the fact that she was in a lot of pain, so much so that when asked to stretch her wrist and fingers, the pain made it impossible (Fig. 1). On the non-affected side she could easily stretch her fingers and make a fist. The pain distribution seemed to be more in the median nerve area than in the ulnar nerve area and electromyography revealed denervation in the median and ulnar nerve. Angiography was normal.

She was operated on at 2.5 months post-trauma. During the operation the median nerve was found adhered to the bone proximally in the forearm. The superficial flexors, the pronator teres, the flexor carpi ulnaris and the flexor pollicis longus all looked healthy. The deep flexors looked browner, and clearly different in colour than the more superficial muscles (Fig. 2). The ulnar nerve was healthy. Extensive neurolysis was performed on the median nerve. The ulnar nerve was explored. Fasciectomy was undertaken proximally at the deep flexor muscles. Apart from the discoloration of the deep flexor muscles and the fibrosis around the proximal

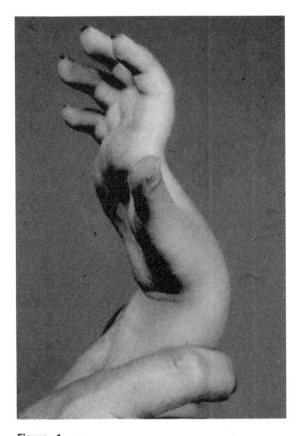

Figure 1

The patient is asked to stretch her fingers, preoperatively, case 1.

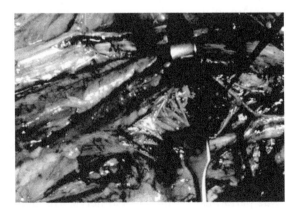

Figure 2

Following fasciectomy of the deep flexor muscles, case 1.

median nerve at the forearm, no infarction was encountered.

Following the operation she was free of pain in a couple of weeks. Post-operatively she was treated with a contracture-preventing splint and physiotherapy. At six months follow-up she was fully recovered with normal flexion and extension at wrist and finger level without any pain (Fig. 3). Grip strength was 80% at the one-year follow-up compared to the healthy side. No further treatment was deemed necessary.

Case 2

A 3.5-year-old boy was seen at our outpatient clinic seven months after a proximal ulnar fracture on the left (dominant) side, treated with

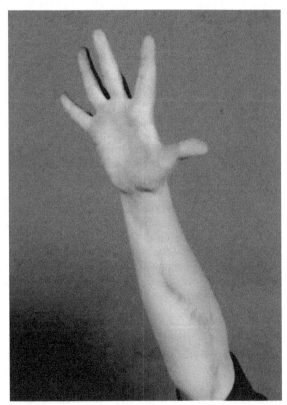

Figure 3

The patient is asked to stretch her fingers, postoperatively, case 1.

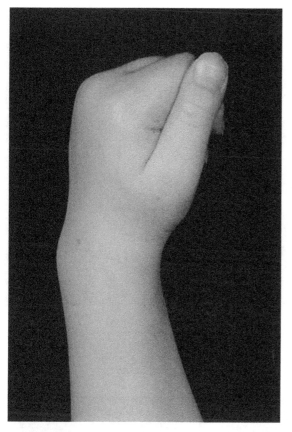

Figure 4

The patient is unable to move his fingers, preoperatively, side view, case 2.

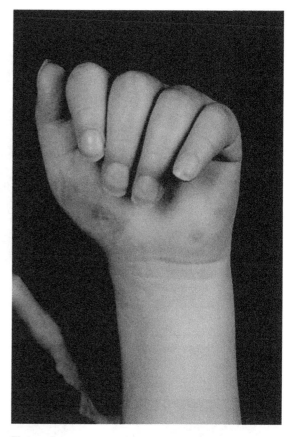

Figure 5

The patient is unable to move his fingers, preoperatively, anterior view, case 2.

a plastercast. After removal of the cast, flexion contractures of the fingers and wrist were encountered. He had been admitted earlier with a pain syndrome, which was considered at the time to be a reflex dystrophy and treated with high dosages of painkillers. He had a closed hand, an extension block at the wrist and he could not supinate (Figs 4 and 5). Sensation was difficult to assess. His left arm was not used, the patient did not tolerate electromyography, angiography showed diminished circulation of the thumb and index, the ulnar artery demonstrated calibre changes in the proximal part, and the brachial artery was intact.

At operation about a year post-trauma the deep finger flexors, the flexor pollicis longus and flexor carpi radialis were adhered. The infarction was mainly at the distal half of the muscles including the superficial flexor muscles (Fig. 6). The infarcted and fibrotic area was excised leaving the distal tendon ends of the deep and superficial flexor muscles unattached. The flexor carpi radialis and flexor pollicis longus were lengthened. The wrist and fingers could be completely stretched at the end of the operation. The median nerve had an hourglass deformity over 3.5 cm in the same area (Fig. 7), and the ulnar nerve had adhesions at the

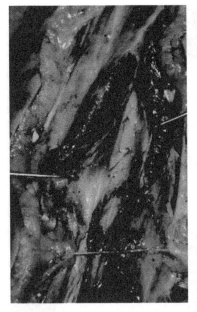

Figure 6

Infarction and fibrosis around the ulnar nerve, case 2

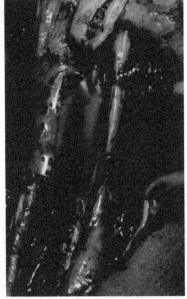

Figure 7

'Hour glass' deformity of the median nerve in the infarction area, case 2

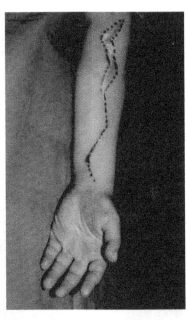

Figure 8

The wrist and fingers are fully released, preoperative view at the second stage, case 2

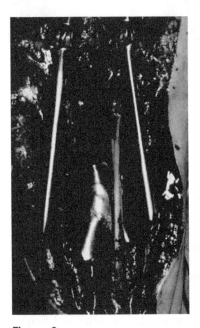

Figure 9

Sural nerve graft repair of the median nerve defect, case 2

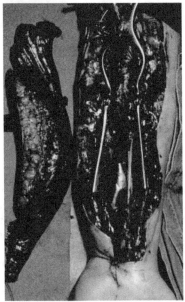

Figure 10

Free innervated vascularized gracilis flap to restore flexor function of fingers, case 2

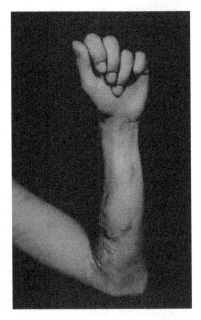

Figure 11

The patient is asked to make a fist, 1 year postoperatively after the second stage, anterior view, case 2

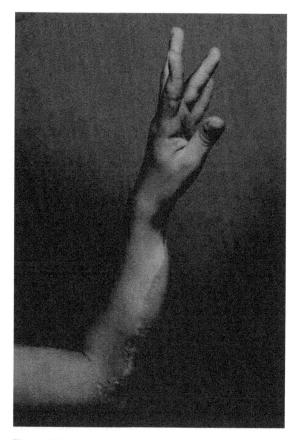

Figure 12

The patient is asked to stretch his fingers 1 year postoperatively, after the second stage, lateral view, case 2

and at six months the fingers could be flexed. At one-year post-operation he had grip strength of 60% when compared to the other hand, with full range of motion in the fingers (Fig. 11 and 12). Sensation in the median nerve area had recovered to near normal in daily use.

Case 3

A 10-year-old boy was seen at our outpatient clinic four years after he had sustained a supracondylar humeral fracture on the right side. Following treatment abroad he developed skin necrosis and infection of the forearm, which subsequently resulted in an ischemic contracture. He had a contracted longitudinal scar from elbow to wrist on the volar side. The palm of the hand was scarred and contracted transversally. The forearm was thin; the wrist had a flexion contracture of 80° without any active movement. The MCP joints were extended by 30°, with active extension to 80°. No flexion was possible in the MCP joints and the PIP joints were flexed to 110° without motion. The IP joint was also extremely flexed. The DIP joints could not be moved and no sensory function was detectable in the median and ulnar nerve distribution area (Figs 13 and 14). Electromyography showed denervation of the median and ulnar nerve and angiography demonstrated no vascular obstruction.

musculotendinous part of the flexor carpi ulnaris muscle.

At the second stage six months later (Fig. 8) the 4 cm section of damaged median nerve was resected and replaced by two strands of sural nerve graft (Fig. 9). Furthermore a free innervated vascularized gracilis musculocutaneous flap was attached from the medial epicondyl to the cut distal ends of the deep flexor tendons, just proximal to the carpal tunnel. The branch of the obburator nerve of the gracilis muscle was repaired end-to-end to the anterior interosseus nerve where it branches of the median nerve. The vessels were hooked up end-to-side to the ulnar artery and comitant vein (Fig. 10). At three months, muscle movements could be detected

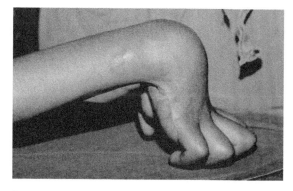

Figure 13

Only movement is possible at the MCP joints, preoperative ulnar view, case 3

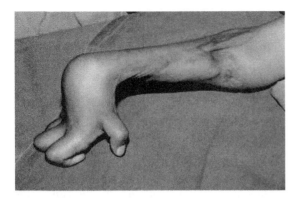

Figure 14

Radial view, case 3.

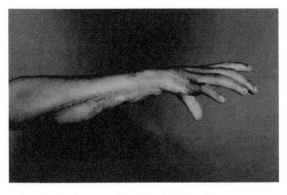

Figure 15

The patient is asked to stretch fingers and wrist 1 year postoperatively following the 3rd stage, case 3.

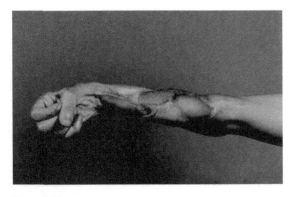

Figure 16

The patient is asked to make a fist 1 year postoperatively following the 3rd stage, case 3.

At operation all volar muscles were found to be completely fibrotic. Excision of the fibrotic area resulted in a disconnection of all the volar tendons. Only following a volar capsulotomy could the wrist and fingers be stretched. The skin defect at the distal forearm was covered with a groin flap. Both the median and ulnar nerve were very thin in the forearm region. At the second stage (a year later) a free innervated vascularized musculocutaneous gracilis flap was attached in a similar way as described in case 2. In a third stage a volar ligamentoplasty of the thumb at the MCP joint and a new capsulolysis of the wrist were performed. This resulted in a range of motion at the wrist of 30° and a normal range of motion at the second to fifth MCP joints.

There was satisfactory flexion and extension in the fingers at the PIP and DIP joints to enable the hand to open and close (Figs 15 and 16). His grip strength was 10% that of the other side and the Semmes-Weinstein test demonstrated sensation to the finest filament in the ulnar and median nerve area.

Discussion

Case 1 shows that although at presentation the case looked bad, only a relatively minor operation was necessary to obtain a nearly 100% recovery. Case 2 started dramatically with a pain syndrome, which completely recovered after extensive neurolysis. The case could have possibly been solved with a muscle slide and tendon transfers from the extensor side, but in the author's experience however, tendon transfers in children with extensive fibrotic areas in the forearm do not work well and there is a preference for a free innervated vascularized musculocutaneous gracilis flap. For case 3, the author believes that a free flap was the only treatment of choice.

References

Benkeddache Y, Gottesman H, Hamidani M (1985) Proposition d'une nouvelle classification du syndrome de Volkmann au stade de sequelles, *Ann Chir Main* **4**:134–42.

Bleton R (1996) Les syndromes des loges au membre superieur. Cahier d' Enseignement de la Soc Franç Chir Main, *Expansion Scientifique* **8**:15–35.

Copley LA, Dormans JP, Davidson RS (1996) Vascular injuries and their sequelae in paediatric supracondylar humeral fractures: towards a goal of prevention, *J Pediatr Orthop* **16**:99–103.

Eaton RG, Green WT (1975) Volkmann's ischaemia: a volar compartment syndrome of the arm, *Clin Orthop* **113**:58–64.

Ercetin O, Akinci M (1994) Free muscle transfer in Volkmann's ischaemic contracture, *Ann Chir Main* **13**:5–12.

Gulgonen A (2001) Invited review article: surgery for Volkmann's ischaemic contracture, *J Hand Surg* **26B**:283–95.

Hargens AR, Mubarak SJ (1998) Current concepts in the pathophysiology, evaluation, and diagnosis of compartment syndrome, *Hand Clin* **14**:371–83.

Holden CEA (1979) The pathology and prevention of Volkmann's ischaemic contracture, *J Bone Joint Surg* **61B**:296–300.

Hovius SER, Ultee J (2000) Volkmann's ischaemic contracture, *Hand Clin* **4**:647–57.

Ikuta Y, Kubo T, Tsuge K (1976) Free muscle transplantation by microsurgical technique to treat severe Volkmann's contracture, *Plast Reconstr Surg* **58**:407–11.

Inoue Y, Taylor GI (1996) The angiosomes of the forearm: anatomic study and clinical implications, *Plas Reconstr Surg* **98**:195–210.

Landi A, De Santis G, Torricelli P, et al (1989) CT in established Volkmann's contracture in forearm muscles, *J Hand Surg* **14B**:49–52.

Lanz U, Felderhoff (2000) Ishaemische Kontrakturen an Unterarm und Hand, *Handchirurgie, Mikrochirurgie und Plastische Chirurgie* **32**:6–25.

Manktelow RT, McKee NH (1978) Free muscle transplantation to provide active finger flexion, *J Hand Surg* **3A**:416–26.

Manktelow RT, Zuker RM, McKee NH (1984) Functioning free muscle transplantation, *J Hand Surg* **9A**:32–9.

Matsen FA III, Mayo KH, Sheridan GW, et al (1976)

Monitoring of intramuscular pressure, *Surgery* **79**:702–9.

Mubarak SJ, Carroll NC (1979) Volkmann's contracture in children: aetiology and prevention, *J Bone Joint Surg* **61B**:285–93.

Page CM (1923) An operation for the relief of flexion contracture in the forearm, *J Bone Joint Surg* **5**:233–34.

Petrolati M, Delaria G, Dell'Antonio A, et al (1978) La rivascolarizzazione distale nelle paralisi ischaemiche di Volkmann, *Chir Mano* **15**:55–64.

Pirone AM, Graham HK, Krajbich JI (1988) Management of displaced extension-type supracondylar fractures of the humerus in children, *J Bone Joint Surg* **70A**:641–50.

Raimondi P, Cavallazzi RM, Spreafico G (1987) Retraccion isquemica de Volkmann; rol de la microcirugia. In: Irisarri C, ed, *Cirugia de la mano traumatica*, (Ene edic: Madrid) 215–28.

Scaglietti O (1957) Sindromi cliniche immediate e tardive da lesioni vascolari nelle fratture degli arti, *Arch Putti di Chir Org di Movimento* **III**: 60–69.

Seddon HJ (1956) Volkmann's contracture: treatment by excision of the infarct, *J Bone Joint Surg* **38B**:152–74.

Seiler JG, Casey P, Binford SH (2000) Compartment syndromes of the upper extremity, *J South Orthop Assoc* 9:233–47.

Seyfer AE (1994) Injection and extravasation injuries. Hand Surgery Update ASSH 1:405–11.

Sheridan GW, Matsen FA III (1976) Fasciotomy in the treatment of the acute compartment syndrome, *J Bone Joint Surg* **58A**:112.

Tsuge K (1975) Treatment of established Volkmann's contracture, *J Bone Joint Surg* **57A**:925.

Tsuge K (1982) Management of established Volkmann's contracture. In: Green D, ed, *Operative hand surgery*, (Churchill Livingstone: Edinburgh) 499–514.

Volkmann R von (1881) Die ischaemischen Muskellahmungen und Kontrakturen, *Zentrolbl Chir* **8**: 801–803.

Whitesides TD, Haney TC, Harada H, et al (1975) A simple method for tissue pressure determination, *Arch Surg* **110**:1311–13.

Zancolli E (1965) Tendon transfers after ischaemic contracture of the forearm. Classification in relation to intrinsic muscle disorders, *Am J Surg* **1098**:356.

Zancolli E (1979) Classification of established Volkmann's contracture and the program for its treatment. In: *Structural and dynamic bases of hand surgery*, (J.B. Lippincott: Philadelphia) 314–24.

15

Replantation and revascularization of the upper extremity in children

Panayotis N Soucacos, Marios Vekris and Alexandros E Beris

Introduction

Even though replantation surgery has now become a routine procedure, it still remains a delicate and demanding surgery requiring adequate training and expertise in microsurgical techniques. Well-defined selection criteria for replantation procedures have evolved over the past few years, including definitive guidelines for thumb, single digit, multiple digit, mid palm amputations and upper extremity amputations. For more complex cases in digital amputations, other alternative techniques, such as transpositional microsurgery and various secondary reconstructive procedures, such as toe-to-hand transfer, are now available. Although replantation procedures have been simplified, a second surgical team can save valuable surgical time by debriding and identifying the vessels in the amputated part, harvesting microvenous grafts, performing bone fixation or tendon repair among other things, while the chief surgeon focuses on revascularization. Overall, the most significant guideline underlining the philosophy of replantation today reflects the aim of not only ensuring the survival of the amputated part, but its functional use as well. Experience dictates that this can be achieved only if the basic principles and indications of replantation surgery are adhered to.

In the 1960s Jacobson and Suarez demonstrated that with the use of the operating microscope and refined techniques, the fine work necessary to facilitate the anastomosis of small vessels less than 1 mm in diameter was possible. The use of magnification along with micro instruments and microsutures opened a new era

in surgery, with the establishment of a new discipline called microsurgery. This marked the end of conventional surgery for cases of major trauma of the upper and lower extremities, such as complete or incomplete non-viable amputations, where a team consisting of both orthopaedic and vascular surgeons was required. Traditionally the orthopaedic surgeon performed bone, tendon and nerve reconstruction, while the vascular or general surgeon was responsible for arterial and venous repair. Initially vascular anastomoses were done with the naked eye without the use of an operating microscope or other means of magnification, and it is in this manner that Malt and McKahnn (1964) performed the world's first arm replantation on a 12–year-old boy. However, with the advent of the era of microsurgery, orthopaedic and pediatric surgeons schooled both in the laboratory and in a variety of clinical cases earned the expertise to manage a wide array of traumatic injuries, particularly amputations.

Thus, it is with the introduction of the operating microscope along with microinstruments and microsutures, the three 'Ms' of microsurgery, that orthopaedic surgeons were able to achieve successful anastomoses of digital arteries in incomplete digital amputations (Kleinert et al 1963, Kutz 1969, Lendvay 1968). It was not until 1965 that the first digital replantation of a completely amputated thumb using microvascular techniques was achieved by Komatsu and Tamai (1968). This was followed by numerous reports from various centres all over the world. Since then, numerous revascularization and replantation procedures for amputated digits have taken place (Buncke et al 1981, MacLoed et al 1978, Merle et al 1991, Morrison et al 1977, Soucacos 1995a, Urbaniak 1987), with assessment of the results according to the type of amputation (Kleinert et al 1977, Soucacos et al 1995a), the severity of the injury (Beris et al 1994, Stevanovic et al 1991, Vlastou and Earle 1986), the number of amputated digits (Soucacos et al 1994b, 1994c) and the various techniques applied (Beris et al 1992, Brown and Wood 1990, Meuli and Meyer 1978, Soucacos et al 1994c).

Although the use of microsurgery by orthopaedic surgeons, at least initially, was almost exclusively applied to replantation, the growing expertise in microsurgical techniques has evolved towards a role in the management of other traumatic injuries including peripheral nerve injuries and type IIIb and IIIc compound fractures. Furthermore, the orthopaedic surgeon has recently been able to apply certain reconstructive microsurgical procedures, particularly free tissue transfers, such as free flaps, free vascularized bone and nerve grafts, in addition to toe-to-hand transfers.

Today, advances in microsurgical techniques have permitted replantation and reconstructive procedures to restore amputated or injured parts with a high degree of success in children. Microsurgery is now at the cutting edge, particularly microsurgical procedures applied to children, whose vessels can be < 0.5 mm in diameter (Gaul and Nunley 1988, Sekijuchi and Ohmori 1979).

The initial tendency to replant virtually every amputated part eventually gave way to attempts to define strict selection criteria and optimize the functional results. Today, the major concern is not 'how to replant an amputated part', but rather 'how to make it functional'. In this regard, replantation without sensation and function is no longer considered acceptable (Shaw and Hidalgo 1987). Fundamental to the success in replantation of a digit is not only a solid microsurgical technique for vascular microanastomosis, nerve coaptation and tendon repair, but also a clear understanding of the selection criteria. The technical limitations encountered in treating children have slowly been overcome with major advances in microsurgical techniques that have made revascularization possible in young children with very small diameter vessels (Devaraj et al 1991, Gaul and Nunley 1988, Gayle et al 1991).

Selection criteria

Although replantation microsurgery has become a routine procedure with vast experience accumulated over the past years, the success rate in replantation procedures in children still varies widely from 42% to close to 90% (Beris et al 1995, Daigle and Kleinert 1991). Nonetheless, there is almost unanimous agreement among surgeons that any amputated part in a child should be replanted.

There is a growing consensus in the literature that replantation at any level is usually better than amputation revision or prosthetic fitting (Taras et al 1991). Among the youngest children reported to have undergone replantation procedures are a 7–month-old with a thumb amputation (0.3 mm vessel diameter) and a 12–month-old (0.4 mm vessel diameter) (Gaul and Nunley 1988, Sekijuchi and Ohmori 1979). Because of the tremendous recuperative ability and despite the small vessel size and the technical difficulties, replantations in children are usually associated with good functional results (Beris et al 1995). Although the functional results after replantation are considerably better in children than in adults, the viability rates in children tend to be lower (Beris et al 1995, Daigle and Kleinert 1991, Taras et al 1991)

Three main types of amputations are recognized based on the viability of the amputated part, including complete amputations, incomplete non-viable amputations, and incomplete viable amputations. Complete amputations are those in which the amputated part is completely detached from the proximal stump with no tissue part interposed between the distal amputated segment and the proximal stump. Amputations in which both neurovascular bundles and the entire or most of the venous network system are severed or severely damaged are incomplete non-viable amputations. Although the distal segment is connected to the proximal stump with either an islet of skin, or a small segment of tendon or nerve, these tissue components are not capable of ensuring the viability of the distal part. In incomplete viable amputations, some arterial blood supply and venous outflow of the distal part are present. Nevertheless, these injuries represent a grey zone which needs to be assessed under the operating microscope to determine whether both the arterial blood supply

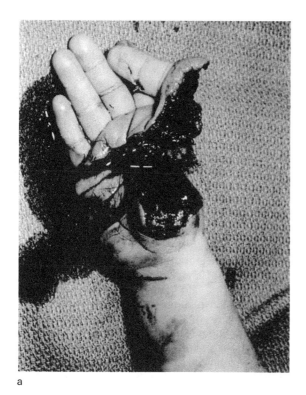

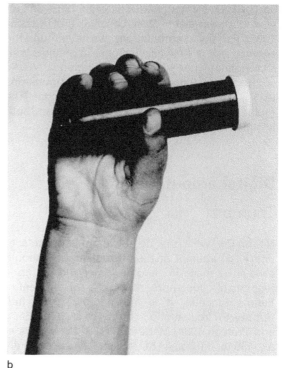

a   b

Figure 1

(a) Preoperative palmer view of an incomplete non-viable amputation of the right thumb and index finger on a 4-year-old girl secondary to a laundry machine injury. (b) Postoperative view 9-months postoperatively showing successful replantation with good grasp function and cosmetic appearance.

and venous outflow of the distal part are adequately served.

Since a complete amputation occurs when a part has been totally severed from the body, this part can be reattached with microvascular repair or replantation. An incomplete non-viable amputation is only partially detached. However, since there is no circulation, microvascular anastomosis is required to restore circulation. This type of procedure is called revascularization. In general, revascularization procedures have a much greater chance of survival than replantations, since there are fewer repaired structures (Saies et al 1994, Soucacos et al 1995b). As in adults, revascularization has a greater chance of survival in children compared to replantations. Moreover, due to the fewer structures requiring repair, it requires less operating time. In some

cases, there may also be better venous drainage (Fig. 1).

The level of injury is an important selection parameter. In general the more proximal the injury is, the greater the concern for failure. This is primarily due to the increased muscle mass in the ischaemic part in proximal amputations. In addition, proximal amputations tend to be associated with more violent mechanisms of injury, and the greater distance which nerves must regenerate in proximal amputations is less favourable for nerve repair. Overall, the functional results following replantation at the shoulder level are comparatively poor, while about one-third of the cases have good replantation results in arm replantations. In contrast, excellent results can be expected in about 40% of proximal forearm replantations and in about 80% of distal forearm and wrist replantations (Beris et al 1995, Jaeger et al 1981, Saies et al 1994, Urbaniak and Forester 1991). For digital amputations, we have found the survival rate is statistically higher in patients with incomplete non-viable amputations (89%) compared to those with complete amputations (81%), while the patient's ability to use the replanted digit was about the same in both groups (Soucacos et al 1995b).

Digital amputations

Thumb

No matter what the degree or mechanisms of injury, an attempt at thumb replantation should always be made in children. Since the thumb is responsible for more than 40% of the entire hand's function, it is indisputably given first priority for replantation (Chow et al 1979, Early and Watson 1984, Merle et al 1991, Soucacos et al 1994b, 1995a). Moreover, a successfully replanted thumb always produces results which are far more favourable than any other reconstructive procedure or prosthetic device. Crucial factors for a functional thumb replantation are length and sensitivity. Compared to complete amputations of the thumb, incomplete non-viable amputations of the thumb are associated with a statistically higher rate of survival (86.2% versus 78.2%) and better sensibility (Soucacos et al 1995a), while motion at the interphalangeal (IP) joint did not differ. The necessity for replantation or reconstruction in bilateral thumb amputations is based not only on the severity of the wound itself which functionally incapacitates the hand, but on the basis that since both hands are critically impaired the patient is prohibited from performing fundamental daily tasks which involve pinching and grasping with the hands (Soucacos et al 1994b). Thus, the indications for bilateral thumb amputations are even greater than for single amputations of the thumb (Fig. 2).

Single digit

There are three major indications for single digit replantation. One primary indication is when the level of the amputation is distal to the insertion of the flexor digitorum sublimis. In a successful replantation, the digit immediately becomes functional as flexion of the middle phalanx by the intact superficialis tendon is possible (Soucacos et al 1995c, Urbaniak 1987, Urbaniak et al 1985).

Amputations at the level of the distal phalanx are also indicated (Foucher et al 1981, Malizos et al 1994, Merle et al 1991, Yomano 1985). Replantation is usually achieved with the anastomosis of one artery, while venous drainage can be provided by provoked bleeding or with the application of leeches (Soucacos et al 1994a).

Ring avulsion injuries represent a specialized category of injury ranging from simple abrasion to complete amputation. In most cases, the mechanism of injury involves the entrapment of a ring or the finger itself in some mechanical device, which results in the complete or incomplete avulsion of the skin combined with crushing of the finger. These types of injuries are fairly common in children. Various classifications of ring avulsion injuries have been proposed in order to assist in making the appropriate decision as to whether or not to replant. Type II injuries which have either isolated arterial or venous compromise can almost always be successfully revascularized. Type IIIa injuries are those with an intact proximal interphalangeal (PIP) joint and flexor digitorum superficialis, while type IIIb injuries are those with complete amputation at the level of the proximal phalanx and severance of both flexor tendons (Beris et al 1994).

A third indication for single digit replantation in children is ring avulsion injuries type II or IIIa. These are defined as combined open hand injuries involving both the dorsal and volar skin and blood supply (arterial inflow and venous return) in an isolated finger (Beris et al 1994, Soucacos and Beris 1998). In this type of injury, the flexor digitorum superficialis tendon remains intact. If the replantation procedure is successful, the digit becomes immediately functional as flexion of the middle phalanx is possible. Since the outcome almost always has good function, they present a strong indication for replantation in children (Fig. 3).

Replantation of a single digit which is amputated at the level of the proximal phalanx or at the PIP joint, particularly in avulsion or crush injuries, is contraindicated. This is because

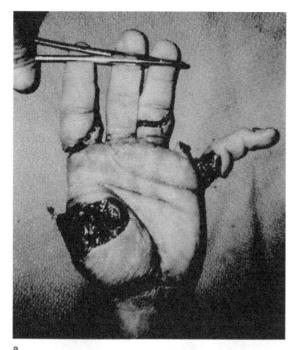

a

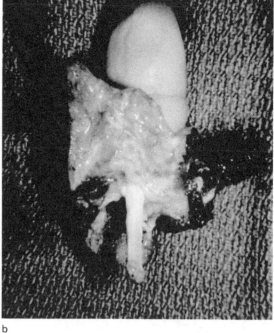

b

Figure 2

Replantation of the thumb is always a prime priority. (a) Preoperative palmer view showing complete amputation of the left thumb, incomplete non-viable amputation of the little finger and incomplete viable amputations of the index and ring fingers on a 15-year-old boy. (b) Volar view showing the completely avulsed thumb. Note the extending flexor policis longis. (c) Postoperative view taken at 3-months showing successful replantation of thumb, and revascularization of little, index and ring fingers.

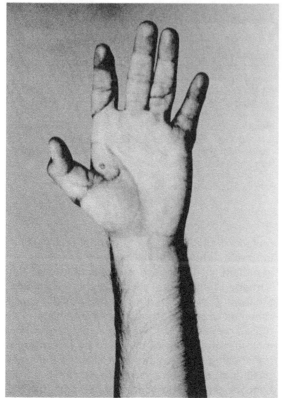

c

the replanted finger almost always results in a non-functioning digit, even after the patient undergoes multiple, mostly unsuccessful reconstructive procedures. However, a relative indication for the replantation of a single digit is found in carefully identified patients who have highly demanding professions, such as musicians.

Multiple digits

Multiple digit amputations have a high priority for replantation. The more digits that can be

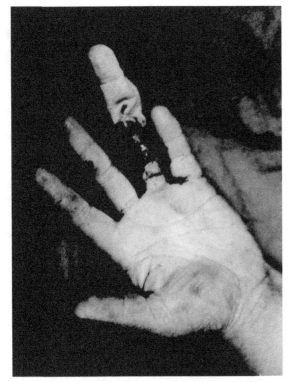

a

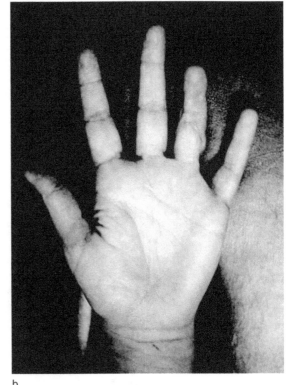

b

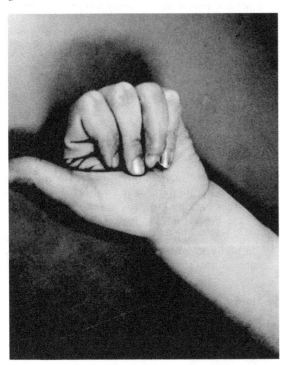

c

Figure 3

Type IIIa ring avulsion injuries are good candidates for replantation in children. (a) Preoperative palmar view showing a type IIIa ring avulsion injury in a 17-year-old girl. Only one digitial artery and one dorsal vein were anastomosed in the replantation procedure. Nonetheless, excellent results were achieved with good extension (b) and flexion (c) 1-year postoperatively. Note that the ring finger was converted to a sublimis digit with flexion only at the PIP joint. However, the slight flexion contracture at the DIP joint is functionally helpful.

replanted, the better the functional results. Thus, in cases where the amputated segments are identified as being too severely mutilated and damaged, efforts are geared towards replanting the least damaged part to the most useful stump. When all of the digits are not replantable and the thumb remains intact, the aim is directed towards restoring the width of the palm by replanting or transposing digits to the ulnar side. By this transpositional procedure, the power grasp of the hand is clearly augmented, while light pinch is maintained (Fig. 4) (Soucacos et al 1994c).

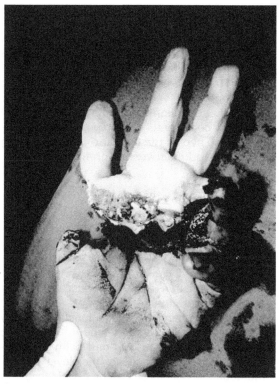

a

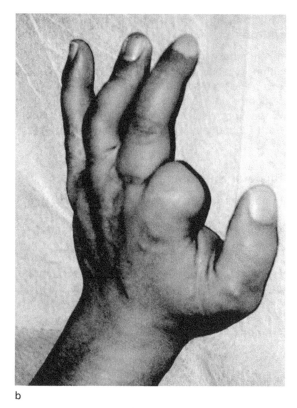

b

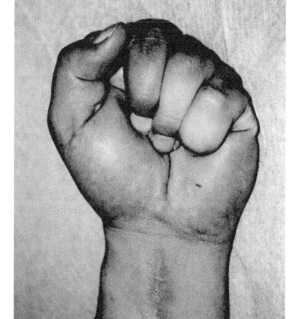

c

Figure 4

(a) Preoperative view of a multiple digit amputation in a 12-year-old boy with complete amputation of the left thumb, index and long fingers and incomplete non-viable amputation of the ring finger. Although replantation was unsuccessful for the index finger, excellent results were achieved with the other digits with good extension (b) and flexion (c) at 1 year postoperatively.

Transpositional microsurgery

Transpositional digital microsurgery refers to the transposition and replantation of any digit to another stump which plays a more significant role in the function of the hand. Five major indications for transpostional digital microsurgery have been identified (Soucacos et al 1994c).

Multiple digit amputations including the thumb

In patients where the thumb is not replantable either because it is too short or has experienced extensive damage, the least damaged digit is replanted in the place of the mutilated thumb. When successful, the patient's hand is usually both functionally and cosmetically acceptable.

Bilateral thumb amputations

In patients who have sustained a bilateral thumb amputation and in whom the thumb of the dominant hand is severely crushed and damaged, the less damaged thumb of the non-dominant hand is transposed to the thumb stump of the dominant hand. This maintains dexterity in the dominant hand. On the other hand, patients who have sustained a bilateral thumb amputation in addition to multiple digital amputations, the least damaged digit is transposed to the stump of the thumb if one or both of the thumbs are badly damaged.

Bilateral, symmetrical amputations

The thumb is intact, and the replantation effort is directed towards increasing the dexterity of the dominant hand by transposing digits over from the non-dominant hand.

Multiple amputations with the thumb intact

Patients with multiple digital amputations in which the thumb remains intact are included in this group. In these patients, an effort is made to replant the digits towards the ulnar side of the hand, so as to preserve the width of the palm and thus, increase the power grasp of the hand.

Amputation of all five digits

The aim is two-fold. First, the goal is to replant and create a functional thumb. Second, an effort is made to transpose the digits ulnarly, thus preserving the width of the palm, as well as the power grip.

Transposition microsurgery appears to have a clear place in the treatment of patients in whom the thumb is not replantable, as well as in patients with multiple digital amputations and in whom the width of the palm and the power grasp of the hand need to be preserved. The fact that arterial and venous anastomoses can be done without tension and on a relatively normal intima are considered advantages of this procedure, which avoids the need for time-consuming interpositioned microvenous grafts.

Mid palm amputations

Mid palm amputations, whether or not they include the thumb, are ideal candidates for replantation and constitute an absolute indication. If replantation efforts are successful, with adequate restoration of both power grasp and light pinch, the hand achieves a functional ability which is superior to any type of prosthetic device. The success rate of mid palm replantations is directly related to the level of the amputation. Specifically, the incidence of successful replantation is significantly higher for amputations located at the level of the superficial or deep palmar arch, compared to those at the level of the common digital arteries (Soucacos 1995a).

Major upper limb amputations

Upper limb amputations are serious compound injuries whose management requires microsurgical skill, compentence in major traumatology, hand surgery, as well as awareness of the dangers of post-ischaemia syndrome. The success rate of major limb replantation in children varies greatly. This is probably related to the fact that most replantation and revascularization series mix children's cases with adult series and only a few series report only on replantation in children (Beris et al 1994). The generally low success rate reported in major limb replantation in children may be related to the mechanism of injury in these cases, which is usually a crush and/or avulsion in injury associated with injury to muscles, nerve and

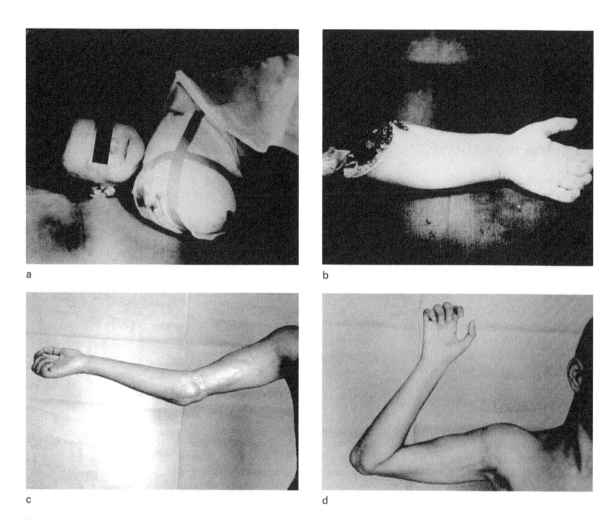

Figure 5

Major upper limb amputation at the level of the distal humerus in a 2-year-old boy. (a) Preoperative view showing child after transport and admittance to the surgical ward with sterile dressing covering the proximal stump. The child had also sustained laceration at the anterior axillary fold with severance of the axillary artery and vein. (b) Preoperative volar view showing the avulsed arm. At 18 years postoperatively, good extension (c) and flexion (d) of the elbow is seen. Cosmetic and functional results were satisfactory with no significant length discrepancy between the upper limbs.

vessels at various levels (Jaeger et al 1981). The level of amputation appears to make a difference to the survival expectation of an amputated part in amputations through the forearm and above. At these levels, the amputated parts contain more muscle which restricts ischaemia times before the onset of muscle necrosis (Fig. 5).

Since the prognosis for nerve regeneration in children is superior compared with adults, the necessity for replantation is made even stronger for upper extremity amputations (Beris et al 1994, Urbaniak and Forster 1991). Children who undergo replantation and/or revascularization procedures, usually require additional procedures to increase the functional outcome of the initial replantation success. In our experience an average of 2.8 additional procedures were required to improve the functional outcome of the initial successful replantation (Beris et al 1994).

General indications

The selection criteria applied to adults do not always apply to children; an attempt at replantation should be made in almost all children. The only contraindications to replantation attempts are severly damaged and mutilated parts, a general condition that may prohibit a long surgical procedure, or the presence of other systemic injuries.

In addition to selection criteria related to the type, level and severity of the amputation, other general factors related to the patient should be considered before replantation is attempted. These include the mechanism of injury, ischaemia, the patient's general health, predicted rehabilitation, and vocation. In children, an attempt should always be made to replant almost any amputated digit.

In children the mechanisms of injury (i.e. guillotine *vs* crush avulsion) is a prognostic factor. Clean-cut 'guillotine' type amputations are good candidates for replantation. Severely crushed or avulsed digits have extensive vascular, nerve and soft tissue damage and the predicted outcome is usually poor. Children tend to have a greater proportion of crush-avulsion injuries compared to adults (Urbaniak and Foster 1991). Avulsion injuries no matter at what level which they occur, tend to give poorer overall results. Segmental injuries at multiple levels are usually associated with severe vascular damage, often too extensive to warrant replantation.

Ischaemia remains a key factor in determining the success of replantation (Brunelli 1988). Since digits consist of mostly skin, bone and subcutaneous tissue and contain no muscles, warm ischaemia is tolerated for a longer period of time. After adequate cooling, we have experienced successful replantation even up to 24-h post-injury and it has been reported up to 36-h. On the other hand, major limbs which consist of a high percentage of muscle can tolerate only 4–6 hours of ischaemia following amputation.

Warm ischaemia or anoxia at 20° to 25°C produces irreversible necrotic changes to the muscle and soft tissues. Because digits lack muscle, the time allowed for warm ischaemia is about 8-h, compared to 6-h for upper or lower extremity parts. By cooling the amputated part to 4°C, ischaemia time for digits can be extended to up to 30-h. The importance of warm or cold ischaemia in survival of the amputated part and success of the procedure, suggests that amputations occurring in warmer countries or even during the warm seasons would have a lower success rate.

If the patient has sustained other major life-threatening injuries at the time of trauma, then replantation of digits may need to be postponed or even cancelled. Certain diseases which can adversely affect peripheral circulation, such as diabetes mellitus, some autoimmune diseases, collagen vascular diseases or atherosclerosis, among others, may also produce a condition which is contraindicated for replantation.

Surgical sequelae and techniques in replantation

Survival is intimately related to the successful anastomosis of arteries without tension and on healthy intima, as well as two veins per patent artery. After thorough cleansing and debridement, structures are identified and repair is performed. In most cases, the repair follows the following sequence: (1) tissue debridement; (2) neurovascular identification in the amputated part and stump; (3) bone shortening and stabilization; (4) tendon repair; (5) arterial anastomoses; (6) venous anastomoses; (7) nerve repair; and (8) soft-tissue and skin coverage. All structures are repaired primarily, including nerves and tendons unless a large nerve gap is present which necessitates a secondary nerve grafting procedure.

Small children are given only general anaesthesia; older children can be given general anaesthesia in combination with an axillary brachial plexus block. Broad-spectrum antibiotics are usually given intravenously, and this is repeated immediately after the reestablishment of circulation to the amputated part. When there is bleeding, the procedure can be done under tourniquet control. Care must be taken, however, not to apply as much tourniquet pressure as used for adults and not to exceed about 1.5-h of tourniquet ischaemia.

Bone fixation

The method of bone fixation used in children depends on the site of the amputation. In digit replantations, usually one or two small Kirschner wires (K-wires) are adequate. (It is preferable to place only one Kirschner wire during the operation, so that the part can be rotated; the second wire can be placed at the end of the procedure, if necessary). Similarly, internal fixation with Kirschner wires is applied with fractures of the metacarpals in children. Plates and screws of various dimensions are reserved for amputations of the upper extremity. In severely contaminated amputations, an external fixator may be applied.

Bone shortening usually preceeds osteosynthesis and vessel anastomosis (Brown and Wood 1990, Meuli and Meyer 1978, Touliatos et al 1995). In general, the procedure entails the careful resection of the bone ends to ensure ease of approximation of the vessels and nerves with minimal stripping of the periosteum. We prefer to remove bone from the amputated part, so that if the replantation fails, the length of the stump has not been sacrificed. In children, the bone should be prepared by minimal shortening far from the epiphyseal growth plate so as not to disturb normal growth (Nunley et al 1987). Bone growth and the development of epiphyseal plates are generally believed to be disturbed after the replantation of amputated extremities in children. In one study of 13 amputated parts of the upper limb, average longitudinal growth was 94.5% in the proximal bone segment directly injured from the initial trauma, and 92.7% in the distal replanted part (Demiri et al 1995). Although it is not clear what parameters affected the prognosis of post-traumatic reactions in the growing cartilaginous plates, the level of amputation seemed to be a significant prognostic factor of epiphyseal growth in the replanted part.

The amount of bone removal depends upon the level of the amputation (Touliatos et al 1995). For amputations of the thumb, the major portion of bone shortening should be done on the amputated part to preserve good bone stock on the stump in case the replantation fails. In amputations through the metacarpal joint, an attempt should be made to obtain a resection arthroplasty by resection of the metacarpal head and leaving the base of the proximal phalanx with the cartilage intact. If the amputation is through the shaft of the phalanges, we usually remove bone from both ends, while in amputations through the interphalangeal joints, bone is removed from both ends and the joint undergoes arthrodesis.

Mini plates with screws, single lag screws, crossed Kirschner wires, a combination of intra-osseous circlage wires and Kirschner wires, as well as intra-medullary Kirschner wires are examples of the materials and techniques suitable for bone fixation (Touliatos et al 1995). Relatively rapid methods for bone fixation include bone or cement pegs. Alternatively, a screw can be inserted in the distal part; the head is subsequently cut off and screwed in the proximal stump. Based on our experience, we have found that intra-medullary Kirschner wires supplemented by a second wire inserted at the end of the procedure is the most effective means for digital bone fixation. This technique is both simple and fast, requires minimal bone exposure, and provides the surgeon with the possibility of intra-operatively realigning the vessels, as needed. The inherent instability of a single intra-medullary K-wire in rotational deformities is avoided by placing the second K-wire at the end of the procedure.

Tendons

Primary repair of extensor tendons is advisable in children. Tendons that were previously isolated, marked and sutured with Tajima-type sutures in the debriding process can be tied together. In digital replantation procedures, the extensor tendons are always repaired first with an end-to-end suture technique directly after bone shortening and fixation. Suturing of the extensor tendons provides additional stability for the replanted digit and in most cases usually presents with no problems. Flexor tendon repair should be done primarily only in very selected clean-cut amputations, otherwise repair should be done as a secondary operation either with tendon grafts or a two-stage reconstruction procedure (Hunter 1984; Soucacos 1995b).

Artery repair

Vascular repair in children follows the same principles for adults. Perhaps the only technical difference is that the very small distal vessels in children will require fewer stitches. On severely crushed or avulsed amputations where vessel damage was severe, intra-venous heparin is given during the operation and for the first postoperative week. Postoperative heparin was used only in severely crushed or avulsed amputation. Otherwise, anticoagulant therapy consisted of aspirin and low molecular dextran for five days, after which only aspirin was given. The generally accepted principles of vascular repair should be followed. Sutures should be only on healthy vessel edges and under normal tension.

Arterial anastomosis takes place after bone shortening and fixation and extensor and flexor tendon repair. It is preferable to repair both digital arteries. Critical for successful microvascular anastomosis are solid microsurgical techniques, and anastomosis on normal intima with no tension. A pneumatic tourniquet around the upper arm should be used for each vascular anastomosis, as it will help decrease blood loss and improve operating time. The artery should be dissected until normal intima is visualized under high-power magnification. If normal intima cannot be approximated without tension, further bone shortening, or preferably the use of a vein graft are indicated. The arterial ends are also assessed for damage to the media or adventitia, which if present needs to be resected further.

In patients with undue tension, a vein graft should be used. Vein grafts can be harvested, according to the diameter of the vessel, from the dorsal aspect of the hand, the volar or dorsal surface of the forearm in upper extremity injuries, or the saphenous vein for larger vessels. Whenever the need for a vein graft is anticipated, veins should be marked before the tourniquet is applied to avoid difficulties finding them later when the veins have collapsed.

In both primary repair and grafting procedures, vessel clamps with an approximator and about nine interrupted sutures were made with 10–0 or 11–0 nylon suture and tapered edge atraumatic needle. A continuous suture was avoided in children because of the stenosing effect that it could produce on the growing vessel. Vessels as small as 0.3 and 0.4 mm have been repaired successfully.

Vein repair

In children, the number of veins repaired is directly porportionate to success, which may explain in part the higher success rate with revascularizations. The need for good venous patency is supported by findings that most failed replantations in children were secondary to venous obstruction. In order to repair two veins for each artery, veins may need to be mobilized or harvested. The most common error is anastomosis under tension or to waste time trying to repair very small veins. Only the largest veins should be anastomosed. The technique of venous anastomosis is similar to arterial anastomosis with a few differences. Fewer sutures are generally required as blood flow is weaker than that of the arteries. In addition, since the venous wall is thinner and more fragile, the use of microclamps during the anastomosis procedure must be kept to a minimum in order to avoid injury by extended pressure which in turn, may lead to necrosis of the venous wall.

Nerves

Repair of the digital nerves adheres to the same guidelines as with the repair of the flexor tendons within the tendon sheath. Thus, in cases with a clean-cut injury, direct end-to-end digital nerve coaptation is indicated. In all other situations, such as crush or avulsion type injuries, secondary procedures using a nerve graft or if the nerve gap is less than 2 cm, using a nerve conduit, are recommended.

Complications

Inadequate perfusion is responsible for acute complications. Following most microvascular procedures used in replantation, the rule of thumb is that when the part or area has developed pallor and loss of turgor (e.g. the area is pale with loss of capillary refill), then arterial insufficiency is present. On the other hand, when the area is cyanotic, congested and turgid, then venous insufficiency is present. The management of any circulatory compromise is dependent upon whether arterial or venous insufficiency is present. If normal perfusion does not return, the patient must be returned to the operating room; if the patient is returned within the first 12–48 hours, some failures can be salvaged by redoing the vein graft, removing the thrombus and grafting a previously unrecognized damaged vessel segment. Congestion can be effectively relieved with the use of medicinal leeches.

Although subacute complications due to infection are fairly frequent in digital replantations, they rarely result in the loss of the replanted part. The most common chronic complications include cold intolerance, tendon adhesions and malunion. Cold intolerance is a common complaint in patients with digital replantation. It is related to the adequacy of digital reperfusion, and provides an argument for maximizing the number of arteries repaired. Cold intolerance improves over time. Tendon adhesions are frequent, resulting in limited motion. In severe cases, tenolysis can be performed after three months.

As in adults, major limb replantation procedures are not without risk in children. The most common complication is sepsis secondary to muscle necrosis. In contrast to adults, in whom replantation procedures can be performed under regional anaesthesia or in combination with general anaesthesia, surgery is always done under general anaesthesia in children.

Incomplete non-viable upper limb amputations have a better success rate compared to complete amputations (Beris et al 1994). Sensibility is generally satisfactory and provides good protective sensation. Growth can be affected in patients with complete amputations of the upper extremity; at five year follow-up, 3 cm shortening was found in replanted forearms and 2.5 cm shortening was observed when the amputation was in the humeral shaft (Beris et al 1994).

Conclusions

Despite some difficulties in replantation of digits, functional re-education appears to be better in children (Beris et al 1995). The better recuperative ability in children compared with adults is noted in their rapid nerve recovery and better sensibility. However, the assessment of static or moving two–point discrimination is often difficult in the very young patient. Muscle function recovery tends to be worse than sensibility, particularly in hand injuries because of the relatively poor reinnervation of the intrinsic muscles of the hand after replantation. Overall, sensory re-education appears to allow the patients to achieve their potential for functional recovery. As such, replanted digits with sensory re-education recover a greater degree of sensation.

In most replantation patients, one or more secondary procedures are required to improve functional results. These include free tissue transfers, tenolyses, nerve grafts, tendon transfers and two-stage tendon reconstruction with a silicone rod.

One of the major factors that determines success in replantation procedures, particularly for digital replantation, appears to be the expertise of the surgeon who using established criteria and techniques should be able to maintain patency in vessels down to 0.4 mm in children. Factors such as age, amputation level, and type of injury do not appear to relate to survival rate. In children, contributing factors to survival appear to be degree of injury and adequacy of venous drainage. Overall, children show a survival rate that is less favourable than that in adults, but have functional results that are uniformly superior.

References

Beris AE, Soucacos PN, Touliatos AS (1992) Experimental evaluation of the length of microvenous grafts under normal tension, *Microsurgery* **13**:195–99.

Beris AE, Soucacos PN, Malizos KN, Xenakis TA (1994) Microsurgical treatment of ring avulsion injuries, *Microsurgery* **15**:459–63.

Beris AE, Soucacos PN, Malizos KN (1995) Microsurgery in children, *Clin Orthop* **314**:112–21

Brown ML, Wood MB (1990) Techniques of bone fixation in replantation surgery, *Microsurgery* **11**:255–60.

Brunelli G (1988) Experimental studies of the effects of ischemia on devascularized limbs. In: Brunelli G, ed, *Textbook of Microsurgery* (Masson: Milan) 89–99.

Buncke HJ, Alpert BS, Hohnson-Giebink R (1981) Digital replantation, *Surg Clin North Am* **61**: 383–94.

Chow JSA, Bilos ZJ, Chunprapaph B (1979) Thirty thumb replantations: indications and results, *Plast Reconstr Surg* **64**:626–30.

Daigle JP, Kleinert JM (1991) Major limb replantation in children, *Microsurgery* **12**:221–31.

Demiri E, Bakhach J, Tsakoniatis N, Martin D, Baudet J (1995) Bone growth after replantation in chidren, *J Reconstr Microsurg* **11**: 113–22.

Devaraj VS, Kay SP, Batchelor AG, Yates A (1991) Microvascular surgery in children, *Br J Plast Surg* **44**:276–80.

Early MJ, Watson JS (1984) Twenty four thumb replantations, *J Hand Surg* **9B**:98–102.

Foucher G, Merle M, Braun JB (1981) Distal digital replantation is one of the best indications for microsurgery, *Int J Microsurg* **3**:263–70.

Gaul JS, Nunley JA (1988) Microvascular replantation in a seven-month old girl: a case report, *Microsurgery* **9**:204–07.

Gayle LB, Lineaveaver WC, Buncke GM et al (1991) Lower extremity replantation, *Clin Plast Surg* **18**:437–47.

Hidalgo DA, Shaw WW, Colen SR (1987) Upper limb replantation. In: Shaw WW, Hidalgo DA, eds, *Microsurgery in trauma*. (Futura Publishing Co., Inc: New York) 71–88.

Hunter JM (1984) Staged flexor tendon reconstruction. In: Hunter JM, Schneider LH, Mackin EJ, Callahan AO, eds, *Rehabilitation of the hand*. (CV Mosby Co: St Louis) 288–313.

Jaeger SH, Tsai TM, Kleinert HE (1981) Upper extremity replantation in children, *Orthop Clin North Am* **12**:897–907.

Kleinert HE, Kasdan ML, Romero JL (1963) Small blood vessel anastomosis for salvage of the severely injured upper extremity, *J Bone Joint Surg* **45A**: 788–96.

Kleinert HE, Juhala CA, Tsai TM, Van Beek A (1977) Digital replantation—selection, technique, and results, *Orthop Clin North Am* **8**:309–18.

Komatsu S, Tamai S (1968) Successful replantation of a completely cut-off thumb: case report, *Plast Reconstr Microsurg* **42**:374–77.

Kutz JE, Hay EL, Kleinert HE (1969) Fate of small vessel repair, *J Bone Joint Surg* **51A**:791.

Lendvay PG (1968) Anastomosis of digital vessels, *Med J Aust* **2**:723–24.

MacLeod AM, O'Brien BM, Morrison WA (1978), Digital replantation: clinical experiences, *Clin Orthop* **133**:26–34.

Malizos KN, Beris, AE, Kabani CT, Soucacos PN (1994) Distal phalanx microsurgical replantation, *Microsurg* **15**: 464–68.

Malt RA, McKhann C (1964) Replantation of severed arms, *JAMA* **198**:716.

Merle M, Dap F, Bour C (1991) Digital replantation. In: Meyer VE, Black MJM, eds, *Microsurgical procedures*. (Churchill Livingstone: London) 21–35.

Meuli HC, Meyer V, Segmuller G (1978) Stabilization of bone in replantation surgery of the upper limb, *Clin Orthop* **33**:179–83.

Morrison WA, O'Brien BM, MacLeod AM (1977) Evaluation of digital replantation: a review of 100 cases, *Orthop Clin North Am* **8**:295–308.

Nunley JA, Spiegle PV, Goldner RD, Urbaniak JR (1987) Longitudinal epiphyseal growth after replantation and transplantation in children, *J Hand Surg* **12A**:274–79.

Saies AD, Urbaniak JR, Nunley JA, Tarasw JS, Goldner RD, Fitch RD (1994) Results after replantation and revascularization in the upper extremity in children, *J Bone Joint Surg Am* **76**:1766–76.

Sekijuchi J, Ohmori K (1979) Youngest replantation with microsurgical anastomoses, *Hand* **11**:64–68.

Shaw WW, Hidalgo DA (1987) Replantation: general consideration. In: Shaw WW, Hidalgo DA, eds, *Microsurgery in trauma*. (Futura Publishing Co., Inc: New York) 59–70.

Soucacos PN, Beris AE, Malizos KN, Kabani CT, Pakos S (1994a) The use of medicinal leeches, *Hirudo medicinalis*, to restore venous circulation in trauma and reconstructive microsurgery, *Int Angiol* **13**:319–25.

Soucacos PN, Beris AE, Malizos KN, Touliatos AS (1994b) Bilateral thumb amputation, *Microsurg* **15**: 454–58.

Soucacos PN, Beris AE, Malizos KN, Vlastou C, Soucacos PK, Georgoulis AD (1994c) Transpositional microsurgery in multiple digital amputations, *Microsurg* **15**: 469–73.

Soucacos PN (1995a) Microsurgery in orthopaedics. In: Casteleyn PP, Duparc J, Fulford P, eds, *European instructional course lectures*, Vol 2, (British Society of Bone and Joint Surgery: London) 149–56

Soucacos PN (1995b) Two-stage flexor tendon recon-struction using silicone rods. In: Vastamaki M, ed, *Current trends in hand surgery*. (Elsevier: Amsterdam) 353–57.

Soucacos PN, Beris AE, Touliatos AS, Korobilias AB, Gelalis J, Sakas G (1995a) Complete versus incomplete nonviable amputations of the thumb: comparison of the survival rate and functional results, *Acta Orthop Scand* **66**:16–18.

Soucacos PN, Beris AE, Touliatos AS, Vekris M, Pakos S, Varitimidis S (1995b) Current indications for single digit replantation, *Acta Orthop Scand* **66**:12–15.

Soucacos PN, Beris AE (1998) S.A.T.T. classification and managment of open hand injuries. In: Roth JR, Richards RS, eds, *International Federation of Societies for Surgery of the Hand*, (Monduzzi Editore: Bologna) 383–88

Stevanovic MV, Vucetic C, Bumbasirevic M, Vuckovic C (1991) Avulsion injuries of the thumb, *Plast Reconstr Surg* **87**: 1099–1104.

Taras JS, Nunley JA, Urbaniak JR, Goldner RD, Fitch RD (1991) Replantation in children, *Microsurgery* **12**:216–20.

Touliatos AS, Soucacos PN, Beris AE, Zoubos AB, Koukoubis TH, Makris H (1995) Alternative techniques for restoration of bony segments in digital replantation, *Acta Orthop Scand* **66**:19–22.

Urbaniak JR (1987) Digital replantation: a 12–year experience. In: Urbaniak JR, ed, *Microsurgery for major limb reconstruction*. (C.V. Mosby Co: St Louis) 12–21.

Urbaniak JR, Forster JS (1991) Replantation in children. In: Meyer VE, Black MJM, eds, *Microsurgical Procedures*. (Churchill Livingstone: London) 69–83.

Urbaniak JR, Roth JH, Nunley JA, Goldner RD, Koman A (1985) The results of replantation after amputation of a single finger, *J Bone Joint Surg* **67A**:611–19.

Vlastou C, Earle AS (1986) Avulsion injuries of the thumb, *J Hand Surg* **11A**:51–56.

Yomano Y (1985) Replantation of the amputated distal part of the fingers, *J Hand Surg* **10A**:211–18.

16

Effect of growth on pediatric hand reconstruction

Alain Gilbert

Introduction

The recent trends in pediatric hand surgery have been to start the reconstructive procedure as early as possible with the aim of an early adaptation in the child, a better result and the positive influence of growth on the end results (Buck-Gramcko 1999). Although these positive influences cannot be denied, one must be aware of some undesired complications due to the influence of growth on the late result after what can be considered as an initially excellent result.

The positive effects of growth

Correction of axial deformities

Mainly true for fractures of the metacarpals and phalanges of the hand. In younger children, axial deviation may correct spontaneously if the deviation is anteroposterior. Lateral deviations rarely correct completely and rotation deformities will not improve (Gilbert 1999). The closer the deformity from the growth plate, and the younger the patient, the better will be the correction. In congenital deformities there may be a spontaneous improvement after treatment for syndactylies with distal fusion or bone grafting (Buck-Gramcko 1999) but there are many cases of such deformities like after distal bone fusion, which will not improve. The clinodactyly and rotation may even increase with time.

Improvement in joint surface anomaly

In cases of articular fractures, slight anomalies will certainly provoke arthritis in adults. In children, providing the deformity is not too severe, the joint may reconstruct with time and although the mobility may be affected, this new joint may hold for many years (Leclercq 2000). However if the deformity is too severe, there is no hope of any functional improvement. In radial club hand after centralization or radialization the head of the ulna will enlarge and progressively cover the carpus like a new radius.

Muscle and tendon adaptation

Growth is very important for the adaptation of the length of the muscles and tendons after various procedures and particularly pollicization. The adequacy of tension between the muscles may take 6–12 months following the operation. Again growth will improve the overall shape of the thumb and after several years the new thumb will look more natural. The abductor digiti minimi transferred to the thumb will hypertrophy and give the shape of a real thenar eminence.

The negative effects of growth

Unfortunately these negative aspects are common and not always predictable. They may be due to several factors.

Impairment or destruction of the growth plate

One of the most well known consequences of growth plate involvement occurs after centralization of the ulna in radial club hand. The shortening of the bone is often severely augmented by the surgical procedure. Another very specific influence can be observed after traumatic amputation and replantation at the level of the growth plate of the proximal or middle phalanges of the fingers. In such a case, an immediate success may slowly become a final failure due to progressive relative shortening of the finger. With sufficient follow-up, it is possible to determine that destruction of one or two growth plates in a young child may be a contraindication for replantation. Pinning through the growth plate has been accused of partial epiphysiodesis. In our experience it is very rare and, looking retrospectively at a large series of toe transfers there were no explanations for some growth defects and no relation was found with pinning. In some osseous syndactylies, or for the treatment of duplications, it is necessary to cut through the epiphysis. This procedure may induce lateral epiphysiodesis, but we have never seen this type of complication when the osteotomy is done on a non-ossified epiphysis.

Limitation of growth due to paralysis and absence of movements

Long-standing extensive paralysis will impair growth and end up with a severe size discrepancy between the two upper extremities. The best example is represented by the consequences of obstetrical brachial palsy. At the end of growth, the difference in size may be up to 8–10 cm. An early repair of the plexus may limit the shortening of the arm but never completely. Absence of repair of the flexor tendons is also a cause of shortening of the finger. Sometimes the tendon is not repaired for several years and there is time for the growth discrepancy to appear. After repair or grafting, the finger grows again normally but will not overcome the established shortening.

Poor planning and calculation

Many of the problems occur because of poor planning. In a congenital absence of fingers, reconstruction may be done by lengthening the first and fifth rays by toe transfer. The toe will grow but sometimes only one of the metacarpals will grow normally and with time the two reconstructed fingers will be of such different sizes that there will soon be no pinch possibilities. Lateral deviation may be due to external factors like in syndactyly of fingers of different sizes or after scars and contractures. Early release will probably allow development without deformity. If the factor is not suppressed, the scar not treated, the syndactyly not released, the apparent bone deviation will become permanent. In the cases where growth is impaired by soft tissue contractures, the treatment must be early. If the situation is not corrected, growth may create severe deviations.

How to manage growth anomalies

Prevention

In many cases growth anomalies can be prevented by early treatment (syndactyly), but in other cases it will be preferable to wait a few years—the delta phalanx can be treated in the first months or years of life but the high incidence of recurrence has led many authors to wait at least three or four years before any attempt is made to correct the deviation. In growth disturbance due to paralysis, an early repair of the nerve may avoid a great part of the length disturbance. However, even an early repair with excellent results will give some length discrepancy. In obstetrical paralysis, the extent of the paralysis is also an important factor. The preventive treatment of shortening is one of the arguments for an early decision and operation of the plexus.

Treatment of growth anomalies

Lengthening is the most common way to treat

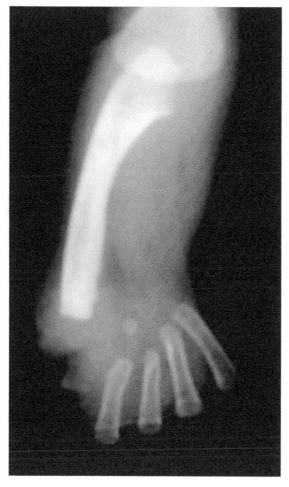

Figure 1

Radial club hand aged 10 months.

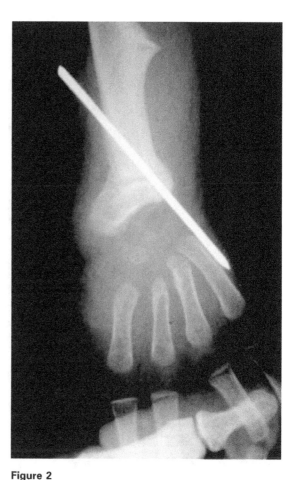

Figure 2

After rotation osteotomy of the lower radius.

lack of growth. In the hand, this procedure is difficult to perform in a very young child since the result is always a percentage of the original size (up to 150% or 200%). If the bone is very small, the gain will be limited and very quickly lost by growth of the other structures. There are few indications for lengthening in young infants; mostly when the growth disturbance prevents pinch and function. In those cases, the family should be aware that further lengthening might be needed in the future. In older children lengthening is done as a final corrective procedure (brachymetacarpal, radial club hand, etc.) using a progressive technique and external fixation. In

the hand, it is usually not necessary to use bone grafting between the extremities and spontaneous callus will heal the defect in one or two months. In the forearm, spontaneous healing, although possible is not the best choice as it is very long (4–6 months) and gives a poor quality of bone. Vascularized fibular grafts, which heal in 6–8 weeks, are in the author's opinion, preferable for forearm reconstruction in the adolescent. In partial closure of the growth plate, techniques such as desepiphysiodesis can be used. This is generally recommended after traumatic disturbance, and although rare, these post-traumatic epiphysiodesis can provoke

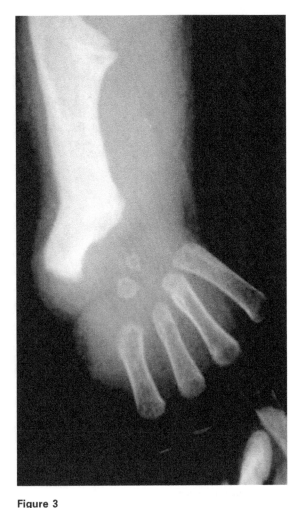

Figure 3

After 8 months recurrence has started.

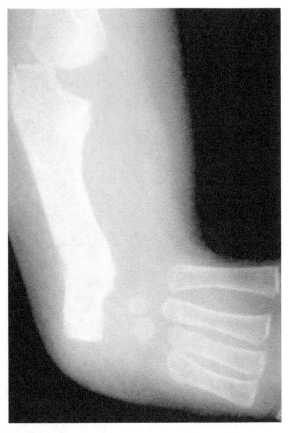

Figure 4

Two years later, there is complete recurrence.

serious desaxations. The procedure has also been used for the treatment of congenital delta-phalanx or Madelung deformity (Vickers 1992), which can be interesting but the results are quite unpredictable. In complete closure of the growth plate, the length discrepancy may become a severe problem and the only solution in the young child is the growth plate transplantation. These transplantations have also been used in congenital disorders such as radial club hand or thumb aplasia. The most common donor site is the upper fibular epiphysis, with its nutrient vessels (Wood and Gilbert 1997) but the iliac crest can also be used. The results of these trans-

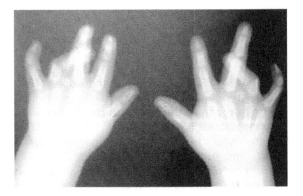

Figure 5

Bilateral delta phalanx.

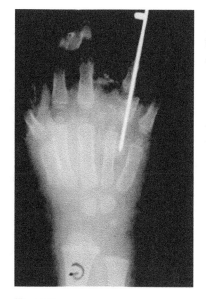

Figure 6

Osteotomy at the age of 22 months.

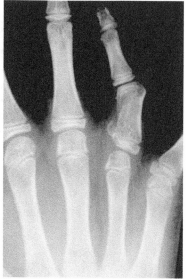

Figure 7

Result 12 years later. Left hand.

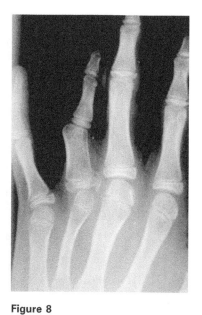

Figure 8

Right hand after remodelling.

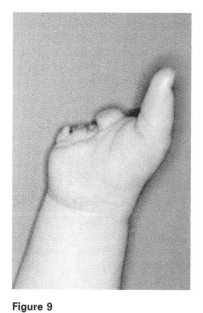

Figure 9

Aplasia of fingers.

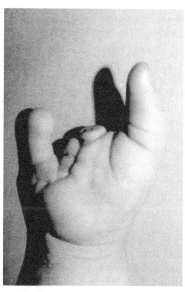

Figure 10

After toe transfer, at the age of 20 months.

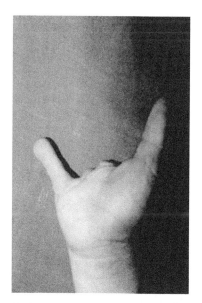

Figure 11

Two years later.

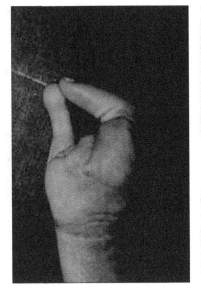

Figure 12

The comparative length is good.

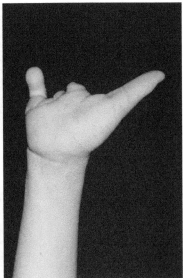

Figure 13

Six years postoperative length is no more balanced.

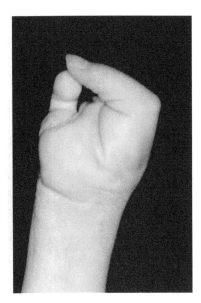

Figure 14

Pinch is now difficult.

plantations seem better in the lower than the upper limb and some very interesting results have been published (Tsai et al 1986). Alternatively, hypergrowth is also a possibility, but its treatment is not always satisfactory. The main possibility is therapeutic epiphysiodesis, which is a difficult operation since destruction of the growth plate without disturbing the stability of the phalanx is not easy. It is often performed for macrodactyly with variable results and it is sometimes necessary to redo the procedure.

Conclusions

The influence of growth in pediatric hand surgery is crucial and this factor should always be taken in account when deciding a procedure in a child. Sometimes growth is a positive factor, but in many cases it is the cause for failure of surgical repairs. Good knowledge of the growth potential of the finger or hand, an atraumatic technique, and adequate follow-up are necessary. It is sometimes better to postpone an operation when the risks of growth interference are too high. In other cases, an early operation may re-establish a normal growth pattern.

References

Buck-Gramcko D (1999) Influence of growth and altered function on bones and muscles. In: Tubiana R, ed, *The Hand*. (Saunders: Philadelphia).

Gilbert A (1999) Fractures of the fingers in children. In: Bruser P, Gilbert A, eds, *Finger Bone and Joint Injuries* (Martin Dunitz: London) 359–64.

Leclercq C, Korn W (2000) Articular fractures of the fingers in children, *Hand Clin* **16**:523–34.

Tsai TM, Ludwig L, Tonkin M (1986) Vascularized fibular epiphyseal transfer, *Clin Orthop* **210**:228–34.

Vickers D, Nielsen G (1992) Madelung deformity: surgical prophylaxis (physiolysis) during the late growth period by resection of the dyschondrostenosis lesion, *J Hand Surg* **17B**:401–7.

Vilkki SK (1998) Distraction and microvascular epiphysis transfer for radial club hand, *J Hand Surg* **23B**:445–52.

Wood M, Gilbert A (1997) *Microvascular Bone Reconstruction* (Martin Dunitz: London)

Index

Printed and bound by CPI Group (UK) Ltd, Croydon, CR0 4YY

23/10/2024

01777691-0005